Middle Range Theory for Nursing

Third Edition

Mary Jane Smith, PhD, RN
Patricia R. Liehr, PhD, RN
Editors

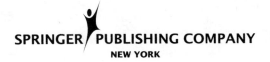

SPRINGER PUBLISHING COMPANY

NEW YORK

Copyright © 2014 Springer Publishing Company, LLC

Springer Publishing Company, LLC
11 West 42nd Street
New York, NY 10036
www.springerpub.com

Acquisitions Editor: Margaret Zuccarini
Production Editor: Michael O'Connor
Composition: diacriTech

ISBN: 978-0-8261-9551-7
e-book ISBN: 978-0-8261-9552-4

13 14 15 16 17 / 5 4 3 2 1

The author and the publisher of this Work have made every effort to use sources believed to be reliable to provide information that is accurate and compatible with the standards generally accepted at the time of publication. The author and publisher shall not be liable for any special, consequential, or exemplary damages resulting, in whole or in part, from the readers' use of, or reliance on, the information contained in this book. The publisher has no responsibility for the persistence or accuracy of URLs for external or third-party Internet websites referred to in this publication and does not guarantee that any content on such websites is, or will remain, accurate or appropriate.

Library of Congress Cataloging-in-Publication Data

Middle range theory for nursing/[edited by] Mary Jane Smith, Patricia R. Liehr. — 3rd ed.
    p. cm.
  Includes bibliographical references and index.
  ISBN 978-0-8261-9551-7 — ISBN 978-0-8261-9552-4 (ebook)
I. Smith, Mary Jane, 1938- II. Liehr, Patricia R.
  [DNLM: 1. Nursing Theory. 2. Nursing Research. WY 86]
  RT84.5
  610.7301—dc23
                                        2013002644

Special discounts on bulk quantities of our books are available to corporations, professional associations, pharmaceutical companies, health care organizations, and other qualifying groups. If you are interested in a custom book, including chapters from more than one of our titles, we can provide that service as well.

For details, please contact:
Special Sales Department, Springer Publishing Company, LLC
11 West 42nd Street, 15th Floor, New York, NY 10036-8002
Phone: 877-687-7476 or 212-431-4370; Fax: 212-941-7842
E-mail: sales@springerpub.com

Printed in the United States of America by Bang Printing.

Contents

v

Contributors

Bradley Aouizerat, PhD
Professor
School of Nursing
University of California,
  San Francisco
San Francisco, CA

Christina Baggott, PhD, RN, PNP
Assistant Professor
School of Nursing
University of California,
  San Francisco
San Francisco, CA

Mary Barger, PhD, RN, CNM
Assistant Professor
School of Nursing
University of California,
  San Francisco
San Francisco, CA

**Virginia Carrieri-Kohlman,
  DNSc, RN, FAAN**
Professor Emeritus
School of Nursing
University of California,
  San Francisco
San Francisco, CA

Heeseung Choi, PhD, RN
Professor
College of Nursing
Seoul National University
Seoul, Korea

DorAnne Donesky, PhD, RN
Assistant Adjunct Professor
School of Nursing
University of California,
  San Francisco
San Francisco, CA

**Kathleen Dracup, FNP, RN,
  FAAN**
Professor
School of Nursing
University of California,
  San Francisco
San Francisco, CA

**Julia A. Faucett, PhD, RN,
  FAAN**
Professor
School of Nursing
University of California,
  San Francisco
San Francisco, CA

Linda Franck, PhD, RN, FAAN
Professor and Chair
School of Nursing
University of California,
   San Francisco
San Francisco, CA

Shelley J. Greif, MPH, RN
Doctoral Student
Florida Atlantic University
Boca Raton, FL

Janice Humphreys, PhD, RN, FAAN
Professor and Vice Chair for
   Academic Personnel
School of Nursing
University of California,
   San Francisco
San Francisco, CA

Eun-Ok Im, PhD, FAAN
Professor
School of Nursing
University of Pennsylvania
Philadelphia, PA

Susan Janson, DNSc, RN, ANP, FAAN
Professor and Harms/Alumnae
   Chair
School of Nursing
University of California,
   San Francisco
San Francisco, CA

Christine Kennedy, PhD, RN, FAAN
Professor
School of Nursing
University of California,
   San Francisco
San Francisco, CA

Kathryn A. Lee, PhD, RN, FAAN
Professor
School of Nursing
University of California,
   San Francisco
San Francisco, CA

Elizabeth R. Lenz, PhD, RN, FAAN
Professor
Ohio State University
   College of Nursing
Columbus, OH

Patricia R. Liehr, PhD, RN
Associate Dean for Nursing
   Research & Scholarship
Christine E. Lynn College
   of Nursing
Florida Atlantic University
Boca Raton, FL

John Lowe, PhD, RN, FAAN
Professor
School of Nursing
Florida Atlantic University
Boca Raton, FL

Christine A. Miaskowski, PhD, RN, FAAN
Professor
School of Nursing
University of California,
   San Francisco
San Francisco, CA

Merle H. Mishel, PhD, RN, FAAN
Professor
School of Nursing
The University of North Carolina
   at Chapel Hill
Chapel Hill, NC

Alvita Nathaniel, PhD, RN, FAANP
Associate Professor
School of Nursing
West Virginia University
Charleston, WV

Linda C. Pugh, PhD, RNC, FAAN
Professor
School of Nursing
York College of Pennsylvania
York, PA

Kathleen Puntillo, DNSc, RN, FAAN
Professor
School of Nursing
University of California,
San Francisco
San Francisco, CA

Anthony R. Ramsey, PhD, FNP-C
Assistant Professor
Waldron College of Health and
Human Services
Radford University
Radford, VA

Pamela G. Reed, PhD, RN, FAAN
Professor
College of Nursing
The University of Arizona
Tucson, AZ

Barbara Resnick, PhD, RN, FAAN
Professor
School of Nursing
University of Maryland
Baltimore, MD

April Lynne Shapiro, MSN, RN
Doctoral Student
School of Nursing
West Virginia University
Morgantown, WV

Marlaine C. Smith, PhD, RN, FAAN
Dean and Professor
Christine E. Lynn College of
Nursing
Florida Atlantic University
Boca Raton, FL

Mary Jane Smith, PhD, RN
Professor of Nursing
School of Nursing
West Virginia University
Morgantown, WV

Patricia L. Starck, DSN, RN, FAAN
Dean and Professor
University of Texas Health
Sciences Center–Houston
School of Nursing
Houston, TX

Lisa Marie Wands, PhD, RN
Postdoctoral Fellow
Tennessee Valley Healthcare
System
Vanderbilt University
Nashville, TN

Loretta A. Williams, PhD, RN, AOCN
Assistant Professor
Department of Symptom Research
The University of Texas
MD Anderson Cancer Center
Houston, TX

Foreword

This third edition of *Middle Range Theory for Nursing* by Mary Jane Smith and Patricia R. Liehr deepens our understandings of the importance of theory development to the scientific enterprise in nursing. Particularly noteworthy is the extent to which the editors and chapter contributors articulate the relevance of the theoretical content for both research and professional nursing practice.

Smith and Liehr were pioneers in nursing knowledge development with the publication of the first edition of this middle range theory book. In that first edition, eight middle range theories for nursing were presented. In this latest edition of the book, 12 theories are included, and each of the chapters exploring these theories includes updated information about the further explication of the theory and its relevance to practice and research. Thus faculty and graduate students will have access to the most recent developments in disciplinary knowledge. The demand for information about middle range theories has substantially increased since the publication of the first edition of this book, and Smith and Liehr have remained in the forefront in expanding the boundaries of knowledge development, sustaining their focus on middle range theories.

Two new theories have been included in this edition, the theory of transitions and the theory of self-reliance—evidence that the discipline has moved forward in the development of theoretical knowledge. It is important to include these new ideas so that, through systematic evaluation, other nurse scholars can assist the theory authors in the refinement of knowledge.

The most significant new content included in this edition is the model of concept building developed by Smith and Liehr. This process of concept building can serve as a complementary process to concept analysis. Yet an important distinguishing factor is the origin of the concept building process in a practice story. Through this rigorous 10-step process, scholars are led from the identification of an important clinical phenomenon to the development and expansion of their conceptual understandings. This process holds great potential for future theoretical and scientific development of the discipline.

It is significant that Smith and Liehr continue to refocus attention on the theory lens of nursing knowledge development, an undertaking that is particularly significant at a time when the focus has drifted to empirical and practical knowledge. As with prior editions, there are key dimensions of the work that make it especially useful to new students of nursing theory, at the graduate and undergraduate levels. Smith and Liehr present their ideas succinctly, and raise important discussions about the nature of theoretical thinking within the discipline. The structured format that is used across all of the chapters that are focused on specific theories provides the reader with a consistent level of explanation and analysis, and is especially useful for those trying to understand the similarities and differences in the theories. This structure facilitates assessment of knowledge development content components, and provides a detailed model for evaluation of the internal and external validity of the theories. And, importantly, each of the chapters includes delineation of the relevance of the theory in research and professional practice.

This third edition is an important contribution to nursing science literature. Smith and Liehr provide depth to our understandings of middle range theory and set the stage for further theory development within the discipline. Nurses in practice, as well as students of nursing at all educational levels, will benefit greatly from this scholarly work. This contribution extends our understandings and presents new opportunities for expanding the science of nursing through research and theory.

Joyce J. Fitzpatrick, PhD, MBA, RN, FAAN
Elizabeth Brooks Ford Professor of Nursing
Frances Payne Bolton School of Nursing
Case Western Reserve University
Cleveland, Ohio

Preface

The interest in middle range theory continues to grow, as demonstrated by the increased number of published theories and the desire among nursing faculty and researchers to use theories at the mid-range level to guide practice and research. This book is based on the premise that students come to know and understand a theory as the meaning of concepts are made clear, and as they experience the way a theory informs practice and research in the everyday world of nursing. Over the years, we continue to hear from students and faculty telling us that the book is user friendly and truly reflects what they need as a reference to move middle range theory to the forefront of research and practice.

Middle range theory can be defined as a set of related ideas that are focused on a limited dimension of the reality of nursing. These theories are composed of concepts and suggested relationships among the concepts that can be depicted in a model. Middle range theories are developed and grow at the intersection of practice and research to provide guidance for everyday practice and scholarly research rooted in the discipline of nursing. We use the ladder of abstraction to articulate the logic of middle range theory as related to a philosophical perspective and practice/research approaches congruent with theory conceptualization.

The middle range theories chosen for presentation in this book cover a broad spectrum—from theories that were proposed decades ago and have been used extensively, to theories that are newly developed and just coming into use. Some of the theories were originated by the primary nurse–author who wrote the chapter, and some were originally created by persons outside of nursing. After much thought and discussion with colleagues and students, we have come to the conclusion that theories for nursing are those that apply to the unique perspective of the discipline, regardless of origin, as long as they are used by nurse scholars to guide practice or research and are consistent with one of the paradigms presented by Newman, Sime, and Corcoran-Perry (1991). These paradigms, which are recognized philosophical perspectives unique to the discipline, present an ontological grounding for the middle range theories in this book. By connecting each theory with a paradigmatic perspective, we offer a view of the middle range theory's place within the larger scope of nursing science. This view was included to create a context for considering theories other than those developed by nurses, which have been used to guide nursing practice and research.

We have structured this book in three sections. The first section includes three chapters that present a meta-perspective on middle range theory, thereby setting the stage for the next sections. The first chapter in this section, "Disciplinary Perspectives Linked to Middle Range Theories," elaborates on the structure of the discipline of nursing as a present and historical context for the development and use of middle range theories. The second chapter, "Understanding Middle Range Theory by Moving Up and Down the Ladder of Abstraction," offers a clear and formal way of presenting the theories. The ladders were created by the editors and represent the editors' view of the philosophical grounding of the theory rather than the chapter authors' view. We have found that a ladder of abstraction can provide a starting place to guide students' thinking when they are trying to make sense of a theory. In addition, moving ideas up and down the ladder of abstraction generates scholarly dialogue. The third chapter in this section is titled "Evaluation of Middle Range Theories for the Discipline of Nursing." Students have told us that understanding the way in which theory is evaluated helps further understanding of the theory. So, we have included this chapter in the first section of the book. Certainly, evaluation of theory is a critical skill required for those who strive to move a theory onward in their own work. A unique feature of the evaluation process described in this chapter is that it is based on postmodern assumptions in which context is appreciated as an essential dimension, creating an always-tentative theory critique.

In the second section of this book, 12 middle range theories are included. Ten of these were presented in the second edition: uncertainty, meaning, self-transcendence, symptom management, unpleasant symptoms, self-efficacy, story, cultural marginality, caregiving dynamics, and moral reckoning. Two new theories are included in this third edition: transitions and self-reliance. The theory of transitions addresses the importance of change in the lives of persons confronting significant health situations. The theory of self-reliance is based on Cherokee core values that have potential for promoting health and well-being across cultures.

Each chapter describing a middle range theory follows a standard format. This includes purpose of the theory and how it was developed, concepts of the theory, relationships among the concepts expressed as a model, use of the theory in nursing research, use of the theory in nursing practice, and conclusion. We believe that this standard format facilitates a complete understanding of the theory and enables a comparison of the theories presented in this book.

The third section contains five chapters that frame a systematic approach for concept development and provides exemplars that highlight the approach. The first chapter in this section, "Concept Building for Research," is one that was first introduced in the second edition. It has been further developed to refine a 10-phase process guiding conceptualization of ideas for research. The process presented in this chapter can be used by faculty who teach courses on concept development and by students who are working to establish their ideas for research. The third section includes two new chapters, written by students, demonstrating use of the concept development process. The chapters, titled "Yearning for Sleep While Enduring Distress" and "Reconceptualizing Normal," provide exemplars that follow the 10-phase process while reflecting unique ways of implementation that bring each phase to life for the students. Finally, in the last two chapters of this section, scholars who wrote about their concept development process in the second edition while they were students, present ideas that they have now taken to research proposal development. These chapters focus on research proposals for studying yearning to be recognized and catastrophic cultural immersion. These students, like many others with whom we have engaged, contributed to our understanding of how to develop structures for research through concept building. Although this structure-developing effort shares some of the processes of concept development, it is distinguished by its foundation in nursing practice stories and the systematic inclusion of inductive and deductive processes that culminate in a newly created model to be used in research.

The reader will notice when reading this book, and comparing the theory descriptions of one edition of this book with the next, that some theories have had ongoing development and use while others have received less attention and use during the past 5 years. The vibrancy of theory is dependent on its use by scholars who critique and apply it, testing its relevancy to real-world practice and research. Proliferation of middle range theory without ongoing critique, application, and development is a concern that requires ongoing attention.

As noted in the second edition of this book, there are beginning clusters of middle range theories around important ideas for the discipline, such as symptoms (theories of unpleasant symptoms and symptom management) and moving through difficult times (theories of meaning, self-transcendence, and transitions). It would be useful to evaluate theory clusters, noting the common ground of guidance emerging from the body of scholarly work documented in the theory cluster. An advantage of this effort would be that the thinking of unique nurse scholars would come together. One might expect that essential dimensions of the discipline could be made explicit by distilling and synthesizing messages from a theory cluster. Although the analysis of theory clusters is not undertaken in this book, the information about middle range theory provided here creates a foundation for considering theory-cluster analysis.

At the end of this book, readers will find a table of middle range theories published from 1988 to 2012 in which the year, full citation, and name of the theory are given. This table is useful as a starting place for scholars who want to find additional middle range theories in the literature.

In conclusion, this third edition presents an organization of chapters by meta-theory, middle range theories for nursing, and concept development through a theoretical lens. The added chapters on transitions and self-reliance contribute to the breadth and depth of the array of middle range theories in this third edition. Chapters elaborating the concept building process contribute exemplars to engage the developing scholar in a meaningful way. As with the previous edition, we have edited and written with the intention of clarifying the contribution of middle range theory. We believe that this clarification serves established and beginning nurse scholars seeking a theoretical foundation for practice and research.

Mary Jane Smith, PhD, RN
Patricia R. Liehr, PhD, RN

REFERENCE

Newman, M. A., Sime, A. M., & Corcoran-Perry, S. A. (1991). The focus of the discipline of nursing. *Advances in Nursing Science, 14,* 1–6.

Acknowledgments

*A*n endeavor such as this book is always the work of many. We are grateful to our students who have prodded us with thought-provoking questions, our colleagues who have challenged our thinking and writing, our contributors who gave willingly of their time and effort, our publisher who believed that we had something to offer, and our families who have provided a base of love and support that makes anything possible.

Middle Range Theory for Nursing

Section One

Setting the Stage for Middle Range Theories

This section describes meta-perspectives that create a context for the middle range theories in this book. In the first chapter, a connection is made between middle range theory and the unique focus of the discipline of nursing, the structure of the discipline, and grand theories in nursing. In the second chapter, middle range theory is described according to philosophical, theoretical, and empirical levels of abstraction along with ladders depicting the assumptions, concepts, and practice/research applications. The editors have created the ladders of abstraction, thereby interpreting each theorist's perspectives and enabling the reader with a means for visualizing, comparing, and contrasting each middle range theory when related to the others. In Chapter 3, a framework for evaluating the substantive foundations, structural integrity, and functional adequacy of middle range theory is provided, emphasizing thoughtful consideration with empathy, curiosity, honesty, and responsibility.

1

Disciplinary Perspectives Linked to Middle Range Theory

Marlaine C. Smith

Each discipline has a unique focus for knowledge development that directs inquiry and distinguishes it from other fields of study. The knowledge that constitutes the discipline has organization. Understanding this organization or the structure of the discipline is important for those engaged in learning the theories of the discipline and for those developing knowledge expanding the discipline. Perhaps this need is more acute in nursing because the evolution of the professional practice based on tradition and knowledge from other fields preceded the emergence of substantive knowledge of the discipline. Nursing knowledge is the inclusive total of the philosophies, theories, research, and practice wisdom of the discipline. As a professional discipline this knowledge is important for guiding practice. Theory-guided, evidence-based practice is the hallmark of any professional discipline. The purpose of this chapter is to elaborate the structure of the discipline of nursing as a context for understanding and developing middle range theories.

The disciplinary focus of nursing has been debated for decades, but now there seems to be some general agreement. In 1978, Donaldson and Crowley stated that a discipline offers "a unique perspective, a distinct way of viewing … phenomena, which ultimately defines the limits and nature of its inquiry" (p. 113). They specified three recurrent themes that delimit the discipline of nursing:

1. Concern with principles and laws that govern the life processes, well-being, and optimum functioning of human beings, sick or well;

2. Concern with the patterning of human behavior in interaction with the environment in critical life situations; and
3. Concern with the processes by which positive changes in health status are affected (p. 113).

Nursing is a professional discipline (Donaldson & Crowley, 1978). Professional disciplines such as nursing, psychology, and education are different from academic disciplines such as biology, anthropology, and economics in that they have a professional practice associated with them. According to the authors, professional disciplines include the same knowledge, descriptive theories, and basic and applied research common to academic disciplines. In addition, prescriptive theories and clinical research are included. So the differences between academic and professional disciplines are the additional knowledge required for professional disciplines. This is important, because many refer to nursing as a practice discipline. This seems to imply that the knowledge is about the practice alone and not about the substantive phenomena of concern to the discipline.

> Failure to recognize the existence of the discipline as a body of knowledge that is separate from the activities of practitioners has contributed to the fact that nursing has been viewed as a vocation rather than a profession. In turn, this has led to confusion about whether a discipline of nursing exists. (Conway, 1985, p. 73)

Although we have made significant progress in building the knowledge base of nursing, this confusion about the substantive knowledge base of nursing lingers with nurses, other professions, and in the public sphere.

Fawcett's (1984) explication of the nursing metaparadigm was another model for delineating the focus of nursing. According to Fawcett, the discipline of nursing is the study of the interrelationships among human beings, environment, health, and nursing. Although the metaparadigm is widely accepted, the inclusion of nursing as a major concept of the nursing discipline is tautological (Conway, 1985). Others have defined nursing as the study of the life process of unitary human beings (Rogers, 1970), caring (Boykin & Schoenhofer, 2001; Leininger, 1978; Watson, 1985), human–universe–health interrelationships (Parse, 1981), and "the health or wholeness of human beings as they interact with their environment" (Donaldson & Crowley, 1978, p. 113). Newman, Sime, and Corcoran-Perry (1991) created a parsimonious definition of the focus of nursing that synthesizes the unitary nature of human beings with caring: "Nursing is the study of caring in the human health experience" (p. 3).

My definition uses similar concepts but shifts the direct object in the sentence: "Nursing is the study of human health and healing through caring" (Smith, 1994, p. 50). This definition can be stated even more parsimoniously: Nursing is the study of healing through caring. Healing comes from the same etymological origin as "health," *haelen*, meaning whole (Quinn, 1990, p. 553). Healing captures the dynamic meaning that health often lacks; healing implies a process of changing and evolving. Caring is the path to healing. In its deepest meaning, it encompasses one's connectedness to all, that is, a person–environment relatedness. Nursing knowledge focuses on the wholeness of human life and experience and the processes that support relationship, integration, and transformation. This is the focus of knowledge development in the discipline of nursing.

Defining nursing as a professional discipline does not negate or demean the practice of nursing. Knowledge generated from and applied in practice is contained within this description. The focus of practice comes from the definition of the discipline. Nursing has been defined as both science and art, with science encompassing the theories and research related to the phenomena of concern (disciplinary focus) and art as the creative application of that knowledge. Newman (1990) and others, perhaps influenced by critical/postmodern scholars, have used the term praxis to connote the unity of theory–research–practice lived in the patient–nurse encounter. Praxis breaks down the boundaries between theory and practice, researcher and practitioner, art and science. Praxis recognizes that the practitioner's values, philosophy, and theoretical perspective are embodied in the practice. Chinn refers to it as "thoughtful reflection and action that occur in synchrony, in the direction of transforming the world" (2013, p. 10). Praxis reflects the embodied knowing that comes from the integration of values and actions and blurs the distinctions among the roles of practitioner, researcher, and theoretician.

Middle range theories are part of the structure of the discipline. They address the substantive knowledge of the discipline by explicating and expanding on specific phenomena that are related to the caring–healing process. For example, the theory of self-transcendence explains how aging or vulnerability propels humans beyond self-boundaries to focus intrapersonally on life's meaning; interpersonally on connections with others and the environment; temporally to integrate past, present, and future; and transpersonally to connect with dimensions beyond the physical reality. Self-transcendence is related to well-being or healing, one of the identified foci of the discipline of nursing. This theory has been examined in research and used to guide nursing practice. With the expansion of middle range theories, nursing is enriched.

Several nursing scholars have organized knowledge of the discipline into paradigms (Fawcett, 1995; Newman et al., 1991; Parse, 1987). The concept of *paradigm* originated in Kuhn's (1970) treatise on the development of knowledge within scientific fields. He asserted that the sciences evolve rather predictably from a preparadigm state to one in which there are competing paradigms around which the activity of science is conducted. The activity of science to which he is referring is the inquiry that examines the emerging questions and hypotheses surfacing from scientific theories and new findings. Paradigms are schools of shared assumptions, values, and views about the phenomena addressed in particular sciences. It is common for mature disciplines to house multiple paradigms. If one paradigm becomes dominant and if discoveries within it challenge the logic of other paradigms, a scientific revolution may occur.

Parse (1987) described nursing with two paradigms: the totality and simultaneity. For her, the theories in the totality paradigm assert the view that humans are bio-psycho-social-spiritual beings responding or adapting to the environment, and health is a fluctuating point on a continuum. The simultaneity paradigm portends a unitary perspective. Unitary refers to the distinctive conceptualization of Rogers (1970, 1992) that humans are essentially whole and cannot be known by conceptually reducing them to parts. Also, the term unitary refers to the lack of separation between human and environment. Health is subjectively defined by the person (group or community) and reflects the process of evolving toward greater complexity and human becoming. Parse locates only two nursing conceptual systems/theories: the Science of Unitary Human Beings (Rogers, 1970, 1992) and the Theory of Human Becoming (Parse, 1981, 1987) in the simultaneity paradigm. For Parse, all nursing knowledge is related to the extant grand theories or conceptual models in the discipline. While she agrees that theories expand through research and conceptual development, she disagrees with the inclusion of middle range theories within the disciplinary structure if they are not grounded in the more abstract theoretical structure of an existing nursing grand theory or conceptual model.

Newman et al. (1991) identified three paradigms. These paradigms are conceptualized as evolving because the more complex paradigms encompass and extend the knowledge in a previous paradigm. The three paradigms are particulate–deterministic, interactive–integrative, and unitary–transformative. From the perspective of the theories within the particulate–deterministic paradigm, human health and caring are understood through their component parts or activities; there is an underlying order and there are predictable antecedents and consequences, and knowledge development progresses to uncover these causal relationships. Reduction and causal inferences are characteristics of this paradigm. The interactive–integrative paradigm acknowledges contextual, subjective, and multidimensional relationships among the phenomena central to the discipline. The interrelationships among parts and the probabilistic nature of change are assumptions that guide the way phenomena are conceptualized and studied. The third paradigm is the unitary–transformative. Here, the person–environment unity is a patterned, self-organizing field within larger patterned self-organizing fields. Change is characterized by fluctuating rhythms of organization disorganization, toward more complex organization. Subjective experience is primary and reflects a pattern of the whole (Newman et al., 1991, p. 4).

Fawcett (1995, 2000) joined the paradigm dialogue with her version of three paradigms. She named them as reaction, reciprocal interaction, and simultaneous action. This model was synthesized from the analysis of views of mechanism versus organism, persistence versus change, and the Parse and Newman and colleagues' nursing paradigm structure. In the reaction worldview, humans are the sum of the biological, psychological, sociological, and spiritual parts of their nature. Reactions are causal and stability is valued; change is a mechanism for survival. In the reciprocal interaction worldview, the parts are seen within the context of the whole, and human–environment relationships are reciprocal; change is probabilistic based on a number of factors. In the simultaneous action worldview, human beings are characterized by pattern and are in a mutual rhythmic open process with the environment. Change is continuous, unpredictable, and moves toward greater complexity and organization (Fawcett, 2000, pp. 11–12).

Each middle range theory has its foundations in one paradigmatic perspective. The philosophies guiding the abstract views of human beings, human–environment interaction, and health and caring are reflected in each of the paradigms. This influences the meaning of the middle range theory, and for this reason, it is important that the theory has a philosophical link to the paradigm clearly identified.

Figure 1.1 illustrates the structure of the discipline of nursing. This is adapted from an earlier version (Smith, 1994). The figure depicts the structure as clusters of inquiry and praxis surrounding a philosophic paradigmatic nexus. The levels of theory within the discipline based on the breadth and depth of focus and level of abstraction are represented. Theory comes from the Greek word, *theoria*, meaning "to see."

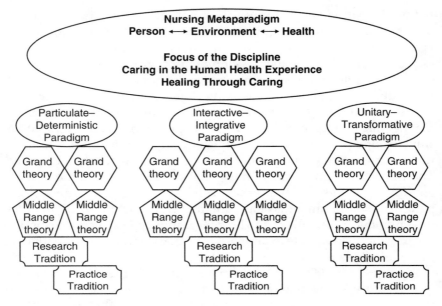

FIGURE 1.1   Structure of the Discipline of Nursing

A theory provides a particular way of seeing phenomena of concern to the discipline. Theories are patterns of ideas that provide a way of viewing a phenomenon in an organized way. Walker and Avant (2010) describe these levels of theory as metatheory, grand theory, middle range theory, and practice theory.

The figure depicts five levels of abstraction. The top oval includes the nursing metaparadigm and focus of the discipline of nursing. This is the knowledge beyond or at a more abstract level than theory per se. Grand theories are at the next level of the figure and include the abstract conceptual systems and theories that focus on the central phenomena of the discipline, such as persons as adaptive systems, self-care deficits, unitary human beings, or human becoming. These grand theories are frameworks consisting of concepts and relational statements that explicate abstract phenomena. In the figure, the grand theories cluster under the paradigms. Middle range theories are more circumscribed, elaborating more concrete concepts and relationships such as uncertainty, self-efficacy, meaning, and the other middle range theories addressed throughout this text. The number of middle range theories is growing. Middle range theory can be specifically derived from a grand theory or can be related directly to a paradigm. At the bottom level of the figure are the research and practice traditions related to the grand and middle range theories. Walker and Avant (2010) refer to this most specific level of theory as practice theory. Practice theories specify guidelines for nursing practice; in fact, the authors state that the word "theory" may be dropped to think of this level as "nursing practices" (p. 12) or what can be considered practice traditions. Both grand theories and middle range theories have practice traditions associated with them.

A practice tradition contains the activities, protocols, guidance, and practice wisdom that emerge from these theories. Models such as the LIGHT model (Andersen & Smereck, 1989) or the attendant nurse caring model (Watson & Foster, 2003) are examples. Smith and Liehr (2008) refer to these as micro-range theories, those that closely reflect practice events or are more readily operational and accessible to application in the nursing practice environment. Research traditions are the associated methods, procedures, and empirical indicators that guide inquiry related to the theory.

Some differentiate between grand theories and conceptual models. Fawcett (2000) differentiates them by how they address the metaparadigm concepts as she has defined them. Those that address the metaparadigm of human beings, environment, health, and nursing are labeled conceptual models, whereas those that do not are considered grand theories. Using her criteria, Human Caring Theory (Watson, 1985, 2008) and Health as Expanding Consciousness (Newman, 1986, 1994) are considered grand theories. Walker and Avant (1995) include conceptual models under the classification of grand theories, and it seems more logical to define conceptual models by scope and level of abstraction instead of their explicit metaparadigm focus. In this chapter, the grand theories will be referred to as theories rather than conceptual frameworks.

The grand theories developed as nursing's distinctive focus became more clearly specified in the 1970s and 1980s. Earlier nurse scholars contributed to theoretical thinking without formalizing their ideas into theories. Nightingale's (1860/1969) assertions in *Notes on Nursing* about caring for those who are ill through attention to the environment are often labeled theoretical. Several grand theories share the same paradigmatic perspective. For example, the theories of Person as Adaptive System (Roy, 1989, 2009), Behavioral Systems (Johnson, 1980), and the Neuman (1989, 1995) Systems Theory share common views of the phenomena central to nursing that might locate them within the interactive–integrative paradigm. Others, such as the Science of Unitary Human Beings (Rogers, 1970, 1992), Health as Expanding Consciousness (Newman, 1986, 1994), and Human Becoming (Parse, 1998), cluster in the unitary–transformative paradigm.

There may be an explicit relationship between some grand theories and middle range theories. For example, Reed's (1991) middle range theory of self-transcendence and Barrett's (1989) theory of power are directly linked to Rogers's Science of Unitary Human Beings. Other middle range theories may not have such direct links to grand theories. In these instances, the philosophical assumptions underpinning the middle range theory may be located at the level of the paradigm rather than of the grand theory. Nevertheless, this linkage is important to establish the theory's validity as a nursing theory. Theoretical work is located in the discipline of nursing when it addresses the focus of the discipline and shares the philosophical assumptions of the nursing paradigms or the grand theories.

Some grand theories in nursing have developed research and/or practice traditions. Laudan (1977) asserts that sciences develop research traditions or schools of thought such as "Darwinism" or "quantum theory," in addition, Laudan's view includes the "legitimate methods of inquiry" open to the researcher from a given theoretical system (p. 79). Research traditions include appropriate designs, methods, instruments, research questions, and issues that are at the frontiers of knowledge development. The traditions reflect logical and consistent linkages between ontology, epistemology, and methodology. Ontology refers to the philosophical foundations of a given theory and is the essence or foundational meaning of the theory. Epistemology is about how one comes to know the theory and incorporates ways of understanding and studying the theory. Methodology is a systematic approach for knowledge generation and includes the processes of gathering, analyzing, synthesizing, and interpreting information. The correspondence among ontology (meaning), epistemology (coming to know), and methodology (approach to study) gives breadth and depth to the theory.

Examples of the connection between ontology, epistemology, and methodology are evident in several grand theories. For instance, the research-as-praxis method was developed by Newman (1990) for the study of phenomena from the Health as Expanding Consciousness perspective, and a research method was developed from the theory of Human Becoming (Parse, 1998). Tools have been developed to measure theoretical constructs such as self-care agency (Denyes, 1982) or functional status within an adaptive systems perspective (Tulman et al., 1991), and debates on the appropriate epistemology and methodology in a unitary ontology (Cowling, 2007; Smith & Reeder, 1998) characterize the research traditions of some extant theories. These examples reflect the necessary relationship between theory, knowledge development, and research methods.

Practice traditions are the principles and processes that guide the use of a theory in practice. The practice tradition might include a classification or labeling system for nursing diagnoses, or it might explicitly eschew this type of labeling. It might include the processes of living the theory in practice such as Barrett's (1998) deliberative mutual patterning, or the developing practice traditions around Watson's theory such as ritualizing hand washing and creating quiet time on nursing units (Watson & Foster, 2003). Practice traditions are the ways that nurses live the theory and make it explicit and visible in their practice.

Middle range theories have direct linkages to research and practice. They may be developed inductively through qualitative research and practice observations, or deductively through logical analysis and synthesis. They may evolve through retroductive processes of rhythmic induction–deduction. As scholarly work extends middle range theories, research and practice traditions continue to develop. For example, scholars advancing uncertainty theory will continue to test hypotheses derived from the theory with different populations. Nurses in practice can take middle range theories and develop practice guidelines based on them. Oncology nurses whose worldviews are situated in the interactive–integrative paradigm may develop protocols to care for patients receiving chemotherapy using the theory of unpleasant symptoms. The use of this protocol in practice will feed back to the middle range theory, extending the evidence for practice and contributing to ongoing theory development. The use of middle range theories to structure research and practice builds the substance, organization, and integration of the discipline.

The growth of the discipline of nursing is dependent on the systematic and continuing application of nursing knowledge in practice and development of new knowledge. Few grand theories have been added to the discipline since the 1980s. Some suggest that there is no longer a need to differentiate knowledge and establish disciplinary boundaries because interdisciplinary teams will conduct research around common problems, eliminating the urge to establish disciplinary boundaries. Even the National Institutes of Health rewards interdisciplinary research enterprises. This emphasis can enrich perspectives through interdisciplinary collaboration, but it is critical to approach interdisciplinary collaboration with a clear view of nursing knowledge to enable meaningful weaving of disciplinary perspectives.

Nursing remains on the margin of the professional disciplines and is in danger of being consumed or ignored if sufficient attention is not given to the uniqueness of nursing's field of inquiry and practice. There are hopeful indicators that nursing knowledge is growing. The blossoming of middle range theories signifies a growth of knowledge development in nursing. Middle range theories offer valuable organizing frameworks for phenomena being researched by interdisciplinary teams. These theories are useful to nurses and persons from other disciplines in framing phenomena of shared concern. Hospitals seeking Magnet status are now required to articulate some nursing theoretic perspective that guides nursing practice in the facility. The quality of the practice environment is important for the quality of care and the retention of nurses. Theory-guided practice elevates the work of nurses leading to fulfillment, satisfaction, and a professional model of practice.

The role of the doctor of nursing practice has the potential to enrich the current level of advanced practice by moving it toward true nursing practice guided by nursing theory. The movement toward translational research and enhanced absorption of research findings into the front lines of care will demand practice models that bring coherence and sense to research findings. Isolated, rapid cycling of findings can result in confusion and chaos if not sensibly synthesized into a model of care that is guided not only by evidence but also by a guiding compass of values and a framework that synthesizes research into a meaningful whole. This is the role of theory. With this continuing shift to theory-guided practice and research, productive scientist–practitioner partnerships will emerge committed to the application of knowledge to change care and to improve quality of life for patients, families, and communities.

REFERENCES

Andersen, M. D., & Smereck, G. A. D. (1989). Personalized nursing LIGHT model. *Nursing Science Quarterly, 2*, 120–130.

Barrett, E. A. M. (1989). A nursing theory of power for nursing practice: Derivation from Rogers' paradigm. In J. Riehl-Sisca (Ed.), *Conceptual models for nursing practice* (3rd ed., pp. 207–217). Norwalk, CT: Appleton & Lange.

Barrett, E. A. M. (1998). A Rogerian practice methodology for health patterning. *Nursing Science Quarterly, 11*, 136–138.

Boykin, A., & Schoenhofer, S. O. (2001). *Nursing as caring.* Sudbury, MA: Jones & Bartlett.

Chinn, P. L. (2013). *Peace and power: New directions for community building* (8th ed.). Burlington, MA: Jones & Bartlett.

Conway, M. E. (1985). Toward greater specificity of nursing's metaparadigm. *Advances in Nursing Science, 7*(4), 73–81.

Cowling, W. R. (2007). A unitary participatory vision of nursing knowledge. *Advances in Nursing Science, 30*(1), 71–80.

Denyes, M. J. (1982). Measurement of self-care agency in adolescents (Abstract). *Nursing Research, 31,* 63.

Donaldson, S. K., & Crowley, D. M. (1978). The discipline of nursing. *Nursing Outlook, 26,* 113–120.

Fawcett, J. (1984). The metaparadigm of nursing: Current status and future refinements. *Image: Journal of Nursing Scholarship, 16,* 84–87.

Fawcett, J. (1995). *Analysis and evaluation of conceptual models of nursing* (3rd ed.). Philadelphia, PA: F. A. Davis.

Fawcett, J. (2000). *Analysis and evaluation of contemporary nursing knowledge: Nursing models and theories.* Philadelphia, PA: F. A. Davis.

Johnson, D. E. (1980). The behavioral system model for nursing. In J. P. Riehl & C. Roy (Eds.), *Conceptual models for nursing practice* (2nd ed., pp. 207–216). New York, NY: Appleton-Century-Crofts.

Kuhn, T. S. (1970). *The structure of scientific revolutions* (2nd ed.). Chicago, IL: University of Chicago Press.

Laudan, L. (1977). *Progress and its problems: Toward a theory of scientific growth.* Berkeley, CA: University of California Press.

Leininger, M. (1978). *Transcultural nursing: Concepts, theories and practices.* New York, NY: Wiley.

Neuman, B. (1989). *The Neuman systems model* (2nd ed.). Norwalk, CT: Appleton & Lange.

Neuman, B. (1995). *The Neuman systems model* (3rd ed.). Norwalk, CT: Appleton & Lange.

Newman, M. A. (1986). *Health as expanding consciousness.* St. Louis, MO: Mosby.

Newman, M. A. (1990). Newman's theory of health as praxis. *Nursing Science Quarterly, 3*(1), 37–41.

Newman, M. A. (1994). *Health as expanding consciousness* (2nd ed.). St. Louis, MO: Mosby.

Newman, M. A., Sime, A. M., & Corcoran-Perry, S. A. (1991). Focus of the discipline of nursing. *Advances in Nursing Science, 14*(1), 1–6.

Nightingale, F. (1969). *Notes on nursing: What it is and what it is not.* London: reprinted by Lippincott, Philadelphia, 1946.

Parse, R. R. (1981). *Man-living-health: A theory of nursing.* New York, NY: Wiley.

Parse, R. R. (Ed.). (1987). *Nursing science. Major paradigms, theories and critiques.* Philadelphia, PA: Saunders.

Parse, R. R. (1998). *The human becoming school of thought: A perspective for nurses and other health professionals.* Thousand Oaks, CA: Sage.

Quinn, J. A. (1990). On healing, wholeness and the haelen effect. *Nursing and Health Care, 10*(10), 553–556.

Reed, P. G. (1991). Toward a nursing theory of self-transcendence: Deductive reformulation using developmental theories. *Advances in Nursing Science, 13*(4), 64–77.

Rogers, M. E. (1970). *An introduction to the theoretical basis of nursing.* New York, NY: F. A. Davis.

Rogers, M. E. (1992). Nursing science and the space age. *Nursing Science Quarterly, 5,* 27–34.

Roy, C. (1989). The Roy adaptation model. In: J. P. Riehl & C. Roy (Eds.), *Conceptual models for nursing practice* (2nd ed., pp. 179–188). New York, NY: Appleton & Lange.

Roy, C. (2009). *The Roy adaptation model* (3rd ed.). Upper Saddle River, NJ: Prentice-Hall Health.

Smith, M. C. (1994). Arriving at a philosophy of nursing. In: J. F. Kikuchi & H. Simmons (Eds.), *Developing a philosophy of nursing* (pp. 43–60). Thousand Oaks, CA: Sage.

Smith, M. C., & Reeder, F. (1998). Clinical outcomes research and Rogerian science: Strange or emergent bedfellows. *Visions: Journal of Rogerian Nursing Science, 6*, 27–38.

Smith, M. J., & Liehr, P. R. (2008). *Middle range theory for nursing* (2nd ed.). New York, NY: Springer Publishing.

Tulman, L., Higgins, K., Fawcett, J., Nunno, C., Vansickel, C., Haas, M. B., & Speca, M. M. (1991). The inventory of functional status-antepartum period: Development and testing. *Journal of Nurse-Midwifery, 36*(2), 117–123.

Walker, L., & Avant, K. (2010). *Strategies for theory construction in nursing* (5th ed.). Upper Saddle River, NJ: Prentice Hall.

Watson, J. (1985). *Nursing: The philosophy and science of caring.* Boulder, CO: Associated University Press.

Watson, J. (2008). *Nursing: The philosophy and science of caring* (2nd ed.). Boulder, CO: University Press of Colorado.

Watson, J., & Foster, R. (2003). The Attending Nurse Caring Model: Integrating theory, evidence and advanced caring-healing therapeutics for transforming professional practice. *Journal of Clinical Nursing, 12*, 360–365.

2

Understanding Middle Range Theory by Moving Up and Down the Ladder of Abstraction

Mary Jane Smith and Patricia R. Liehr

*E*very discipline has a process of reasoning that is rooted in the philosophy, theories, and empirical generalizations that define it. The reasoning process is logical when all levels come together and make sense in an orderly and coherent manner. The ladder of abstraction is a logical system for locating and relating three different and distinct levels of discourse: the philosophical, theoretical, and empirical. The aim of this chapter is to describe the ladder of abstraction as central to understanding and using middle range theory in research and practice. The philosophical, theoretical, and empirical dimensions of the middle range theories presented in this book are considered relative to the ladder of abstraction. The ladder of abstraction is a structure that maps the connection between levels of discourse (Figure 2.1).

If one pictures a ladder with three rungs, the highest is the philosophical, the middle the theoretical, and the lowest is the empirical. These rungs represent levels of discourse or distinct ways of describing ideas. The philosophical is the highest level, representing beliefs and assumptions that are accepted as true and fundamental to the theory. The philosophical level represents belief systems essential to the reasoning found in the theoretical and empirical expression of middle range theories.

The theoretical is in the realm of the abstract, consisting of symbols, ideas, and concepts. Many of the theories in this book are known by a central abstraction. For instance, uncertainty, meaning, and self-transcendence are some of the theoretically abstract ideas that will be discussed in this book. Implicit in abstraction is an outer shadow of vagueness that enables the ongoing development of the idea. This bit of vagueness can throw a person off guard and engender confusion

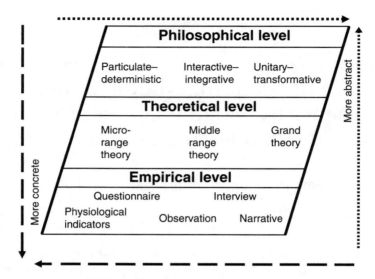

FIGURE 2.1   Ladder of Abstraction

about the meaning of an idea. However, the abstract nature of theory is not intended to be confusing or abstruse. In deciphering the abstract and differentiating ideas according to the philosophical, theoretical, and empirical, one figures out meaning and comes to know what is explicit about an abstract idea.

The empirical is the lowest rung on the ladder, at a concrete level of discourse. For instance, the gathering of a practice story is low on the ladder. The empirical represents what can be observed through the senses and moves beyond to include perceptions, symbolic meanings, self-reports, observable behavior, biological indicators, and personal stories (Ford-Gilboe, Campbell, & Berman, 1995; Reed, 1995).

Ideas are put into language to explain and describe their essence. Ideas at the theoretical level are concepts specific to a theory. Concepts are the building blocks of theory and characterize properties that describe and explain the theory at a middle range level of discourse. Levels of discourse are differing ways of expressing, defining, and specifying an idea. If one idea is more abstract than another, then it is more encompassing, enveloping a broader scope. On the other hand, if an idea is less abstract, it is more concrete. This notion of the relationship between levels of abstraction is key to understanding and making sense of the theoretical. Levels of abstraction apply to each rung of the ladder in relation to the other rungs. That is to say, the philosophical is at a higher level than the theoretical. When one is grappling with understanding the theoretical or middle level on the ladder, the process is to move the idea up to evaluate the philosophical premise and move down to its empirical indicators where the theory connects to the world of practice and research. The concepts defining the structure of theory are learned by thinking through meaning in the context of nursing practice and research. To have a complete understanding, one moves the theoretical idea back and forth, along and within the rungs of the ladder. For example, if trying to understand a theory, a start at the middle rung of the ladder would lead to the question: How is the theory defined conceptually? What are the concepts, and what do the concepts mean? Then, given the answers to the first set of questions, a move to a lower ladder rung would lead to this question: What does this mean to me and how does it connect with what I already know, namely my experience? Then one might look at how personal experience fits with the description of the theory. One might also question what values and beliefs are included in the assumptions of the theory, thus moving the theory up the ladder of abstraction. The point is that in coming to know the realm of the theoretical, one thinks through the theory by moving up and down the rungs of the ladder. The theory becomes understandable through discourse with self and with others through reading, thinking, and dialogue. Such discourse is always both tacit and explicit. This means that a person can begin to describe in words the meaning of an abstract idea and at the same time hold more knowledge about the idea than can be made explicit. Each time the idea is described through talking, writing, and discussion, a greater grasp is achieved. A thorough understanding of the theory is essential to applying the theory in practice and research.

It should be pointed out that staying on one rung deters understanding and limits the ability to use the theory in practice or research. Persons may choose to stay on the rung that is most comfortable. For example, theorists may stay at the theoretical, and researchers may stay at the empirical, while meta-theorists may be more comfortable at the philosophical level. It is a premise of this work on middle range theory that to move nursing science to the front lines of practice and research, nurses must be skilled in moving up and down and back and forth on the ladder of abstraction when studying, practicing, and researching the science of nursing.

When all levels of an idea can be mapped on the ladder of abstraction and the levels cohere with each other, the theoretical is guided by a logical process that provides clarity and facilitates understanding and use of the theory in research and practice. To understand a theory at all levels of abstraction requires a process of reasoning. By moving from the lower rung of the ladder to the middle and then the upper rung, one is making sense of phenomena through inductive reasoning. Conversely, movement from the upper philosophical rung to the theoretical and then to the empirical is deductive reasoning. The substantive knowledge of the discipline structured by logic guides thinking through nursing research and advanced nursing practice. This point flies in the face of the notion that theory is bewildering logic, abstruse, and rather incomprehensible. There is logic to the abstract that can be reasoned through with the ladder of abstraction. Each level of the ladder will be discussed in the context of the middle range theories presented in this book.

PHILOSOPHICAL LEVEL

The philosophical level includes assumptions, beliefs, paradigmatic perspectives, and points of view. Reasoning through a nursing situation for practice and research is based on assumptions, which are beliefs accepted as true about what constitutes reality. Assumptions about how individuals change are at the backbone of a theory. A paradigm is a worldview that includes disciplinary values and perspectives that are at the philosophical level.

Multiple paradigmatic schemas have been developed in nursing, and several of these are discussed in the first chapter. The schema used to guide discussion in this book is the one developed by Newman, Sime, and Corcoran-Perry (1991), who identified caring in the human health experience as the focus of the discipline of nursing. They also identified three paradigms that guide the discipline: the particulate–deterministic, interactive–integrative, and unitary–transformative. Each paradigm incorporates unique values about health and caring and how change comes about. In the particulate–deterministic paradigm, the person is viewed as an isolated entity, change as primarily linear and causal, and the knowledge base grounded in the perspective of the biophysical sciences. The interactive–integrative paradigm describes persons as reciprocal interacting entities, change as probabilistic and related to multiple factors, and knowledge as grounded in the perspective of the social sciences. In the unitary–transformative paradigm, the person is viewed as unitary, evolving in a mutual and simultaneous process where change is creative and unpredictable, and the knowledge base grounded in the human sciences.

One can clearly see that the three paradigms, all of which hold assumptions, values, and point of view, are at differing levels of abstraction. The most abstract is the unitary–transformative, next is the interactive–integrative, and lowest in level of abstraction is the particulate–deterministic. These are examples of levels of abstraction within the philosophical rung of the ladder. Although theorists may not explicate their assumptions or paradigmatic perspectives, a careful reading of the theory will lead to understanding where the theorists stand in relation to a point of view and what makes up the philosophical underpinnings of the proposed theory.

The ladder of abstraction (Figure 2.1) depicts the philosophical level as the highest level of abstraction, which includes the particulate–deterministic, interactive–integrative, and unitary–transformative paradigms. The middle range theories presented in this book have been placed by the editors in one of these paradigms on the philosophical rung of the ladder. This was a judgment reflecting the view of two people that occurred through scholarly discourse. It is important for the reader to understand that different judgments may be made by different people who have different understandings of the theory and the paradigms. There isn't a "right" way to link a theory with a paradigm, but there are always substantiated reasons for the linking decisions that are based on logical coherence. The editors made the decision about the theory–paradigm link based on an understanding of the knowledge roots of the middle range theories.

The middle range theories of uncertainty, unpleasant symptoms, self-efficacy, symptom management, cultural marginality, care giving dynamics, transitions, and moral reckoning are rooted primarily in the social sciences and relate to a multidimensional and contextual reality. These eight theories have substantiated links to the interactive–integrative paradigm. The middle range theories of story, meaning, self-transcendence, and self-reliance are primarily rooted in the human sciences and relate to reality as a process of mutual and creative unfolding. These four theories describe values consistent with the unitary–transformative paradigm. There is value in understanding the paradigmatic perspective of a theory because it helps one to lay out a starting point for a theory by establishing its philosophical foundation where there is meaning for the theory's content, structure, and use in practice and research.

THEORETICAL LEVEL

The reader will note that the middle range theories found in this book are presented in the historical order of publication. This ordering decision was made based on the year the author introduced ideas relevant to the theory in a peer-reviewed publication. All theories in the book comply with the focus of nursing as presented by Newman et al. (1991), who say that nursing "is the study of caring in the human health experience" (p. 3). They go on to say "A body of knowledge that does not include caring and human health experience is not nursing knowledge" (p. 3). Caring is described as a moral imperative having a service identity. All 12 middle range theories described in this work have a focus of caring in the human health experience. Application of any one of these theories in practice or research aims at facilitating change in the human health experience.

The human health experience is explicit in each of the theories as experiencing uncertainty; suffering; vulnerability; symptoms; decisions to make behavioral change; a complicating health challenge; life transitions; being responsible, disciplined and confident; living at the margin of cultures; giving care to another; and situation binds that demand moral reckoning. It is noteworthy that two of the middle range theories, Unpleasant Symptoms and Symptom Management, share the common human experience of symptoms. There is also common ground for the theories of Meaning and Self-Transcendence through their respective focus on suffering and vulnerability, which are intricately connected human health experiences. Furthermore, the theories of cultural marginality and self-reliance are rooted in unique cultural perspectives.

Caring in the human health experience requires consideration of how the nurse lives relationships with people regarding their health. Based on these theories, some of the ways that caring transpires in the context of nursing are through promoting structure and order, inviting and engaging in dialogue, supporting inner resources, understanding symptom experience and offering relief, tailoring information, responding to struggle, counseling caregivers, and discussing situational binds.

The middle range theories in this book add to the body of knowledge about nursing regardless of their discipline of origin. All the theories have been applied in nursing practice and research to enhance caring in the human health experience. Theories belong to many disciplines. What is important to nursing science is that the research and practice based on a theory can be grounded in the focus and paradigmatic perspective of the discipline of nursing.

The theoretical rung on the ladder of abstraction includes concepts, frameworks, and theories. A theoretical concept is different from an everyday concept because it is a mental image of an aspect of reality that is put into words to describe and explain the meaning of a phenomenon significant to the discipline of nursing. A theoretical framework is a structure of interrelating concepts that describe and explain the meaning of a phenomenon. Then what is a theory? Theory is described in the literature at all levels of abstraction. The accepted definition of a theory rests in the eye of the beholder. Chinn and Kramer (1999, p. 258) define theory as "a creative and rigorous structuring of ideas that project a tentative, purposeful and systematic view of phenomena." Im and Meleis (1999, p. 11) define theory as "an organized, coherent and systematic articulation of a set of statements related to significant questions in a discipline that are communicated in a meaningful whole to describe or explain a phenomenon or set of phenomena." On the other hand, McKay (1969) describes theory as a logically interrelated set of confirmed hypotheses. Chinn and Kramer's definition of theory is at the highest level of abstraction, next is Im and Meleis, and at the lowest level is McKay. Given this array of theory definitions, it is easy to understand why one could argue several ways about whether a particular theory is indeed a theory: It all depends on the way theory is defined.

Furthermore, there are levels of theory within the theoretical rung of the ladder. At the most abstract level, there are the grand theories. These are theories that have a very broad scope. The conceptual focus of some of these grand theories includes goal attainment (King, 1996), self-care (Orem, 1971), adaptation (Roy & Andrews, 1991), becoming (Parse, 1992), and unitary human field process (Rogers, 1994). Each of these grand theories shares the common ground of offering a structure that enables description and explanation of essential conceptualizations of nursing. However, even on the common ground of grand theory, some are more abstract than others. For instance, becoming is more abstract than goal attainment.

Middle range theories, the subject of this book, are described by Merton (1968, p. 9) as those theories "that lie between the minor but necessary working hypotheses that evolve in abundance during day-to-day research and the all-inclusive systematic efforts to develop unified theory." He goes on to say that the principal ideas of middle range theories are relatively simple. Here, simple means rudimentary, straightforward ideas that stem from the focus of the discipline. Thus, middle range theory is a basic, usable structure of ideas, less abstract than grand theory, and more abstract than empirical generalizations or micro-range theory.

Micro-range theories, described as situation specific by Im and Meleis (1999, p. 13) are theories that focus on "specific nursing phenomena that reflect clinical practice and that are limited to specific populations or to particular fields of practice." These theories "offer a blueprint that is more readily operational and/or has more accessible utility in clinical situations" (p. 19). It can be seen that this level of theory is lower on the ladder of abstraction than middle range theory. While Im's theory of transitions (see Chapter 11) is at the middle range level of abstraction, the population-specific theories that emerge from it are at a lower level of abstraction. Examples of situation-specific theories are menopausal transition of Korean immigrant women, learned response to chronic illness of patients with rheumatoid arthritis, and women's responses when dealing with their multiple roles (Im & Meleis, 1999). In this case, a middle range theory has spawned situation-specific theories that have direct application to specific nursing practice situations. The ladder of abstraction depicts micro-range theory, middle range theory, and grand theory on ascending levels of discourse (Figure 2.1). The ladders for each theory presented here show a description of the philosophical, conceptual, and empirical connections. The author of each chapter has specifically identified theory concepts, so the inclusion of concepts on the ladder thus became a straightforward process. Sometimes the authors of published articles on middle range theory do not clearly identify concepts. In that instance, the reader is left to decipher what the concepts of the theory are and how they are defined. For some middle range theories, it may be necessary to differentiate concepts by a very careful reading of the manuscript and examination of the model. When this interpretative process is needed, there is always a risk that the concepts identified by the reader are not exactly what the author of the theory intended.

EMPIRICAL LEVEL

The empirical level represents discourse that brings a theory to research and practice. Empirics include physiologic indicators, questionnaires, observation, interview, and narrative (Figure 2.1). Like other rungs on the ladder, the empirical level of discourse moves from the most concrete (physiologic indicators) to the most abstract (narrative). Even at this lowest level of discourse, there is a range of abstraction.

Whether practicing or doing research, the nurse connects with the empirical level. The advanced practice nurse may use physiologic indicators, interview, and observation while applying theory to caring in the human health experience. The nurse researcher may use observation and narrative in a single study while applying theory to examine caring in the human health experience. Decisions about empirics are guided by philosophy and theory. It is important that the nurse chooses empirics that fit with philosophic and theoretical perspectives, thus providing a match between all levels of abstraction.

MIDDLE RANGE THEORIES ON THE LADDER OF ABSTRACTION

There are 12 middle range theories in this book, presented in a chronological order according to when the chapter author introduced the idea in a refereed publication. For instance, although the Theory of Meaning was first presented by Starck as a theory in 2003, she began using Viktor Frankl's ideas in her dissertation research, where she studied perception of meaning and purpose in life for people who had suffered spinal cord injury. The first date noted in her chapter citing this work is 1979 in *Dissertation Abstracts*. In 1985, she published an article on logotherapy, which we identified as the first related work published in a refereed journal. Starck's place in the order of chapters reflects the 1985 citation. This approach to ordering the chapters places explicit emphasis on the continued work necessary to grow ideas over time; implicit emphasis suggests that nursing scholars must be willing to persist with the sometimes tedious work of theory building, and this work occurs with spurts and stalls, usually over decades.

The first middle range theory presented encompasses both Uncertainty in Illness and Reconceptualized Uncertainty in Illness. Mishel and Clayton address both of these theories in Chapter 4. The original uncertainty theory pertains to acute illness, while the reconceptualized theory pertains to the continual uncertainty experienced in chronic illness. On the ladder, the reconceptualization is represented in bold print at the philosophical and theoretical level. The theories are consistent with beliefs associated with the interactive–integrative paradigm.

Persons experience uncertainty during diagnosis and treatment and when illness has a downward trajectory, and persons experience continual uncertainty in ongoing chronic illness and also with the possibility of recurrence of an illness. Concepts at the theoretical level in both theories are antecedents of uncertainty, appraisal of uncertainty, and coping with uncertainty. Concepts added in the reconceptualized theory include self-organization and probabilistic thinking. Moving to the empirical level with practice is offering information and explanation, providing structure and order, and focusing on choices and alternatives. An instrument has been developed that is directly related to the theory, the uncertainty in illness scale (Figure 2.2).

The second middle range theory presented is Starck's Theory of Meaning, based on the work of Viktor Frankl. This theory is grounded in the unitary–transformative paradigm. It is assumed that through a transformative process, persons find meaning. When confronted with a hopeless situation, meaning can be freely and responsibly realized in every moment. Concepts at the theoretical level include life purpose,

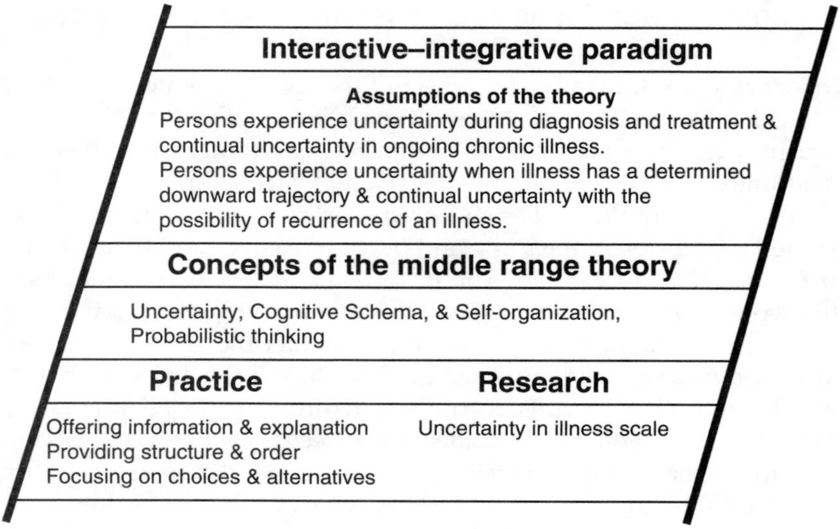

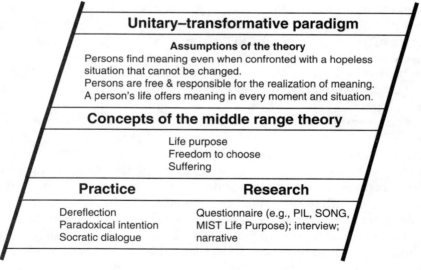

FIGURE 2.2   Ladder of Abstraction: Uncertainty in Illness

FIGURE 2.3   Ladder of Abstraction: Meaning

freedom to choose, and suffering. Practice approaches at the empirical level include dereflection, paradoxical intention, and Socratic dialogue. Empirical indicators for research include questionnaires, interviews, and other narrative approaches (Figure 2.3).

The third middle range theory, Self-Transcendence developed by Reed, is grounded in assumptions of the unitary–transformative paradigm. Self-transcendence is a unitary process. The theory assumes that persons are integral and coextensive with their environments and capable of an awareness that extends beyond physical and temporal dimensions. Concepts at the theoretical level of discourse include vulnerability, self-transcendence, and well-being. Taking the theory to the empirical level with practice includes integrative spiritual care, support of inner resources, and expansion of intrapersonal, interpersonal, temporal, and transpersonal boundaries. Like the theory of uncertainty, a research instrument has been developed that is directly related to the theory, the self-transcendence scale (Figure 2.4).

The fourth theory presented in this book is Symptom Management Theory by Humphreys, Janson, Donesky, Dracup, Lee, Puntillo, Faucett, Aouizerat, Miaskowski, Baggott, Carrieri-Kohlman, Barger, Franck, and Kennedy. This theory is grounded in assumptions of the interactive–integrative paradigm, in which persons manage their symptoms in interaction with the environment. The specific assumptions of the theory include that health and illness affect symptom management, improvement in symptoms extends beyond personal health, and symptoms are subjective and experienced in clusters. There are three concepts at the middle range level of discourse. The concepts are symptom experience,

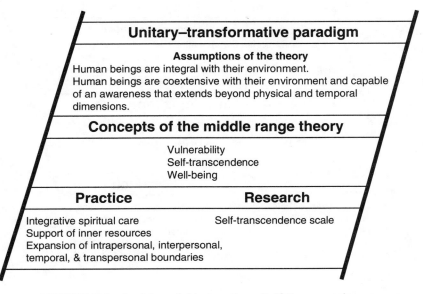

FIGURE 2.4 Ladder of Abstraction: Self-Transcendence

symptom management strategies, and symptom status outcomes. At the empirical level, practice application occurs with patient–provider communication marked by an understanding of the symptom experience and the implementation of effective strategies. Research application includes measurement of symptom-specific outcomes and contextual factors related to the symptom under study (Figure 2.5).

The fifth middle range theory is Unpleasant Symptoms by Lenz and Pugh. This theory is grounded in the beliefs and assumptions associated with the interactive–integrative paradigm. Specific beliefs of the theory are that there are commonalities across different symptoms experienced by persons in varied situations, and that symptoms are subjective phenomena occurring in family and community contexts. Concepts at the theoretical level include symptoms, influencing factors, and performance. Practice application at the empirical level includes assessment of the symptom, symptom management, and relief intervention. Empirical measurements are gathered through scales and observations that capture the symptom experience (Figure 2.6).

The sixth middle range theory is Self-Efficacy by Resnick, which is grounded in the assumptions of the interactive–integrative paradigm. Persons change in a reciprocal interactive process when they exercise influence over what they do and decide how to behave. Concepts at

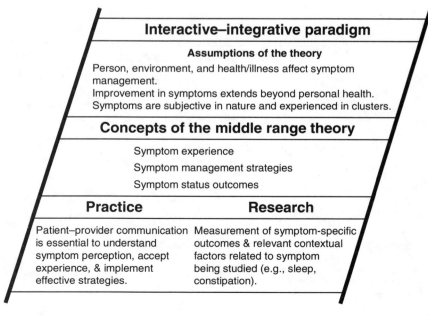

FIGURE 2.5 Ladder of Abstraction: Symptom Management

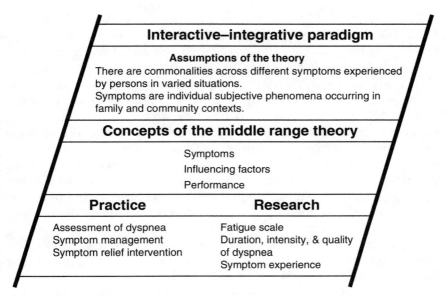

FIGURE 2.6   Ladder of Abstraction: Unpleasant Symptoms

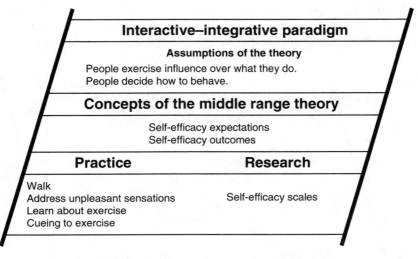

FIGURE 2.7   Ladder of Abstraction: Self-Efficacy

the theoretical level include self-efficacy expectations and self-efficacy outcomes. Examples of practice applications at the empirical level include learning about exercise, addressing unpleasant sensations, and cueing to exercise. Research based on this middle range theory uses self-efficacy scales (Figure 2.7).

The seventh middle range theory presented is Liehr and Smith's Story Theory, which is grounded in the assumptions of the unitary–transformative paradigm where change is viewed as creative and unpredictable. Story is a narrative happening that enables transformative experience in the unitary nurse–person process. The specific assumptions of the theory include that persons change in interrelationship with their world as they live an expanded present and experience meaning. There are three concepts at the theoretical level: intentional dialogue, connecting with self-in-relation, and creating ease. At the empirical level, the health story is the basis for both practice and research. Examples of empirical approaches in practice include creation of a story path and family tree. Health story data may be analyzed using phenomenological, linguistic, case study, or story inquiry methods (Figure 2.8).

The eighth theory found in the book is the Theory of Transitions presented by Im. This theory is in keeping with the assumptions of the interactive–integrative paradigm and describes circumstances related to change in health/illness, life situations, and developmental stages. Assumptions include the centrality of transitions to nursing practice, the reciprocity of the nurse–client relationship, and the fact that patterns and processes of transitions are complex. Nursing therapeutics incorporate the phases of assessment of readiness, preparation for transition, and role supplementation. Research studies have produced

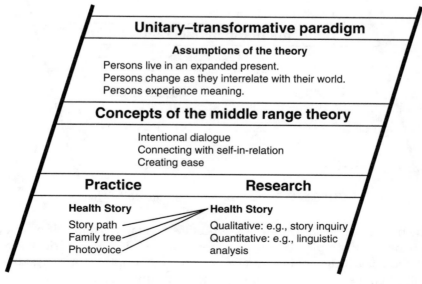

FIGURE 2.8 Ladder of Abstraction: Story

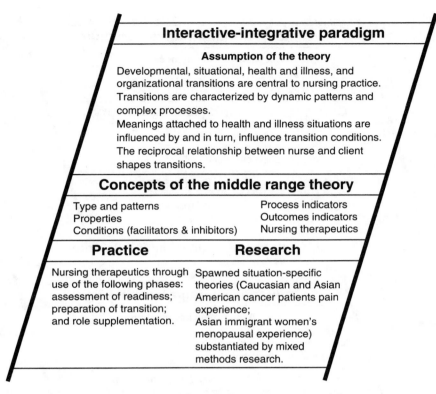

FIGURE 2.9 Ladder of Abstraction: Transitions

three situation-specific theories on the pain experience of Caucasian and Asian American cancer patients and the menopausal experience of Asian women (Figure 2.9).

The ninth theory is the Theory of Self-Reliance developed by Lowe. This theory is in keeping with the unitary–transformative paradigm and is rooted in the author's Cherokee values. Assumptions specific to the theory are the value of being true to oneself and being connected with others. This theory articulates a process for promoting well-being with attention to appreciation for one's culture. The talking circle offers an approach to nursing practice through honoring the process of life and growth. A 24-item self-reliance instrument has been developed and used in intervention studies (Figure 2.10).

The tenth theory presented in this book is the Theory of Cultural Marginality developed by Choi. This theory is embedded in the interactive–integrative paradigm, and it describes the experience of people who are caught between two cultures. Assumptions specific

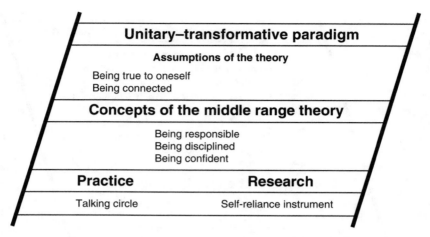

FIGURE 2.10   Ladder of Abstraction: Self-Reliance

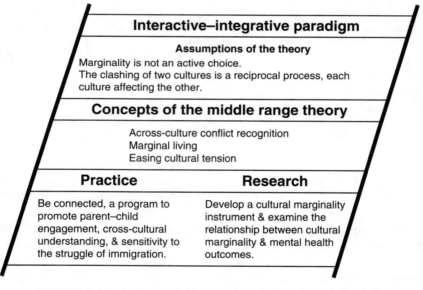

FIGURE 2.11   Ladder of Abstraction: Cultural Marginality

to the theory include across-cultural conflict recognition, marginal living, and easing cultural tension. Examples of practice applications include promoting parent–child engagement through cross-cultural understanding and being sensitive to the struggle of immigration. Research activities are aimed at developing an instrument to measure cultural marginality and studying mental health outcomes of persons living through across-culture conflict (Figure 2.11).

The eleventh theory found in this book is the Theory of Caregiving Dynamics by Williams. This theory is in keeping with the assumptions of the interactive–integrative paradigm and holds that the interactive caregiving relationship extends over time. Specific assumptions include recognition of the coexistence of negative and positive aspects of caregiving, distinction between informal and formal caregiving, and the emerging nature of the caregiving relationship over time. Concepts descriptive of the theory are commitment, expectation management, and role negotiation. Application of the theory in practice consists of caregiver classes with tailored information, attention to exercise and nutrition, and counseling. Research based on the theory focuses on the care recipient's view and testing interventions that enhance the caregiving relationship (Figure 2.12).

The twelfth theory is Nathaniel's Theory of Moral Reckoning, which is grounded in the interactive–integrative paradigm. According to this theory, persons engage in a social process of deliberating when faced with a moral dilemma. Assumptions supporting the theory include facing a moral dilemma where no one choice is right or wrong and experiencing situational binds that are inherent to being human. Concepts in the theory are ease, situational bind, resolution, and reflection. Practice based on the theory includes providing structured

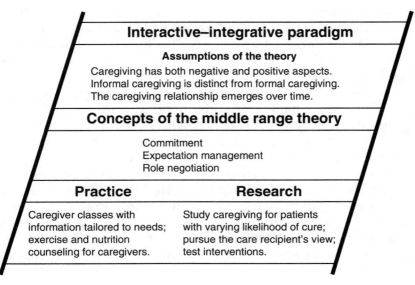

FIGURE 2.12   Ladder of Abstraction: Caregiving Dynamics

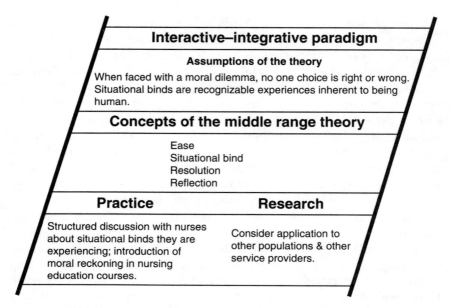

FIGURE 2.13   Ladder of Abstraction: Moral Reckoning

discussion with nurses about situational binds and introduction of moral reckoning in nursing education courses. Research guided by the theory includes study of moral reckoning with nurses. Because moral reckoning is a human experience that is increasingly common in this day and age, it warrants consideration for guiding nursing practice and structuring study for people who are in a moral bind (Figure 2.13).

There is one final ladder of abstraction on Evaluation of Middle Range Theory in Chapter 3. Smith offers a process for understanding and evaluating middle range theories based on postmodern beliefs (Figure 2.14). Overall, the ladders of abstraction provide a structure to guide the student in deciphering theory so that it can be used productively in advanced nursing practice and research. So, we urge you to begin climbing the ladders … stay long enough on each rung to get comfortable and spend enough time on all three rungs to get the whole picture of any theory. Also, expect to be uncomfortable when a rung is new to you. Discomfort is a space for growing and connecting what you know with what you are learning.

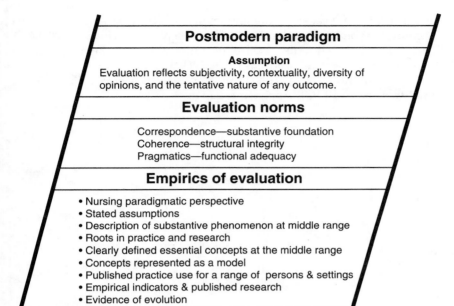

FIGURE 2.14   Ladder of Abstraction: Evaluation

REFERENCES

Chinn, P., & Kramer, M. K. (1999). *Theory and nursing: Integrated knowledge development*. St. Louis, MO: Mosby.

Ford-Gilboe, M., Campbell, J., & Berman, H. (1995). Stories and numbers: Coexistence without compromise. *Advances in Nursing Science, 18*(1), 14–26.

Im, E., & Meleis, A. I. (1999). Situation-specific theories: Philosophical roots, properties, and approach. *Advances in Nursing Science, 22*(2), 11–24.

King, I. (1996). The theory of goal attainment in research and practice. *Nursing Science Quarterly, 9*, 61–66.

McKay, R. P. (1969). Theories, models, and systems for nursing. *Nursing Research, 18*, 393–399.

Merton, R. K. (1968). *Social theory and social structure*. New York, NY: Free Press.

Newman, M., Sime, A. M., & Corcoran-Perry, S. A. (1991). The focus of the discipline of nursing. *Advances in Nursing Science, 14*(1), 1–6.

Orem, D. (1971). *Nursing: Concepts of practice*. New York, NY: McGraw-Hill.

Parse, R. R. (1992). Human becoming: Parse's theory of nursing. *Nursing Science Quarterly, 5*(1), 35–42.

Reed, P. (1995). A treatise on nursing knowledge development for the 21st century: Beyond postmodernism. *Advances in Nursing Science, 17,* 70–84.

Rogers, M. E. (1994). The science of unitary human beings: Current perspectives. *Nursing Science Quarterly, 7,* 33–35.

Roy, C., & Andrews, H. A. (1991). *The Roy adaptation model: The definitive statement.* Norwalk, CT: Appleton & Lange.

3

Evaluation of Middle Range Theories for the Discipline of Nursing

Marlaine C. Smith

Theories are patterned ideas that provide a coherent way of viewing complex phenomena. Middle range theories have a more limited view of circumscribed phenomena than do grand theories. However, because nursing is a professional discipline, all the theories within it should be evaluated from a perspective that considers the salient elements of the discipline in the evaluation. Although there are many sets of criteria for evaluating nursing conceptual models and grand theories (Chinn & Kramer, 2010; Fawcett, 2004; Fitzpatrick & Whall, 2004; Parse, 1987; Stevens, 1998), few focus particularly on theories at the middle range. In addition, there has been little guidance for beginning nursing scholars on the purpose and the process of critical analysis and evaluation of theories. A common course assignment on the evaluation of nursing theory becomes a pedantic exercise, ending in a rather cynical view of theory development. One is reminded of the aphorism: When our only tool is a hammer, all we see are nails. In other words, the tool of critical evaluation taught to students is often weighted toward finding the faults, errors, and inconsistencies within the theoretic structures. It is no wonder that there is evidence of some devaluation of nursing theory and a reticence to engage in its development.

The theoretical measurement of outcomes of practice, while a worthy endeavor, has eclipsed the compelling need to create systems of thought with potential to describe and explain the nature of phenomena of concern to nursing science. The nursing scholars who contribute to the development of theory for the discipline—including those who are featured in this text—are innovative pioneers who courageously offer their ideas for the advancement of the discipline and the betterment of health care. It is important, then, to balance the identification of theoretic weaknesses with the aspects of appreciation, recognition, and affirmation of strengths. The purpose of this chapter is to provide tools for a balanced and reasoned evaluation of middle range theory for the discipline of nursing. Describing the purposes of theory evaluation, articulating a set of criteria to guide evaluation of middle range theory, and elaborating a process for conducting this evaluation organize this chapter.

THE PURPOSE OF THEORY EVALUATION: TOWARD A POSTMODERN VIEW

Evaluation is one of the most popular indoor sports of the organizations in which we live. Because these organizations are accountable to various stakeholders, evaluation is used as a measure of assurance and accountability. The meaning of evaluation carries an onerous tone because of the baggage that is often attached to it. Students receive grades that reflect evaluation of achievement in a course. A score or category is received when one is evaluated for job performance. Often this evaluation is attached to some reward. The memory of the evaluation of papers, projects, and practice may be more often marked by the red ink of what was done wrong than by what was achieved or done well.

The common, modern definition of evaluation is a process of determining or fixing the value, worth, or significance of something. This definition reflects the anxieties that are experienced surrounding evaluation, connoting the determination of a static and absolute outcome of worth or value. A postmodern meaning of evaluation is quite different. It reflects the presence of subjectivity and contextuality, the diversity of opinions from a community, and, ultimately, the tentative nature of any outcome. It becomes an informed and flawed opinion rendered at a particular moment in time by a person with inherent biases and values. This opinion, which one hopes is not arbitrary or capricious, is based on some sound, reasonable measures or criteria that can be applied consistently. However, it is important to note that the criteria and the evaluator's application of them are value laden. In this way, they should be viewed not as absolute judgments of worth, but as one honest examination by a member of a community.

The evaluation of theory, then, is a process of coming to an opinion about its worth or value. Kaplan (1964)—in his discussion of the validation of theory—states that its purpose is to examine a theory's value or worth for advancement by the scientific community. When evaluating nursing theory, we ask questions about its worthiness to be used as a guide for inquiry and practice and to be taught to students.

Theory, by its definition in any paradigm of science, is a creative constellation of ideas, offered as a possible explanation or description of an observed or experienced phenomenon. In the process of evaluation, one is not determining the truth of the theory, but rather its value for further exploration within the scientific community. History affirms the tentative nature of theory evaluation. Theories that were judged by the scientific community as valid were often later abandoned. Ptolemaic theory on the geocentric nature of the planetary system was abandoned later for the Copernican theory that the Earth and the planets revolve around the Sun.

Many revolutionary ideas of our time were evaluated initially as worthless. Rogers's (1970) conceptual system—describing the integral nature of human–environment energy fields—was an object of ridicule in the early 1970s. Thirty years later, its correspondence to burgeoning contemporary thought is stunning.

Members of a disciplinary community bear the responsibility to participate in authentic dialogue around ideas within the field of study. The purpose of evaluation of theory in this context is to share in the evolution of the discipline through reflection and comment on the ideas offered within the community. The greater value of evaluating theory is to participate as individuals in the community's structuring of ideas. Although the theory is given to the community, the community reforms it through critique, testing, and application. The life of any theory is determined by the scientific community's engagement with it. Evaluation of theory is essential to the life of the theory, leading to its extension, revision, and refinement. Based on the preceding discussion, it is important that the evaluator stay true to the purpose of evaluation of theory. The stance of one who is evaluating theory from a postmodern perspective is characterized by intellectual empathy, curiosity, honesty, and responsibility. The empathic stance is the attempt to understand the perspective of the theorist and is defined by Paul (1993) as "to imaginatively put oneself in the place of others in order to understand them" (p. 261). Here, the evaluator listens carefully to the point of view. Listening is being aware of one's own biases but trying to put them aside to thoughtfully consider others' ideas, even if the evaluator does not share them. The stance of empathy requires an appreciation of others' points of view and a seeking out of the origin and context of those points of view. Curiosity is the second characteristic of the critical stance. Here, the evaluator raises questions in the process of studying the theory that are born from a quest to understand. The evaluator plays with the theory in different circumstances and imagines ways of testing or understanding it more deeply. The evaluator engages fully in trying to understand and acquire a range of sources on the theory and its application. The third stance is one of honesty. The evaluator trusts individual inner wisdom and recognizes the need to honor that wisdom in sharing the evaluation. Knowing personal biases and limitations, the evaluator is still willing to share reflections on the theory. One of the major hurdles in learning to evaluate theory is to rely on one's own opinions rather than jumping on the bandwagon of others who are considered wiser or more learned. From the postmodern perspective, each evaluation should stand on its own, one voice among many diverse ones in the community. It may be difficult to publish negative comments, but it is important to remember that these may be the needed stimuli to make important clarifications or changes in the theory. Finally, the evaluator must be a responsible steward of the discipline. As a member of the scientific community, the evaluator has an obligation to care about the nature of evolution of nursing knowledge. That responsibility entails a thoughtful and scholarly response to the critique, applying the criteria fairly and drawing conclusions that can be useful in the revision or extension of the theory as others use it. Once a theory is published, it no longer belongs to the theorist. The voice of the theorist becomes one of many in the community using the theory to guide processes of knowledge development and practice.

In summary, the purpose of a postmodern approach to the evaluation of middle range theory in nursing is to come to a decision about the merits and limitations of the theory for nursing science. The evaluator approaches the evaluation from a stance of empathy, curiosity, honesty, and responsibility. Evaluation of theory is acknowledged as necessary to the evolution of the theory in the context of the scientific community.

THE ORIGIN OF EVALUATIVE FRAMEWORKS

Theories are the language of science. "Science is the process of systematically seeking an understanding of phenomena through creating some unifying or organizing frameworks about the nature of those phenomena. In addition, science involves the evaluation of these frameworks for their credibility and empirical honesty" (Smith, 1994, p. 50). The organizing or unifying frameworks of science are theories. Rigorous and systematic standards of inquiry govern the development and testing of theories. Theories are evaluated for their credibility and empirical honesty by judging them against established standards.

The nature of science and, therefore, the theories of science have undergone change. Philosophies of science have evolved from a sole reliance on the assumptions of logical–positivist views toward expanding philosophies of the postpositivist or postmodern era (Smith, 1998). For example, the traditional or empirical–analytic view of science defines theories as sets of interrelated propositions that describe, explain, or predict the nature of phenomena (Kerlinger, 1986). In the human science view, which encompasses phenomenology, hermeneutics, and critical and poststructural perspectives, the purpose of theory is to create an understanding of phenomena through description and interpretation. Therefore, the structural rules, which apply to traditional science, do not apply to human science. For this reason, the frameworks used to evaluate theories must be inclusive enough to encompass these differences.

Kaplan's (1964) perspective on the "validation" of theories is open enough to encompass a diversity of theoretic forms. He emphasizes that the evaluation of any theory is not a matter of pronouncement of its truth. "At any given moment a particular theory will be accepted by some scientists, for some of their purposes, and not by other scientists, or not for other contexts of possible application" (p. 311).

The evaluation of theory involves the exercise of good judgment in determining a relative and tentative truth, and is by its nature normative in that the community ultimately determines the outcome. "The validation of a theory is not the act of granting an imprimatur but the act of deciding that the theory is worth being published, taught, and above all, applied—worth being acted on in contexts of inquiry or of other action" (Kaplan, 1964, p. 312). Kaplan identifies three major philosophical conceptions or norms of truth that can be exercised in the process of evaluating theory: correspondence or semantic norms, coherence or syntactic norms, and pragmatics or functional norms.

The norm of correspondence refers to the substantive meaning of the theory. Through application of this norm, one judges the degree to which the theory fits the facts. Although facts are in themselves understood through a theoretic lens, Kaplan argues that this does not necessarily present a tautology. Any theory must in some way pass the test of common sense. Although he acknowledges that significant discoveries have flown in the face of common sense, these discoveries in some way could be explained through their relationship to accepted knowledge or some convergence of evidence that supported the plausibility of the theory. Through the norm of correspondence, one evaluates the extent to which the theory fits comfortably within the nexus of existing knowledge.

The norm of coherence relates to the integrity of the theory's structure. Kaplan describes the experience of the "click of relation, when widely different and separate phenomena suddenly fall into a pattern of relatedness, when they click into position" (p. 314). This experience of truth or wholeness occurs when all the fragments of the theory come together to form an integrated whole. Simplicity is the most widely applied norm of coherence. Descriptive simplicity is the quality of expressing the complex ideas of the theory parsimoniously. Inductive simplicity refers to the phenomenon being described by the theory. The theory must encompass a manageable number of ideas; too many will overwhelm the capacity of the theory to serve its purpose to provide a framework for understanding. Kaplan warns that a theory can be too simple in that it goes too far in reducing the complexities. Theories should introduce the degree of complexity necessary for clear understanding, nothing more. He quotes Whitehead's axiom: "Seek simplicity and distrust it" (p. 318). Another norm of coherence is aesthetics, that is, the beauty perceived upon the contemplation of the theory. The beauty of the theory involves some sense of symmetry and balance, but Kaplan warns, "Beauty is not truth" (p. 319). The process of developing theory is creative and that creativity is expressed in a product that possesses an aesthetic quality.

The final norm is pragmatics and refers to the effectiveness or functional capability of the theory. In a professional discipline, the norm of pragmatics instructs us to consider the degree to which the theory can guide practice and research to advance the goals of the discipline. On the other hand, Kaplan states that the theory is not judged by the extent to which it makes some external difference alone; he acknowledges that other factors might interfere with or enhance the success of application. The theory is also judged by what it can do for science, "how it guides and stimulates the ongoing process of scientific inquiry" (pp. 319–320). So the degree to which the theory has spawned research questions is relevant. "The value of the theory lies not only in the answers it gives but also in the new questions it raises" (p. 320).

A theory is validated when it is put to good use in the application of concerns to the discipline. The evaluative framework for middle range theories is based on these norms. Criteria will be clustered into the following three categories: substantive foundation, structural integrity, and functional adequacy.

An abundance of evaluative frameworks for nursing theories have evolved over the past several decades (Chinn & Kramer, 2010; Fawcett, 2004; Fitzpatrick & Whall, 2004; Parse, 1987; Stevens, 1998). Some of these frameworks are applicable to middle range theories, whereas others are not. Liehr and Smith (1999) summarized the literature about the nature of middle range theories and concluded that middle range theories are identified by their scope, level of abstraction, and proximity to empirical findings. Scope refers to the breadth of phenomena addressed by the theory. Compared to conceptual models and grand theories, middle range theories offer constellations of ideas or concepts about more circumscribed phenomena of concern to the discipline. In this way, they are intermediate in scope, focusing on a limited number of concepts focused on a limited aspect of reality (Liehr & Smith, 1999). Level of abstraction locates middle range theories between the abstract level of conceptual models and grand theories and situation-specific theories. The language of middle range theories describes concepts and relationships between them more concretely. Finally, middle range theories are more proximal to empirical findings than conceptual models and grand theories. They are developed through an analysis of empirical findings or at a level of immediate testability. These three qualities of middle range theories should be represented in the evaluative frameworks for them.

The following criteria (Table 3.1) have been developed from Kaplan's norms for validating theories and are informed by the essential qualities of middle range theories to create an evaluative framework specific to theories of the middle range.

TABLE 3.1
Framework for the Evaluation of Middle Range Theories

Substantive Foundations

1. The theory is within the focus of the discipline of nursing.
2. The assumptions are specified and congruent with focus.
3. The theory provides a substantive description, explanation, or interpretation of a named phenomenon at the middle range level of discourse.
4. The origins are rooted in practice and research experience.

Structural Integrity

1. The concepts are clearly defined.
2. The concepts within the theory are at the middle range level of abstraction.
3. There are no more concepts than needed to explain the phenomenon.
4. The concepts and relationships among them are logically represented with a model.

Functional Adequacy

1. The theory can be applied to a variety of practice environments and client groups.
2. Empirical indicators have been identified for concepts of the theory.
3. There are published examples of use of the theory in practice.
4. There are published examples of research related to the theory.
5. The theory has evolved through scholarly inquiry.

Substantive Foundation

Substantive foundation is the first category of criteria for the evaluation of middle range theory in nursing. This category includes criteria based on Kaplan's norm of correspondence and leads to questions about the meaning or semantic elements of the theory. A middle range theory in nursing contributes to the knowledge of the discipline of nursing and is developed from assumptions that are clearly specified. The theory provides knowledge that is at the middle range level of abstraction. There are four major criteria related to substantive meaning: (1) the theory is within the focus of the discipline of nursing; (2) the assumptions are specified and are congruent with the focus of the discipline of nursing; (3) the theory provides a substantive description, explanation, or interpretation of a named phenomenon at the middle range level of discourse; and (4) the origins are rooted in practice and research experience. Each of these criteria and the questions that guide the application of the criteria in evaluating the theory will be discussed. The first criterion emphasizes that a middle range theory in nursing is judged by its location in and contribution to the discipline of nursing. The question, "What makes a middle range theory in nursing a *nursing* theory?" is interesting to consider. Some (Fawcett, 2004; Parse, 1987) assert that nursing theories are only those identified as the conceptual models and grand theories developed by nurses in the 1960s through the 1980s. From this perspective, legitimate middle range theories in nursing are those deduced from or inductively developed within existing conceptual models and grand theories of nursing. This is problematic in that it fixates theory development in what has been considered legitimate in the past. It is important to leave space for the possibility of emergent conceptual models or grand constructions that may be articulated as sets of foundational assumptions on which middle range theories are constructed. The evaluator should expect that a middle range theory in nursing contributes to knowledge about human–environment health relationships, caring in the human health experience, and/or health and healing processes (Fawcett, 2004; Newman, Sime, & Corcoran-Perry, 1991; Smith, 1994). It should be possible to locate the theory within a paradigmatic perspective endorsed by nursing, such as the particulate–deterministic, interactive–integrative, unitary–transformative schemas (Newman et al., 1991), the totality or simultaneity paradigm (Parse, 1987), or the reaction, reciprocal interaction, or simultaneous action worldview (Fawcett, 2004).

The second criterion regarding the specification of assumptions in the category of substantive foundations is that the origins and ontological foundations of the theory are specified. The developer of the middle range theory holds philosophical assumptions that are either explicitly stated or implied by the meaning of the theory. Fawcett (2004) argues that the belief that middle range theory is developed outside the context of a conceptual frame of reference is absurd. She emphasizes the contextual nature of theory building. The assumptions of a middle range theory identify the context for theory building and should be identifiable. A stronger middle range theory would explicate the assumptions.

The ideas of parent theories or models should be clearly identified in the explication of the meaning of the theory. The developers should cite primary sources from any parent theories that may be accessed for greater depth in understanding. Although some middle range theories will not be explicitly derived from nursing conceptual models, parent ideas that shaped theory development would be clearly described.

Finally, the meaning of the theory should be consistent with its foundational assumptions. This consistency is essential. If Rogers's Science of Unitary Human Beings (SUHB) forms the assumptions of a middle range theory, the meaning of the concepts within the theory should not violate these assumptions. One would not use the language of adaptive responses in a theory purportedly derived from the SUHB. If the assumptions are not derived from an existing conceptual model/grand theory, one is left to analyze inferred foundations about how the assumption corresponds with the meaning of the middle range theory.

The third criterion related to substantive foundations states that the middle range theory provides substantive knowledge about a named circumscribed phenomenon of concern to nursing. Liehr and Smith (1999) contend that a middle range theory is known by the way it is named and that it should be "named in the context of the disciplinary perspective and at the appropriate level of discourse" (p. 86). Middle range theory is defined by its focus on providing knowledge about a specific phenomenon of concern to nursing. The theory should offer a substantive description, explanation, or interpretation of this particular phenomenon that leads to a new understanding or different way of considering the phenomenon. It is incumbent on the developer of the theory to provide adequate explanation substantiated by logical reasoning and reference to existing knowledge sources that lead to a full understanding of the meaning of the concepts and their relationships to each other.

Finally, the theory should capture the complexities of the phenomenon that it addresses. A theory is a map of some aspect of reality; like a map, it cannot capture the landscape. However, to the extent possible, the theory should approximate the fullest range of conceptual relationships that it addresses.

The fourth criterion deals with the rooting of the origins of the theory in practice and research experience. Middle range theory grows out of the research and practice experiences of nurses, who articulate a set of concepts to describe and explain a phenomenon that they have observed in their work. The evaluator will seek out the practice and research roots of the theory. It may be that one set of roots (practice or research) is sturdier than the other. This assessment may indicate a next direction for further application of the theory. Well-developed middle range theory will have documented development related to both practice and research that evolves over time.

Structural Integrity

A middle range theory is a framework that organizes ideas. Like any framework, it has a structure. The structure provides strength, balance, and the aesthetic qualities that ensure its integrity. Structural integrity is the category that was derived from Kaplan's (1964) norm of coherence. There are four criteria for evaluation of the structural integrity of middle range theories: (1) the concepts are clearly defined, (2) the concepts of the theory are at the middle range level of abstraction, (3) there are no more concepts than are needed to explain the phenomenon, and (4) the concepts and relationships among them are logically represented with a model. The four criteria for structural integrity and their application are discussed below.

The first criterion is that the ideas and the relationships among them are clearly presented within the theory. Concepts are the names given to the abstract ideas that constitute the theory. The relationships among the ideas are developed into statements or propositions. In any middle range theory, the concepts within it should be clearly defined. Any neologisms (newly coined terms) should be adequately defined. The relationship statements, whether called propositions or not, should articulate the relationships among the central ideas or concepts within the theory. Concepts, even within the context of middle range theory, are abstractions, and, as such, it takes some willingness to understand them. However, the definitions should lead to this understanding and provide precise meaning.

The second criterion related to structural integrity is that the ideas of the theory are at the middle range level of abstraction. All concepts should be on the ladder of abstraction at a similar level. For example, health may be considered a concept at the metaparadigm level; adaptation, at the level of grand theory; and anxiety, at the level of the middle range. Mixing these as concepts within one theory would be an example of concepts at differing levels of abstraction. Similarly, the concepts in the theory should consistently be presented at the middle range level, more concrete and circumscribed than concepts at a higher level of abstraction. The deductive or inductive processes of theory development should be transparent in the presentation of the theory. Movement up the ladder of abstraction to paradigms or down the ladder to empirical indicators should be logical, reasoned, and clear.

The third criterion is that there should be no more concepts than necessary to describe the theory as named. The theory should be organized and presented parsimoniously. That means that the ideas should be synthesized and communicated in the simplest, most elegant way possible. Extraneous concepts or unclear differentiation of concepts creates complexity that confuses rather than clarifies.

The fourth or final criterion is that the ideas of the theory are integrated to create an understanding of the whole phenomenon, which is presented in a model. This criterion leads to consideration of the internal consistency, balance, and aesthetics of the theory. The concepts and statements of the theory should be logically ordered so that they lead to an appreciation and apprehension of the theory's meaning. The relationships among the ideas can be represented in a schema, a model, or a list of logically ordered statements. In any case, it is the responsibility of the developer to make these relationships accessible. All ideas (concepts and related statements) in the theory should have semantic congruence, that is, the meanings should not be contradictory. Middle range theories are creative products of science. As such, there should be balance and harmony in the way they are presented.

Functional Adequacy

For a professional discipline, functional adequacy is arguably the acid test of a middle range theory. Middle range theories are closely tied to research and practice. They may be generated from research findings or deduced from larger models to form a set of testable hypotheses. They may have been developed in relation to a practice dilemma and can be used to create practice guidelines. Middle range theories build nursing knowledge and are valuable in and of themselves for this contribution. There are five criteria for functional adequacy of middle range theories: (1) the theory can be applied to a variety of practice environments and client groups, (2) empirical indicators have been identified for concepts of the theory, (3) there are published examples of use of the theory in practice, (4) there are published examples of research related to the theory, and (5) the theory has evolved through scholarly inquiry. Each of these criteria will be described below.

The first criterion of functional adequacy is that the theory provides guidance for a variety of practice population and environments. One would expect literature that documents use of the theory with more than one population and in more than one setting. Because the theory is middle range rather than situation specific, this generality criterion is important and limited to the central phenomenon of the theory.

The second criterion is that there are empirical indicators identified for the concepts of the theory. Empirical adequacy is an essential aspect of middle range theory. Empirics are meant to go beyond empiricism and include perceptions, symbolic meanings, self-reports, observable behavior, biological indicators, and personal stories (Ford-Gilboe, Campbell, & Berman, 1995; Reed, 1995). Researchers working with the middle range theory may have selected empirical indicators for measurement of theoretical constructs, or they may have developed the middle range theory from descriptions and stories. Both of these examples support the theory's empirical adequacy. Empirical adequacy is an indication of the maturity of the theory.

The third criterion is that there are published examples of how the theory has been used in practice. This criterion offers evidence to support that the theory makes a difference in the lives of people. Published reports of the theory should demonstrate that use of the theory enhances well-being and quality of life. When the middle range theory is taken to practice there are expectations about emergent outcomes. These outcomes may be identified and tested by those conducting evaluation studies on theory-guided practice.

The fourth criterion is that there are published examples of research related to the theory. This criterion is a strong indicator of functional adequacy. The research findings can be examined for the level of support of the theory. In addition, middle range theories may generate hypotheses or research questions. Any refinements to the theory based on research findings should be examined; this indicates that the theory is open enough to change through the incorporation of further testing or development of ideas. In the process of evaluating this criterion, it is important to examine the evolution of the theory over time through inquiry and reflection.

The fifth criterion is that the theory has evolved through scholarly inquiry. Theories should evoke thinking, raise questions, invite dialogue, and urge us toward further exploration. This engaging quality of the theory is a hallmark of its potential for advancing the discipline. In order for the theory to grow, a community of scholars must engage with it in practice and research. Middle range theories build the discipline of nursing through expanding knowledge related to specific phenomena. The speculations offered by the theory push the boundaries of what is currently known and invite continuing systematic inquiry. In this way, the theory evolves and contributes to the development of nursing science and art.

APPLYING THE FRAMEWORK TO THE EVALUATION OF MIDDLE RANGE THEORIES

The evaluation of middle range theory involves preparation, judgment, and justification. In the preparation phase, those evaluating the theory should spend time understanding the theory as fully as possible through dwelling with it. Dwelling with is investing time in reading and reflecting on the theory. The elements of the critical stance—empathy, curiosity, honesty, and responsibility, as articulated earlier in this chapter—are applied during preparation. It is important to gather a variety of sources on and about the theory, including primary sources written by the author of the theory, research reports, critiques, and practice papers. Reading the theory repeatedly to understand the ideas is the first step. In this process of beginning analysis, it is important to identify the central ideas and the structure of the theory. Middle range theories are developed from parent theories, empirical findings, or practice insights. Depth in understanding a theory may require going to the source documents that were critical to its development. Critical evaluation requires attending to questions and reactions to the theory that surface during the reading. It is important to record these questions and reactions. The next step in preparation is studying the practice and research reports related to the theory. Note how the theory was tested or extended through research. Examine how the theory has been applied in practice and any outcome studies that relate to the application of practice approaches or models based on the theory. Written critiques by others will provide another source of information. Because they may interfere with or unduly influence one's own evaluation, it is preferable to read those critiques or evaluations after one's own is completed.

The judgment phase is the heart of the evaluative process. In this phase, the evaluator reads and reflects on the criteria in the evaluative framework. The evaluator trusts him- or herself as the instrument of judgment, one who has seriously and rigorously engaged in studying the theory. The evaluator reflects on and refers to the notes and responses created during the analysis process. The criteria in the evaluative framework are a guide toward making decisions about the meaning, structure, practice, and research applications. The strengths and weaknesses of the theory should receive equal weight in the judgment phase. Both of these elements of the evaluation can contribute to the development of the theory. In the justification phase, the evaluator supports judgments with explicit reasons for the decisions and with examples that illustrate points. In this phase, the evaluator can refer to other written critiques that may support or refute judgments about the theory. The evaluation is written in a narration structured by the criteria in the framework. Each criterion is addressed through weaving judgments and support of those judgments. A balanced evaluation identifies both the strengths and limitations of the theory and suggests specific recommendations for clarification, extension, or revision.

The goal of this chapter was to explicate the purpose, structure, and process of evaluating middle range theories. Middle range theories are at the frontier of nursing science. The development of substantive knowledge through middle range theories promises movement toward disciplinary maturity. These theories will direct and spawn new inquiry and will stimulate the development of nursing practice approaches to enhance health and well-being. The evaluation of nursing theory is an essential activity within the scientific community. It leads to the advancement, refinement, and extension of substantive knowledge in the discipline. It is a critical skill of any scholar and is honed through practice and mentoring.

REFERENCES

Chinn, P. L., & Kramer, M. K. (2010). *Integrated knowledge development in nursing* (8th ed.). St. Louis, MO: Mosby.

Fawcett, J. (2004). *Analysis and evaluation of contemporary nursing knowledge*. Philadelphia, PA: F. A. Davis.

Fitzpatrick, J. J., & Whall, A. L. (2004). *Conceptual models of nursing*. Stamford, CT: Appleton & Lange.

Ford-Gilboe, M., Campbell, J., & Berman, H. (1995). Stories and numbers: Coexistence without compromise. *Advances in Nursing Science, 18*, 14–26.

Kaplan, A. (1964). *The conduct of inquiry*. San Francisco, CA: Chandler.

Kerlinger, F. N. (1986). *Foundations of behavioral research* (3rd ed.). New York, NY: Holt, Rinehart & Winston.

Liehr, P., & Smith, M. J. (1999). Middle range theory: Spinning research and practice to create knowledge for the new millennium. *Advances in Nursing Science, 21*(4), 81–91.

Newman, M. A., Sime, A. M., & Corcoran-Perry, S. A. (1991). Focus of the discipline of nursing. *Advances in Nursing Science, 14*(1), 1–6.

Parse, R. R. (1987). *Nursing science: Major paradigms, theories, and critiques.* Philadelphia, PA: W. B. Saunders.

Paul, R. (1993). *Critical thinking: How to prepare students for a rapidly changing world.* Santa Rosa, CA: Foundation for Critical Thinking.

Reed, P. (1995). Treatise on nursing knowledge development for the 21st century: Beyond postmodernism. *Advances in Nursing Science, 17,* 70–84.

Rogers, M. E. (1970). *An introduction to the theoretical basis of nursing.* Philadelphia, PA: F. A. Davis.

Smith, M. C. (1994). Arriving at a philosophy of nursing: Discovering? constructing? evolving? In J. Kikuchi & H. Simmons (Eds.), *Developing a philosophy of nursing* (pp. 43–60). Thousand Oaks, CA: Sage.

Smith, M. C. (1998). Knowledge building for the health sciences in the twenty-first century. *Journal of Sport and Exercise Psychology, 20,* S128–S144.

Stevens, B. (1998). *Nursing theory: Analysis, application, evaluation.* Boston, MA: Little, Brown.

Section Two

Middle Range Theories Ready for Application

Twelve middle range theories are presented in this section. Each theory is organized by the following topics: purpose of the theory and how it was developed, concepts of the theory, a model showing relationships among the concepts, and use of the theory in research and practice. Therefore, the organizational structure of each theory provides consistent information relevant to developing a deepened understanding of a theory. We have found that a consistent organization structure provides a strong foundation for scholars wishing to compare, contrast, and understand theories. A reader will notice connections between some of the middle range theories in this book. For instance, the theories of self-transcendence and meaning not only share the same unitary–transformative paradigmatic perspective but also share a common spirit of finding ways to move on in the midst of difficult circumstances. Several middle range theories in this book have cultural roots or links; these include cultural marginality, transitions, and self-reliance. The theories of unpleasant symptoms and symptom management provide two approaches to the important topic of symptoms. Scholars wishing to choose a theory to guide research and practice will appreciate the organizational structure of the chapters, where one theory can be readily considered in relation to another. Middle range theories are human constructions rooted in extant literature, personal knowing, and research/practice experience of the authors. The theories have been explicated through defined concepts, modeled to show logical relationships, and applied directly to practice and research.

4

Theories of Uncertainty in Illness

Merle H. Mishel

In this chapter, two theories of uncertainty in illness are described. The original uncertainty in illness theory (UIT) was developed to address uncertainty during the diagnostic and treatment phases of an illness or an illness with a determined downward trajectory (Mishel, 1988). The reconceptualized uncertainty in illness theory (RUIT) was developed to address the experience of living with continuous uncertainty in either a chronic illness requiring ongoing management or an illness with a possibility of recurrence (Mishel, 1990).

The UIT proposes that uncertainty exists in illness situations, which are ambiguous, complex, and unpredictable. Uncertainty is defined as the inability to determine the meaning of illness-related events. It is a cognitive state created when the individual cannot adequately structure or categorize an illness event because of insufficient cues (Mishel, 1988). The theory explains how patients cognitively structure a schema for the subjective interpretation of uncertainty with treatments and outcomes. The theory is composed of three major themes: (1) antecedents of uncertainty, (2) appraisal of uncertainty, and (3) coping with uncertainty. Uncertainty and cognitive schema are the major concepts of a theory.

The RUIT retains the definition of uncertainty and major themes as in the UIT. The two concepts of self-organization and probabilistic thinking are added. The RUIT addresses the process that occurs when a person lives with unremitting uncertainty found in chronic illness or in illness with a potential for recurrence. The desired outcome from the RUIT is a growth to a new value system, whereas the outcome of the UIT is a return to the previous level of adaptation or functioning (Mishel, 1990).

PURPOSE OF THEORIES AND HOW THEY WERE DEVELOPED

The purpose of each theory is to describe and explain uncertainty as a basis for practice and research. The UIT applies to the prediagnostic, diagnostic, and treatment phases of acute and chronic illnesses. The RUIT applies to enduring uncertainty in chronic illness or illness with the possibility of recurrence that requires self-management. The theories focus on the ill individual and on the family or parent of an ill individual. Usage of theory within groups or communities is not consistent.

The finding that uncertainty was reported to be common among people experiencing illness or receiving medical treatment led to the creation of the UIT (Mishel, 1988). Although the concept was cited in the literature, there was no substantive exploration of how uncertainty developed or was resolved. It was a personal experience with my ill father that catalyzed the concept for me. He was dying from colon cancer, and his body was swollen and emaciated. He didn't understand what was happening to him so he focused on whatever he could control to provide some degree of predictability. The effort he spent on achieving some understanding brought the significance of uncertainty home to me. Although I had explored the concept of uncertainty, it was not until I entered doctoral study in psychology that I focused in earnest on the concept.

Developing the UIT included a synthesis of the research on uncertainty, cognitive processing, and managing threatening events. The UIT was revised from the original measurement model published in 1981, to the theory published in 1988. During my doctoral study, I focused on the development and testing of a measure of uncertainty. At that time, I was influenced by the literature on stress and coping that discussed uncertainty as one type of stressful event (Lazarus, 1974). As I began to explore the literature, I discovered the work of Norton (1975), who identified eight dimensions of uncertainty. His work—along with that of Moos and Tsu (1977)—formed a framework leading to the development of the Mishel Uncertainty in Illness Scale.

My early ideas were further influenced by Bower (1978) and Shalit (1977), who described uncertainty as a complex cognitive stressor, and by Budner (1962), who described ambiguous, novel, or complex stimuli as sources of uncertainty. The ideas of these cognitive psychologists influenced my view of uncertainty as a cognitive state rather than as an emotional response. This distinction directed ongoing theory development. Uncertainty as a stressor or threat was based on the work of both Shalit (1977) and Lazarus (1974). The descriptions of coping as a primary appraisal of uncertainty and response to uncertainty as a secondary appraisal were adapted from the work of Lazarus (1974). The Uncertainty in Illness Scale (Mishel, 1981) incorporated the work of these primary sources to conceptualize uncertainty in illness.

When the Uncertainty in Illness Scale was published, a body of findings on uncertainty quickly emerged in the nursing literature (Mishel, 1983, 1984; Mishel & Braden, 1987, 1988; Mishel, Hostetter, King, & Graham, 1984; Mishel & Murdaugh, 1987). Research findings on uncertainty substantiated the antecedents of the theory. The stimuli frame variable, composed of familiarity of events and congruence of events, was formed from research on uncertainty in illness and research in cognitive psychology. Symptom pattern was developed from qualitative studies (Mishel & Murdaugh, 1987) describing the importance of consistency of symptoms to form a pattern. The antecedent of cognitive capacities was based on cognitive psychology (Mandler, 1979) and practice knowledge about instructing patients when cognitive processing abilities were compromised. The final antecedent of structure providers was developed from research on uncertainty in illness.

The appraisal section of the theory was developed using sources from the 1981 model and based on clinical data and discussions with colleagues. Colleagues identified personality variables as important in the evaluation of uncertainty, and clinical data indicated that uncertainty could be a preferred state under specific circumstances. This led to inclusion of inference and illusion as two phases of appraisal (Mishel & Braden, 1987; Mishel & Murdaugh, 1987).

The RUIT was developed through discussion with colleagues, qualitative data from chronically ill individuals, and an awareness of the limitations of the UIT. The UIT was linear and explained uncertainty in the acute and treatment phases of illness, but did not address life changes over time expressed by persons with chronic illness. Qualitative interviews with chronically ill individuals revealed continuous uncertainty and a new view of life that incorporated uncertainty. From the perspective of critical social theory (Allen, 1985), the patient's desire for certainty may reflect the goals of control and predictability that form the sociohistorical values of Western society (Mishel, 1990). Clinical data revealed that those who chose to incorporate uncertainty into their lives were living a value system on the edge of mainstream ideas. To explain the clinical data, a framework that conceptualized uncertainty as a preferred state was initiated using the process of theory derivation described by Walker and Avant (1989). Chaos was chosen as the parent theory to reconceptualize uncertainty. Chaos theory emphasizes disorder, instability, diversity, disequilibrium, and restructuring as the healthy variability of a system. The reconceptualized theory included ideas of disorganization and reformulation of a new stability to explain how a person with enduring uncertainty emerges with a new view of life.

Drawing from chaos theory (Prigogine & Stengers, 1984), uncertainty is viewed as a force that spreads from illness to other areas of a person's life and competes with the person's previous mode of functioning. As uncertain areas of life increase, pattern disruption occurs and uncertainty feeds back on itself and generates more uncertainty. When uncertainty persists, its intensity exceeds a person's level of tolerance. There is a sense of disorganization that promotes personal instability. With a high level of disorganization comes a loss of a sense of coherence (Antonovsky, 1987). A system in disorganization begins to reorganize at an imperceptible level that represents a gradual transition from a perspective of life oriented to predictability and control to a new view of life in which multiple contingencies are preferable.

CONCEPTS OF THE THEORIES

Uncertainty is the central concept in the theory and is defined as the inability to determine the meaning of illness-related events inclusive of inability to assign definite value and/or to accurately predict outcomes. Another concept central to the uncertainty theory is cognitive schema, which is defined as the person's subjective interpretation of illness-related events (see Figure 4.1). The UIT is organized around three major themes related to the concepts: antecedents of uncertainty, appraisal of uncertainty, and coping with uncertainty.

The ideas included in the antecedent theme of the theory include stimuli frame, cognitive capacity, and structure providers. Stimuli frame is defined as the form, composition, and structure of the stimuli that the person perceives. The stimuli frame has three components: symptom pattern, event familiarity, and event congruence. Symptom pattern refers to the degree to which symptoms are present with sufficient consistency to be perceived as having a pattern or configuration. Event familiarity is the degree to which the situation is habitual, repetitive, or contains recognized cues. Event congruence refers to the consistency between the expected and the experienced illness-related events. Cognitive capacity and structure providers influence the three components of the stimuli frame. Cognitive capacity is the information-processing ability of the individual.

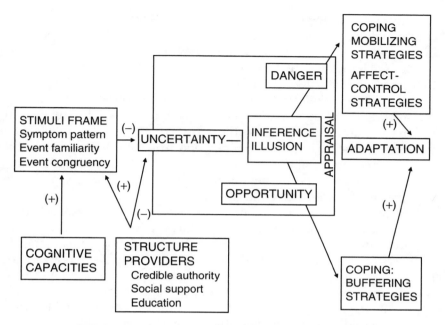

FIGURE 4.1   Perceived Uncertainty in Illness
Source: Reprinted with permission from Mishel, M. H. (1988).
Uncertainty in illness. *The Journal of Nursing Scholarship, 20*(4),
225–232.

Structure providers are the resources available to assist the person in the interpretation of the stimuli frame. Structure providers include education, social support, and credible authority.

The second major theme in the UIT is appraisal of uncertainty, which is defined as the process of placing a value on the uncertain event or situation. There are two components of appraisal: inference or illusion. Inference refers to the evaluation of uncertainty using related examples and is built on personality dispositions, general experience, knowledge, and contextual cues. Illusion refers to the construction of beliefs formed from uncertainty that have a positive outlook. The result of appraisal is the valuing of uncertainty as a danger or an opportunity.

The third theme in the UIT is coping with uncertainty and includes danger, opportunity, coping, and adaptation. Danger is the possibility of a harmful outcome. Opportunity is the possibility of a positive outcome. Coping with a danger appraisal is defined as activities directed toward reducing uncertainty and managing the emotion generated by a danger appraisal. Coping with an opportunity appraisal is defined as activities directed toward maintaining uncertainty. Adaptation is defined as biopsychosocial behavior occurring within the person's individually defined range of usual behavior.

The RUIT includes the antecedent theme in the UIT and adds the two concepts of self-organization and probabilistic thinking. Self-organization is the reformulation of a new sense of order, resulting from the integration of continuous uncertainty into one's self-structure in which uncertainty is accepted as the natural rhythm of life. Probabilistic thinking is a belief in a conditional world in which the expectation of certainty and predictability is abandoned. The RUIT proposes four factors that influence the formation of a new life perspective: prior life experience, physiological status, social resources, and health care providers. In the process of reorganization, the person reevaluates uncertainty by gradual approximations, from an aversive experience to one of opportunity. Thus, uncertainty becomes the foundation for a new sense of order and is accepted as the natural rhythm of life. There is an ability to focus on multiple alternatives, choices, and possibilities; reevaluate what is important in life; consider variation in personal investment; and appreciate the impermanence and fragility of life. The theory identifies conditions under which the new ability is maintained or blocked.

The concepts of both theories tie clearly to nursing by describing and explaining human responses to illness situations. Uncertainty crosses all phases of illness from prediagnosis symptomatology to diagnosis, treatment, treatment residuals, recovery, potential recurrence, and exacerbation. Thus, the theories are pertinent to the health experience for all age groups. Uncertainty is experienced by ill persons, caregivers, and parents of ill children.

The theories incorporate a consideration of the health care environment as a component of the stimuli frame and the broader support network. Nursing care is represented under the concept of structure providers. Because an important part of nursing involves explaining and providing information, it follows that nursing actions are interventions to help patients manage uncertainty. The outcomes of both theories are directly related to health. The health outcome is to regain personal control, as in adaptation (UIT) or consciousness expansion (RUIT).

RELATIONSHIPS AMONG THE CONCEPTS: THE MODELS

As seen in Figure 4.1, the UIT is displayed as a linear model with no feedback loops. According to the model, uncertainty is the result of antecedents. The major path to uncertainty is through the stimuli frame variables. Cognitive capacities influence stimuli frame variables. If the person has a compromised cognitive capacity due to fever, infection, pain, or mind-altering medication, the clarity and definition of the stimuli frame variables are likely to be reduced, resulting in uncertainty. In such a situation, it is assumed that stimuli frame variables are clear, patterned, and distinct, and only become less so because of limitations in cognitive capacity. However, when cognitive capacity is adequate, stimuli frame variables may still lack a symptom pattern or be unfamiliar and incongruent due to lack of information, complex information, information overload, or conflicting information. The structure provider variables then come into play to alter the stimuli frame variables by interpreting, providing meaning, and explaining. These actions serve to structure the stimuli frame, thereby reducing or preventing uncertainty. Structure providers may also directly impact uncertainty. The health care provider can offer explanations or use other approaches that directly reduce uncertainty. Similarly, uncertainty can be reduced by one's level of education and resultant knowledge. Social support networks also influence the stimuli frame by providing information from similar others, providing examples, and offering supportive information.

Uncertainty is viewed as a neutral state and is not associated with emotions until evaluated. During the evaluation of uncertainty, inference and illusion come into play. Inference and illusion are based on beliefs and personality dispositions that influence whether uncertainty is appraised as a danger or as an opportunity. Because uncertainty renders a situation amorphous and ill defined, positively oriented illusions can be generated from uncertainty, leading to an appraisal of uncertainty as an opportunity. Uncertainty appraised as an opportunity implies a positive outcome, and buffering coping strategies are used to maintain it. In contrast, beliefs and personality dispositions can result in uncertainty appraised as danger. Uncertainty evaluated as danger implies harm. Problem-focused coping strategies are employed to reduce it. If problem-focused coping cannot be used, then emotional coping strategies are used to respond to the uncertainty. If the coping strategies are effective, adaptation occurs. Difficulty in adapting indicates inability to manipulate uncertainty in the desired direction.

The RUIT (Figure 4.2) represents the process of moving from uncertainty appraised as danger to uncertainty appraised as an opportunity and resource for a new view of life. As noted earlier in this chapter, the reconceptualized theory builds on the original theory at the appraisal portion. The RUIT describes enduring uncertainty that is initially viewed as danger due to its invasion into broader areas of life resulting

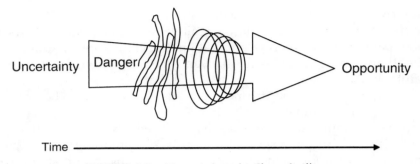

FIGURE 4.2   Uncertainty in Chronic Illness
Source: Reprinted with permission from Bailey, D. E., & Stewart, J. L.
(2001). Mishel's theory of uncertainty in illness. In A. M. Mariner-Tomey &
M. R. Alligood (Eds.), *Nursing theorists and their work* (5th ed.,
pp. 560–583). St. Louis, MO: Mosby.

in instability. The jagged line within the arrow represents both the invasion of uncertainty and the growing instability. The patterned circular portion of the line represents the repatterning and reorganization resulting in a revised view of uncertainty. The bottom arrow indicates that this is a process that evolves over time.

USE OF THE THEORIES IN NURSING RESEARCH

Beginning with the publication of the Uncertainty in Illness Scale (Mishel, 1981), there has been extensive research into uncertainty in both acute and chronic illnesses. The research on uncertainty includes studies in nursing and other disciplines. Several comprehensive reviews of research have summarized and critiqued the current state of the knowledge on uncertainty in illness (Bailey & Stewart, 2001; Barron, 2000; Mast, 1995; McCormick, 2002; Mishel, 1997a, 1999; Neville, 2003; Stewart & Mishel, 2000). Other authors have attempted to develop an expanded definition of uncertainty (Penrod, 2001) or have critiqued the current work based on a misunderstanding of the reconceptualized uncertainty theory (Parry, 2003). In this chapter, the research review will be limited to studies that directly address components of the UIT and the RUIT and will not include studies that use the uncertainty scales but do not consider aspects of the theories in study design, literature review, or discussion of findings.

Although some studies focus on components of the UIT or RUIT, in the past few years, more studies have used uncertainty as the conceptual framework for the study and directly tested major sections of the UIT, elaborated on the UIT, or elaborated on selected antecedents and outcomes adding richness to the theory (Caroll & Arthur, 2010; Jurgens, 2006; Kang, 2005, 2006, 2011; Kang, Daly, & Kim, 2004; McCormick, Naimark, & Tate, 2006; Sammarco, 2001; Sammarco & Konency, 2010; Santacroce, 2003; Stewart, Mishel, Lynn, & Terhorst, 2010; Wonghongkul, Dechaprom, Phumivichuvate, & Losawatkul, 2006). Mishel's Uncertainty in Illness Scale–Community Form has demonstrated validity and reliability for measuring uncertainty in men undergoing active surveillance for early stage prostate cancer (Bailey, Wallace, Latini, et al., 2011) and ethnically diverse female breast cancer survivors (Sammarco & Konecny, 2010). The theory has also been used as the basis for revising the Parent's Perception of Uncertainty Scale (Santacroce, 2001). In a study by Kang et al. (2004), researchers operationalized and tested the antecedents of social support and education as structure providers along with the stimuli frame variable of symptom pattern on uncertainty in patients with atrial fibrillation. Symptom severity was the strongest predictor of uncertainty, whereas the structure provider variables of education and social support reduced uncertainty. An unusual grounded theory study explored children's perception of uncertainty during treatment for cancer, citing the uncertainty theory as the sensitizing theory (Stewart, 2003). A study in children and adolescents with cancer used the uncertainty theory to guide a conceptual model that served as the study framework; a strong relationship was found between children's uncertainty and psychological distress (Stewart, Mishel, Lynn, & Terhorst, 2010). The uncertainty theory has grown through research studies in the areas of credible authority and social support as the theory has been used by investigators in nursing and health communication (Brashers et al., 2003; Brashers, Neidig, & Goldsmith, 2004; Clayton, Mishel, & Belyea, 2006).

Many studies have focused on the antecedents of stimuli frame and structure providers. Three aspects of illness have been found to cause uncertainty: (1) severity of illness, (2) erratic nature of symptoms, and (3) ambiguity of symptoms. Severity of illness and ambiguity of symptoms correspond to the stimuli frame component of symptom pattern, whereas the erratic nature of symptoms corresponds to the stimuli component of event congruence.

Studies that focus on severity of illness and uncertainty are classified as those that address the theoretical link between symptom pattern and uncertainty. Severity of illness refers to symptoms with such intensity that they do not clearly reflect a discernable, under-standable pattern. Several studies have shown that severity of illness is a predictor of uncertainty, although the indicators of severity of ill-ness have varied across studies (Mishel, 1997a). Among patients in the acute or treatment phase of illnesses such as cardiovascular disease (Christman et al., 1988), cancer (Galloway & Graydon, 1996; Hilton, 1994), fibromyalgia (Johnson, Zautra, & Davis, 2006), and severe pedi-atric illness (Tomlinson, Kirschbaum, Harbaugh, & Anderson, 1996), including pediatric cancer (Santacroce, 2002), severity of illness was positively associated with uncertainty in patients and/or family mem-bers. According to the UIT, the nature of the severity presents diffi-culty delineating a symptom pattern about the extent of the disease, resulting in uncertainty.

Stimuli Frame: Symptom Pattern

Studies that address the process of identifying symptoms of a dis-ease or condition and reaching a diagnosis are classified as address-ing symptom pattern. The process of receiving a diagnosis requires that a symptom pattern exists and can be labeled as an illness or a condition. In the UIT, absence of the symptom pattern is associ-ated with uncertainty. Uncertainty levels have been reported to be highest in those without a diagnosis and undergoing diagnostic examinations (Hilton, 1993; Mishel, 1981). In studies where patients' symptoms are not clearly distinguishable from those of other comor-bid conditions, or where symptoms of recurrence can be confused with signs of aging or other natural processes and not recognizable as signs of disease, such as in lupus, breast cancer, and cardiac dis-ease, symptoms are associated with uncertainty (Hilton, 1988; Mishel & Murdaugh, 1987; Nelson, 1996; Winters, 1999). In a study of long-term breast cancer survivors, it was not the symptoms that elicited uncertainty but events that triggered thoughts of recurrence or the meaning of physical symptoms from long-term treatment side effects (Gil et al., 2004). High levels of symptoms such as pain are associated with uncertainty when one does not know how to manage the symp-toms (Johnson et al., 2006). Similarly, research has demonstrated the association between uncertainty and physical symptoms of breast cancer survivors, demonstrating that unpredictable physical symp-toms that may come and go, such as fatigue and arm problems, can create uncertainty about breast cancer recurrence (Clayton, Mishel, et al., 2006; Wonghongkul et al., 2006). Other research has focused on understanding the ambiguity of symptom experience associated with preterm labor (Weiss, Saks, & Harris, 2002). Even previous experience with preterm labor did not reduce the ambiguity associated with this condition.

The erratic nature of symptom onset and disease progression is a major antecedent of uncertainty in chronic illness (Mishel, 1999). Symptoms that occur unpredictably fit the description of the stimuli frame component of event incongruence because there is no congruity between the cue and the outcome. The timing and nature of symptom onset, duration, intensity, and location are unforeseeable, characterized by periods of stability, erratic flares of exacerbation, or unpredictable recurrence resulting in uncertainty (Brown & Powell-Cope, 1991; Mast, 1998; Mishel & Braden, 1988; Sexton, Calcasola, Bottomley, & Funk, 1999). Similarly, difficulty being aware of physical symptoms and determining their meaning in acute heart failure patients has also been found to be related to greater uncertainty (Jurgens, 2006). Among parents of ill children, unpredictable trajectories with few markers of illness are positively associated with uncertainty (Cohen, 1993b). Difficulty in determining cause of illness has been found to be associated with uncertainty (Cohen, 1993a; Sharkey, 1995; Turner, Tomlinson, & Harbaugh, 1990). Recent work on patients with endometriosis found that because no cure exists and treatment effectiveness varies, patients experience uncertainty surrounding the relationship of diagnosis to treatment outcomes (Lemaire, 2004). In young adults with asthma, uncertainty has been proposed to occur due to episode severity and/or frequency, which is not contingent upon the person's attempt to manage the illness (Mullins, Chaney, Balderson, & Hommel, 2000).

Stimuli Frame: Event Familiarity

Studies that focus on the health care or home environment for treatment of illness fit under the stimuli frame component of event familiarity. Although fewer studies have addressed this component of stimuli frame, the studies that have been conducted support that unfamiliarity with health care environment, organization, and expectations is associated with uncertainty. Health care environments characterized by novelty and confusion where the rules and routines are unknown and equipment and treatments are unfamiliar are associated with uncertainty (Horner, 1997; Stewart & Mishel, 2000; Turner et al., 1990).

Structure Providers: Social Support

In the UIT, social support from friends, family, and those with similar experiences are proposed to reduce uncertainty directly and indirectly by influencing the stimuli frame. Those with similar experience have been found to influence the stimuli frame by providing information about illness-related events and symptom pattern (Van Riper & Selder, 1989; White & Frasure-Smith, 1995). There are a number of studies that support the role of social support in reducing uncertainty among parents of ill children, adult and adolescent patients, and their care providers (Bennett, 1993; Davis, 1990; Mishel & Braden, 1987; Neville, 1998; Tomlinson et al., 1996). However, when the illness is stigmatized, the questionable acceptance by others limits the use of social support to manage uncertainty (Brown & Powell-Cope, 1991; Weitz, 1989). Social interaction also may not always be supportive. Unsupportive interactions serve to heighten uncertainty (Wineman, 1990). The dual impact of social support has also been investigated in men with HIV or AIDS. Brashers et al. (2004) reported that other individuals help HIV patients manage uncertainty by providing instrumental support, facilitating skill development, giving acceptance or validation, allowing ventilation, and encouraging a perspective shift. They also report that there are problems associated with social support and uncertainty management including a lack of coordination in managing uncertainty, the addition of relational uncertainty, and the burden of caregiver uncertainty. Other investigators have found that family members experience high levels of uncertainty, which may impair their ability to provide support for the patient (Brown & Powell-Cope, 1991; Mishel & Murdaugh, 1987; Wineman, O'Brien, Nealon, & Kaskel, 1993). In a study of uncertainty in African American and White family members of men with localized prostate cancer, uncertainty was associated with family members feeling less positive about treatments and patient recovery, feeling more psychological distress, and engaging in less active problem solving (Germino et al., 1998). These findings bring into question the ability of family members to be supportive of the patient when family members are trying to deal with their own uncertainties. Among younger breast cancer survivors, both social support and uncertainty together explained 27% of the variance in quality of life, with higher levels of social support functioning to reduce uncertainty (Sammarco, 2001). Current research supports the theoretical relationship between social support and uncertainty and provides information on factors that influence effective social support.

Structure Providers: Credible Authority

Credible authority refers to health care providers who are seen as credible information givers by the patient or family member. As experts, health care providers have been proposed to reduce uncertainty by providing information and promoting confidence in their clinical judgment and performance. Trust and confidence in the health care provider's ability to make a diagnosis, to control the illness, and to provide adequate treatment has been reported to be related to less uncertainty across a variety of acute and chronic illnesses (Mishel & Braden, 1988; Santacroce, 2000). On the other hand, patients' lack of confidence in the provider's abilities increases uncertainty (Becker, Janson-Bjerklie, Benner, Slobin, & Ferdetich, 1993; Smeltzer, 1994). Uncertainty has also been found to increase when patients report that they are not receiving adequate information from health care providers (Galloway & Graydon, 1996; Hilton, 1988; Nyhlin, 1990; Small & Graydon, 1993; Weems & Patterson, 1989).

Clayton, Mishel, et al. (2006) report the testing of a model based on the UIT with an emphasis on the role of doctor–patient communication in older breast cancer survivors. The findings did not support the role of doctor–patient communication in relation to uncertainty or to well-being. Various explanations for the lack of influence of doctor–patient interaction in the model may be that the need for information from the physician may decrease over time from diagnosis through recovery unless there is a recurrence. This idea is supported by the work of Brashers, Hsieh, Neidig, and Reynolds (2006), who found that patients with an enduring chronic illness such as HIV held beliefs and attitudes about health care providers in a variety of dimensions. Brashers and colleagues describe the criteria used by these patients to evaluate the provider and strategies for managing their relationship with the provider. This work clearly contributes to the theory; however, further research is needed to determine whether the information is applicable to individuals with other diagnoses.

Appraisal of Uncertainty

According to the UIT, appraisal of uncertainty involves personality dispositions, attitudes, and beliefs, which influence whether uncertainty is appraised as a danger or an opportunity. There is support for the impact of uncertainty on reducing personality dispositions such as optimism, sense of coherence, and level of resourcefulness

(Christman, 1990; Hilton, 1989; Mishel et al., 1984). Certain dispositions such as generalized negative outcome expectancies interact with uncertainty to predict psychological distress (Mullins et al., 1995). However, selected cognitive and personality factors have been reported to mediate the relationship between uncertainty and danger or opportunity. Mediators that decrease the impact of uncertainty on danger and adjustment include higher enabling skill, self-efficacy, mastery, hope, challenge, and existential well-being (Braden, Mishel, Longman, & Burns, 1998; Landis, 1996; Mishel, Padilla, Grant, & Sorenson, 1991; Mishel & Sorenson, 1991; Wonghongkul et al., 2006; Wonghongkul, Moore, Musil, Schneider, & Deimling, 2000). Some studies where appraisals were found to be positive are of population that are a number of years posttreatment. Others have reported that positive appraisals of uncertainty can be found along with negative appraisals, enabling both to exist simultaneously. This has been reported for patients awaiting coronary artery bypass surgery where uncertainty can be seen as a source for hope (McCormick et al., 2006). However, recent work by Kang (2006) with a sample of patients with atrial fibrillation reported that appraisal of uncertainty as an opportunity had a negative relationship with depression, and appraisal of uncertainty as a danger was positively associated with depression. As uncertainty increased, so did the danger appraisal, which was related to a decrease in mental health (Kang, 2005).

Coping With Uncertainty

Numerous investigators who have studied the management of uncertainty have found that higher uncertainty is associated with danger and resultant emotion-focused coping strategies such as wishful thinking, avoidance, and fatalism (Christman, 1990; Hilton, 1989; Mishel & Sorenson, 1991; Mishel et al., 1991; Redeker, 1992; Webster & Christman, 1988). Severe symptoms such as high levels of pain in interaction with uncertainty have been reported to reduce one's ability to cope with symptoms (Johnson et al., 2006). Others report more varied coping strategies for managing uncertainty including cognitive strategies such as downward comparison, constructing a personal scenario for the illness, use of faith or religion, and identifying markers and triggers (Baier, 1995; Mishel & Murdaugh, 1987; Wiener & Dodd, 1993). Mishel (1993) offered a review of major uncertainty management methods; however, there is little evidence for the use of any of these coping strategies mediating the relationship between uncertainty and emotional distress (Mast, 1998; Mishel & Sorenson, 1991; Mishel et al., 1991). Although there has not been much study of the role of hopefulness in managing uncertainty, findings from a study of participation in a clinical drug trial revealed that uncertainty was related to a decrease in hope during time in the trial. Those with more uncertainty and less hopefulness reported more negative moods (Wineman, Schwetz, Zeller, & Cyphert, 2003). Research with Thai patients being treated for head and neck cancer used the uncertainty theory as a framework to study factors that contribute to quality of life as a way to address coping approaches for this population. Findings indicated that symptom experience had a positive impact on uncertainty and uncertainty had a negative impact on quality of life (Detprapon, Sirapo-ngam, Mishel, Sitthimongkol, & Vorapongsathorn, 2009), leading the authors to suggest that coping with symptoms and uncertainty is critical to optimizing quality of life. In the area of uncertainty in children, Stewart (2003) reported that children emphasized the routine and ordinariness of their lives despite their cancer diagnosis and treatment as a way of coping.

Uncertainty and Adjustment

According to the UIT, adjustment refers to returning to the individual's level of preillness functioning. However, most of the research has interpreted this as emotional stability or quality of life. Few studies have tested the complete outcome portion of the theory, including uncertainty, appraisal, coping strategies, and adjustment. Most studies examine the relationship between uncertainty and an outcome and relate these findings to the theory. The findings from these studies have consistently shown positive relationships between uncertainty and negative emotional outcomes (Bennett, 1993; Mast, 1998; Mishel, 1984; Mullins et al., 2001; Sanders-Dewey, Mullins, & Chaney, 2001; Small & Graydon, 1993; Taylor-Piliae & Molassiotis, 2001; Wineman, Schwetz, Goodkin, & Rudick, 1996). Further evidence for the significant effect of uncertainty on depression was reported by Mullins et al. (2000) in young adults with asthma. The effect of uncertainty on depression was at its maximum under conditions of increased illness severity. Uncertainty has also been related to poorer psychosocial adjustment in the areas of less life satisfaction (Hilton, 1994), negative attitudes toward health care, family relationships, recreation and employment (Mishel et al., 1984; Mishel & Braden, 1987), less satisfaction with health care services (Green & Murton, 1996), and poorer quality of life (Carroll, Hamilton, & McGovern, 1999; Padilla, Mishel, & Grant, 1992). Santacroce (2003) has identified the linkage between uncertainty and negative outcomes in her literature review on parental uncertainty and posttraumatic stress in serious childhood illness.

There has been extensive study of uncertainty in illness based on the UIT, and most of the research supports components of the theory. Overall, the theory has been very useful in guiding research with a variety of clinical populations and caregivers.

Research on RUIT

Less attention has been given to the study of the RUIT, possibly due to difficulty in studying a process that evolves over time. Support for the RUIT has been found in qualitative studies that favor a transition through uncertainty to a new orientation toward life with acceptance of uncertainty as a part of life (Mishel, 1999). The samples for these studies included long-term diabetic patients (Nyhlin, 1990), chronically ill men (Charmaz, 1994), HIV patients (Brashers et al., 2003; Katz, 1996), persons with schizophrenia (Baier, 1995), spouses of heart transplant patients (Mishel & Murdaugh, 1987), family caregivers of AIDS patients (Brown & Powell-Cope, 1991), breast cancer survivors (Mishel et al., 2005; Nelson, 1996; Pelusi, 1997), adolescent survivors of childhood cancer (Parry, 2003), and women recovering from cardiac disease (Fleury, Kimbrell, & Kruszewski, 1995). Bailey, Wallace, and Mishel (2007), using the RUIT as an organizing framework, interviewed men who were undergoing watchful waiting as their treatment for prostate cancer. Although the findings were not totally supportive of the RUIT, men did express that they had generated options, created opportunities for themselves, and remained hopeful of a positive outcome. Parry's (2003) study of childhood cancer survivors suggests that uncertainty can be a catalyst for growth, for a greater appreciation for life, and for greater awareness of life purpose. However, in another study of survivors of childhood cancer, findings showed that uncertainty mediated the relationship between posttraumatic stress disorder and health promotion behaviors, indicating that uncertainty exists over time and reduces health promotion activities (Santacroce & Lee, 2006).

Findings supporting the RUIT seem to differ by subject population and methodology where more qualitative studies—compared with quantitative studies—support the RUIT. The transition through uncertainty toward a new view of life was framed differently by each investigator and included themes such as a revised life perspective, new ways of being in the world, growth through uncertainty, new levels of self-organization, new goals for living, devaluating what is worthwhile, redefining what is normal, and building new dreams (Bailey & Stewart, 2001). All the investigators described the gradual acceptance of uncertainty and the restructuring of reality as major components of the process, both of which are consistent with the RUIT.

An instrument to measure the change theoretically proposed in the RUIT was developed by Mishel and Fleury and is being tested for construct validity. The scale addresses growth through uncertainty toward a new view of life and was developed to address the discrepancy noted above between qualitative and quantitative approaches to study the RUIT. Initial use of the scale was reported by Mast (1998), and further testing of the scale is occurring before it is available for general use. The Growth Through Uncertainty Scale (GTUS) has been used in a few clinical investigations. In an intervention study guided by the RUIT, baseline analysis of the data included use of the GTUS. The analysis was to identify variables that would predict either negative mood state or personal growth (GTUS) in older African American and White long-term breast cancer survivors. Of the variables found to be significant predictors, negative cognitive state, which included uncertainty, was a significant predictor of both outcomes. The overall findings were supportive of the RUIT because cognitive reappraisal, defined as the tendency to address concerns from a positive point of view, predicted 40% of the variance in personal growth (GTUS) (Porter et al., 2006). Also, in findings from this intervention study, at 10 months and 20 months postintervention, older long-term African American breast cancer survivors in the treatment group maintained or increased scores on the GTUS over time, while scores for subjects in the control group declined over time (Gil, Penckofer, Maurer, & Bryant, 2006; Mishel et al., 2005).

Interventions to Manage Uncertainty

An uncertainty management intervention has been developed and tested in four clinical trials for breast cancer patients and patients with localized or advanced prostate cancer (Braden et al., 1998; Mishel, 1997b; Mishel et al., 2002, 2003). The intervention was structured to follow the UIT and was delivered by weekly phone calls to cancer patients. All studies included equal numbers of White and minority samples. The intervention was effective in teaching patients skills to manage uncertainty including improvements in problem solving, cognitive reframing, treatment-related side effects, and patient–provider communication. Improvement was also found in the ability to manage the uncertainty related to side effects from cancer treatment. Religious participation and education were found to be moderators of the treatment outcomes of cancer knowledge and patient–provider communication in the intervention trial for men with localized prostate cancer. Education was a covariate in the study of older women during treatment for breast cancer. Using the UIT and RUIT as frameworks for study of an intervention for older long-term African American and White breast cancer survivors, a self-delivered uncertainty management intervention with nurse assistance was tested and results indicated that the intervention at 10 months and 20 months follow-up produced significant differences in experimental and control groups in cognitive reframing, cancer knowledge, patient–provider communication, and a variety of coping skills. The most important results were the improvement in the treatment groups' pursuit of further information along with declines in uncertainty and stable effects in personal growth over time (Gil et al., 2006; Mishel et al., 2005).

Further intervention work based on the UIT and RUIT was conducted by Bailey, Mishel, Belyea, Stewart, and Mohler (2004) among men selecting watchful waiting in prostate cancer. The results from this clinical trial showed that men in the intervention improved on the GTUS on the subscale of living life in a new light and believing that their future would be improved. In another study with the same population, a pilot study with nine participants (Kazer, Baily, Sanda, Colberg, & Kelly, 2011) supported use of an Internet intervention to improve quality of life while uncertainty remained consistent.

In a study of an intervention program that incorporated uncertainty reduction for women with recurrent breast cancer and their family members, factual information about cancer recurrence and treatments encouraged assertive approaches with health care providers; participants focused on learning to live with uncertainty in preference to negative certainty (Northouse et al., 2002). An intervention trial for newly diagnosed breast cancer patients in Taiwan used the UIT framework and provided information to questions raised by patients. This continual supportive care was given at four points during treatment. The findings indicated that support was increased and uncertainty was decreased 1 month after surgery and 4 months after diagnosis (Liu, Li, Tang, Huang, & Chiou, 2006). Other intervention studies included uncertainty as a variable but did not use either the UIT or RUIT as a framework for the study or intervention (Kreulen & Braden, 2004;

McCain et al., 2003; Taylor-Piliae & Chair, 2002). The number of intervention studies using the uncertainty theory or including intervention to address uncertainty is continually increasing in the literature.

USE OF THE THEORIES IN NURSING PRACTICE

Nurses are included in the UIT as part of the antecedent variable of structure providers. The clinical literature supports delivery of information as the major method to help patients manage uncertainty. Nurses provide information that helps patients develop meaning from the illness experience by providing structure to the stimuli frame. When considering the RUIT, nurses help patients manage chronic uncertainty by assisting with patients' reappraisal of uncertainty from stressful to hopeful in addition to providing relevant information.

Understanding the sources of patient uncertainty can help nurses plan for effective information giving and may greatly assist nurses to help patients manage or reduce their uncertainty. In one of the few articles to address the environmental component of the stimuli frame, Sharkey (1995) discussed how family coping could be enhanced by home care nurses normalizing health care into the familiar routines of families caring for a terminally ill child at home. Among cardiac patients, White and Frasure-Smith (1995) suggested that nurses promote the use of patient-solicited social support to manage uncertainty in percutaneous transluminal coronary angioplasty (PTCA) patients. These researchers suggested that the benefit from the social support received by PTCA patients was due to direct requests tailored to specific needs versus unsolicited social support due to simply being ill. In addition, information from nurses about the potential long-term success of this procedure might help reduce the higher uncertainty found in PTCA patients 3 months after surgery. Among breast cancer survivors, Gil et al. (2004, 2005) suggested that nurses can help women identify their personal triggers of uncertainty about recurrence and then teach coping skills such as breathing relaxation, pleasant imagery, calming self-talk, and distraction to help survivors manage their uncertainty.

The RUIT has also been used to inform clinical practice and help nurses understand sources of patient uncertainty. An example of how mental health nurses can assist patients by understanding sources of uncertainty is found in research by Brashers et al. (2003) describing the medical, social, and personal forms of uncertainty for persons living with HIV/AIDS. Further, this research suggests nurses should be aware that subgroups of this population such as women, drug users, gay men, and parents can experience different sources of uncertainty based on social stigma, role and/or identity confusion, and lack of familiarity with the medical system. Other research using the RUIT indicates that childhood cancer survivors often have late emerging side effects that impact quality of life and the experience of uncertainty similar to other long-term cancer survivors (Lee, 2006; Santacroce & Lee, 2006). These studies suggest that childhood cancer survivors who lack effective coping and uncertainty management skills may be unable to reappraise uncertainty and are at risk for the development of posttraumatic stress symptoms (PTSS) as a way of avoiding uncertainty when life demands become excessive (Lee, 2006). Health professionals who are aware of the increased risk of PTSS created by an inability to reappraise uncertainty can offer developmentally appropriate information, thereby clarifying the ambiguity of future survivorship and helping childhood cancer survivors manage the continual uncertainty in their lives (Santacroce & Lee, 2006).

Recognizing uncertainty and then providing contextual cues to reduce ambiguity and increase understanding is one approach that nurses can use when communicating with patients to decrease uncertainty. Contextual cues provide explanations of what patients will see, hear, and feel during procedures and tests, as well as what signs and symptoms they will experience at various points in their illness trajectory. Providing information and explanations about treatments and medications has been proposed to be the most important and frequent approach to reducing patient uncertainty (Mishel et al., 2002; Wineman et al., 1996). Galloway and Graydon (1996), who based their findings on recently discharged colon cancer patients, noted that nurses could provide information to alleviate the uncertainty of being discharged to the home environment. Correspondingly, Mitchell, Courtney, and Coyer (2003) found that nurses provide beneficial contextual cues and information to both families and patients on transfer from the intensive care unit to a general hospital floor. Families of patients who received clear information were more able to make decisions for patients, reported less anxiety, and were better able to provide emotional and physical patient support. Other effective methods for reducing patient uncertainty can include encouraging communication with patients who have successfully managed their uncertainties. Weems and Patterson (1989) suggest sharing the uncertainties of waiting for a renal transplant with someone who has already received a transplant, or sharing uncertainties of how to live with chronic obstructive pulmonary disease with someone who is successfully managing this chronic disease (Small & Graydon, 1993). This type of communication provides information to patients for structuring the stimuli and also functions as a source of social support.

Offering comprehensive information allows the nurse to function as a credible authority, strengthening the stimuli frame by enhancing disease predictability and reducing symptom ambiguity. Righter (1995) used the UIT to describe the role of an enterostomal therapy (ET) nurse as a credible authority for the ostomy patient. She describes the ET nurse as providing structure and order to the experience of the new ostomy patient through clinical expertise and experience. The ET nurse reduces the ambiguity of the ostomy experience by providing information, counseling, and support. This facilitates ostomy patients' adaptation to their newly altered perception of themselves and helps them regain a sense of control and mastery by creating order and predictability. Other ideas on changing clinical practice to reduce patient uncertainty include educational interventions delivered in person, by telephone, or by individualized patient information packets delivered through the mail (Calvin & Lane, 1999; Mishel et al., 2002). Research by Bailey et al. (2004) found that nurses can clarify information about treatment options that create confusion for men who have selected watchful waiting as their treatment choice for prostate cancer. Nurses can answer patient questions about variations in prostate-specific antigen values, thus reducing uncertainty about both disease progression and future events. Understanding the meaning of laboratory values helped men sort out the confusion associated with mixed messages given to them by family who promoted aggressive treatment and urologists who promoted watchful waiting. Mishel et al. (2002) found that prostate cancer patients immediately postsurgery or during radiation therapy felt reassured when their questions were answered by a nurse, resulting in reduced anxiety and uncertainty. These men also expressed appreciation for the concern of a health professional and subsequently reported feeling less alone in their battle with cancer.

When considering the predictability of illness trajectories, Sexton et al. (1999) found that advanced practice nurses helped patients manage a diagnosis of asthma by implementing nursing actions that helped patients predict and manage their asthma attacks. Similarly, among breast cancer survivors, unpredictable physical symptoms, such as fatigue and arm problems, that may come and go can create uncertainty about breast cancer recurrence (Clayton, Mishel et al., 2006; Wonghongkul et al., 2006). Thus, providers—including advanced practice nurses—should try to communicate in a manner that fully explains existing symptoms and their relationship or lack thereof to cancer recurrence (Clayton, Dudley, & Musters, 2006).

Clinical journals are increasingly identifying patient uncertainty as an important part of the illness experience and provide suggestions for nursing actions to reduce patient uncertainty or facilitate a new outlook by focusing on choices and alternatives. Suggestions for managing uncertainty in clinical practice include work by Crigger (1996), who suggests that nurses can help women adapt positively to multiple sclerosis by shifting the emphasis from the management of physical disability to the management of uncertainty, thereby helping women achieve mastery over their daily lives. Similarly, Calvin and Lane (1999) suggested incorporating preoperative psychoeducational interventions to reduce uncertainty as part of orthopedic preadmission visits. Other examples of using the UIT to develop and implement nursing interventions to reduce uncertainty and regain control in clinical settings are suggested by Allan (1990) for HIV-positive men; Sterken (1996) for fathers of pediatric cancer patients; Northouse, Mood, Templin, Mellon, and George (2000) for patients with colon cancer; and Sharkey (1995) for homebound pediatric oncology patients. Ritz et al. (2000) report another nursing intervention to manage uncertainty in clinical practice. These clinicians investigated the effect of follow-up nursing care by the advanced practice nurse after discharge of newly treated breast cancer patients. Six months after diagnosis, uncertainty was reduced and quality of life was improved.

On the basis of the antecedent variables of UIT, Northouse et al. (2000) suggested that health professionals keep in mind individual characteristics of patients, social environments, and methods of illness appraisal when caring for patients with colon cancer. They suggested that nurses provide patients with a framework of expectations about the physical and emotional illness trajectory associated with the first year of managing this diagnosis. Thus, use of the UIT can help nurses recognize groups of patients and/or caregivers that may be at risk for increased uncertainty. For example, Sterken (1996) found that younger fathers did not understand the information given to them about their child's treatment and disease patterns as well as older fathers, illustrating how cognitive capacity influences uncertainty. Santacroce (2002) found that African American parents of children newly diagnosed with cancer experienced greater uncertainty than White parents. She posits that past experiences with the health care system can impact parental uncertainty. These studies illustrate the difficulty as well as the potential benefit in using demographic characteristics to identify persons at risk for heightened uncertainty.

Current investigators have explained how the theory can be applied to understanding a clinical situation, clinical diagnosis, or clinical practice. For example, it is important to realize when increased uncertainty can place patients at risk for additional illnesses, such as recognizing that uncertainty is a major factor contributing to depression in patients with hepatitis C (Saunders & Cookman, 2005). Some clinical areas such as women's health and cardiovascular disease have been studied in depth. In the area of women's health, Sorenson (1990) discusses the concepts of symptom pattern, event familiarity and congruency, cognitive capacity, structure providers, and credible authority, using examples from normal pregnancy to help nurses relate the theory to women who are experiencing difficulty adapting to the uncertainties of pregnancy. For women experiencing high-risk pregnancy, they preferred the coping strategy of avoidance as a means for managing uncertainty and preserving their sense of well-being (Giurgescu, Penckofer, Maurer, & Bryant, 2006). Suggestions are made about how perinatal nurses can help women accept impending motherhood and utilize more effective coping mechanisms to reduce uncertainty and improve psychological well-being. Lemaire and Lenz (1995) applied the UIT to the condition of menopause. The stimuli frame for menopause was defined as the symptoms that indicate approaching menopause, including mood swings, hot flashes, dry skin, and memory changes. If women received factual information from a source deemed credible, such as nurses and health care providers, it was thought that familiarity with the event of menopause would be increased and uncertainty about this normal life event would be decreased. Consistent with predictions of UIT, uncertainty declined after receipt of understandable information delivered by a credible source, allowing women to construct meaning from the ambiguity and unpredictability of their symptoms surrounding the normal process of menopause. Similarly, Lemaire (2004) suggests that nurses who understand the uncertainty associated with the symptoms of endometriosis are better able to care for women experiencing this condition. Nursing actions such as providing informational material, offering referrals to support groups, and sharing electronic resources can help women better understand and manage the ambiguity and unpredictability of symptoms such as cramping, nonmenstrual pain, and fatigue. Other research has focused on understanding the ambiguity of symptoms associated with preterm labor (Weiss et al., 2002). Weiss et al. found that women lacked familiarity with the symptom pattern of preterm labor. They suggest that language used by women in describing preterm labor be incorporated into educational materials available to all pregnant women to help them recognize preterm labor as differentiated from term labor. They stress that every expectant woman needs education about the cues to use in recognizing preterm labor.

In patients diagnosed with atrial fibrillation, UIT can help nurses identify patients at risk for increased uncertainty (Kang et al., 2004). Focusing on the antecedents of uncertainty, findings showed that patients with more severe symptoms and those with less education experienced greater uncertainty, helping nurses to be more aware of which patients may be at risk. Other research has found that those patients who receive an implantable cardioverter defibrillator experience great uncertainty, never knowing when their arrhythmias may reoccur and when the device may "fire" (Flemme et al., 2005). Carroll and Arthur (2010) studied uncertainty, optimism and anxiety in patients receiving their first implantable defibrillator. Further, hospital nurses may have little time to prepare these patients for discharge as there is no need for further hospitalization postimplantation of the device. Therefore, outpatient clinic and office nurses can provide key information and support to these patients, recognizing that the high levels of uncertainty frequently experienced by these patients put them at risk for poorer quality of life. Similarly, Rydström Dalheim-Englund, Segesten, and Rasmussen (2004) note the uncertainty that affects the whole family when a child has asthma, suggesting education for both parents and siblings about asthma as well as the impact of asthma on family dynamics. Further, these authors stress the importance of communicating to families that their nurse is approachable about both disease issues and family dynamics issues as part of holistic disease management.

Another approach to improving patient care is recognizing the importance of professional education on uncertainty to effect change in clinical practice. Wunderlich, Perry, Lavin, and Katz (1999) suggested that critical care nurses would benefit from staff development sessions on how to address the uncertainty that patients experience during the process of weaning from mechanical ventilation. Dombeck (1996) commented that health care professionals need to increase their own tolerance for ambiguity and uncertainty to effectively listen to clients who are experiencing ambiguity and uncertainty. Similarly, Light (1979) noted that health care professionals have been socialized to minimize uncertainty; this socialization may make it difficult to effectively address patient uncertainty until health care workers learn more about it (Baier, 1995). Recognizing the importance of integrating UIT into a management strategy for asthma patients, the American Nurses Credentialing Center's Commission on Accreditation offered 3 credit hours for successful completion of a continuing education unit (CEU) quiz following the published article (Sexton et al., 1999) about coping with uncertainty. Other CEU offerings incorporating uncertainty theory have been offered following a case study on spiritual disequilibrium (Dombeck, 1996) and an article on weaning a patient from mechanical ventilation (Wunderlich et al., 1999).

CONCLUSION

The uncertainty in illness theories have been used in multiple ways to inform clinician understanding of patients, families, and illness situations. Clinical research guided by both the original UIT (1988) and the RUIT (1990) for those coping with both acute and chronic illnesses will continue to help identify appropriate nursing interventions for many types of illnesses and patients. Ultimately the recognition of the importance of uncertainty can change clinical practice, allowing the development of nursing interventions that facilitate a positive patient adaptation to the illness experience.

REFERENCES

Allan, J. D. (1990). Focusing on living, not dying: A naturalistic study of self-care among seropositive gay men. *Holistic Nursing Practice, 4*(2), 56–63.

Allen, D. G. (1985). Nursing research and social control: Alternative models of science that emphasize understanding and emancipation. *Image: Journal of Nursing Scholarship, 17,* 58–64.

Antonovsky, A. (1987). *Unraveling the mystery of health: How people manage stress and stay well.* San Francisco, CA: Jossey-Bass.

Baier, M. (1995). Uncertainty of illness for persons with schizophrenia. *Issues in Mental Health Nursing, 16,* 201–212.

Bailey, D. E., Mishel, M. H., Belyea, M., Stewart, J. L., & Mohler, J. (2004). Uncertainty intervention for watchful waiting in prostate cancer. *Cancer Nursing, 27*(5), 339–346.

Bailey, D. E., & Stewart, J. L. (2001). Mishel's theory of uncertainty in illness. In A. M. Mariner-Tomey & M. R. Alligood (Eds.), *Nursing theorists and their work* (5th ed., pp. 560–583). St. Louis, MO: Mosby.

Bailey, D. E., Wallace, M., & Mishel, M. H. (2007). Watching, waiting and uncertainty in prostate cancer. *Journal of Clinical Nursing, 16*(4), 734–741.

Bailey, D. E., Wallace, M., Latini, D. M., Hegarty, J., Carroll, P. R., Klein, E. A., & Albertsen, P. C. (2011). Measuring illness uncertaintly in men undergoing active surveillance for prostate cancer. *Applied Nursing Research, 24,* 193–199.

Barron, C. R. (2000). Stress, uncertainty, and health. In V. H. Rice (Ed.), *Handbook of stress, coping and health: Implications for nursing research, theory, and practice* (pp. 517–539). Thousand Oaks, CA: Sage.

Becker, G., Janson-Bjerklie, S., Benner, P., Slobin, K., & Ferdetich, S. (1993). The dilemma of seeking urgent care: Asthma episodes and emergency service use. *Social Science and Medicine, 37,* 305–313.

Bennett, S. J. (1993). Relationships among selected antecedent variables and coping effectiveness in postmyocardial infarction patients. *Research in Nursing and Health, 16,* 131–139.

Bower, G. H. (1978). *The psychology of learning and motivation: Advances in research and theory.* New York, NY: Academic Press.

Braden, C. J., Mishel, M. H., Longman, A. J., & Burns, L. (1998). Self-help intervention project: Women receiving breast cancer treatment. *Cancer Practice, 6*(2), 87–98.

Brashers, D. E., Hsieh, E., Neidig, J. L., & Reynolds, N. R. (2006). Managing uncertainty about illness: Health care providers as credible authorities. In R. M. Dailey & B. A. Le Poire (Eds.), *Applied interpersonal communication matters.* New York, NY: Peter Lang.

Brashers, D. E., Neidig, J. L., & Goldsmith, D. J. (2004). Social support and the management of uncertainty for people living with HIV. *Health Communication, 16,* 305–331.

Brashers, D. E., Neidig, J. L., Russell, J. A., Cardillo, L. W., Haas, S. M., Dobbs, L. K., … Nemeth, S. (2003). The medical, personal, and social causes of uncertainty in HIV illness. *Issues in Mental Health Nursing, 24*(5), 497–522.

Brown, M. A., & Powell-Cope, G. M. (1991). AIDS family caregiving: Transitions through uncertainty. *Nursing Research, 40,* 337–345.

Budner, S. (1962). Intolerance of ambiguity as a personality variable. *Journal of Personality, 30,* 29–50.

Calvin, R., & Lane, P. (1999). Perioperative uncertainty and state anxiety of orthopaedic surgical patients. *Orthopedic Nursing, 18*(6), 61–66.

Carroll, D., Hamilton, G., & McGovern, B. (1999). Changes in health status and quality of life and the impact of uncertainty in patients who survive life-threatening arrhythmias. *Heart and Lung, 28*(4), 251–260.

Carroll, S. L., & Arthur, H. M. (2010). A comparative study of uncertainty, optimism and anxiety in patients receiving their first implantable defibrillator for primary and secondary prevention of sudden cardiac death. *International Journal of Nursing Studies, 47,* 836–845.

Charmaz, K. (1994). Identity dilemmas of chronically ill men. *The Sociological Quarterly, 35*(2), 269–288.

Christman, N. J. (1990). Uncertainty and adjustment during radiotherapy. *Nursing Research, 39*(1), 17–20.

Christman, N. J., McConnell, E. A., Pfeiffer, C., Webster, K. K., Schmitt, M., & Ries, J. (1988). Uncertainty, coping, and distress following myocardial infarction: Transition from home to hospital. *Research in Nursing and Health, 11,* 71–82.

Clayton, M. F., Dudley, W. N., & Musters, A. (2006). Communication with breast cancer survivors. *Health Communication, 39,* 175.

Clayton, M. F., Mishel, M. H., & Belyea, M. (2006). Testing a model of symptoms, communication, uncertainty, and well-being, in older breast cancer survivors. *Research in Nursing and Health, 29*(1), 18–39.

Cohen, M. H. (1993a). Diagnostic closure and the spread of uncertainty. *Issues in Comprehensive Pediatric Nursing, 16*, 135–146.

Cohen, M. H. (1993b). The unknown and the unknowable—Managing sustained uncertainty. *Western Journal of Nursing Research, 15*(1), 77–96.

Crigger, N. J. (1996). Testing an uncertainty model for women with multiple sclerosis. *Advances in Nursing Science, 18*(3), 37–47.

Davis, L. L. (1990). Illness uncertainty, social support, and stress in recovering individuals and family caregivers. *Applied Nursing Research, 3*(2), 69–71.

Detprapon, M., Sirapo-ngam, Y., Sitthimongkol, Y., Mishel, M. H., & Vorapongsathorn, T. (2009). Testing uncertainty in illness theory to predict quality of life among Thais with head and neck cancer. *Thai Journal of Nursing Research, 13*(1), 1–15.

Dombeck, M. (1996). Chaos and self-organization as a consequence of spiritual disequilibrium. *Clinical Nurse Specialist, 10*(2), 69–73; quiz 74–75.

Flemme, I., Edvardsson, N., Hinic, H., Jinhage, B. M., Dalman, M., & Fridlund, B. (2005). Long-term quality of life and uncertainty in patients living with an implantable cardioverter defibrillator. *Heart and Lung, 34*(6), 386–392.

Fleury, J., Kimbrell, L. C., & Kruszewski, M. A. (1995). Life after a cardiac event: Women's experience in healing. *Heart and Lung, 24*, 474–482.

Galloway, S., & Graydon, J. (1996). Uncertainty, symptom distress, and information needs after surgery for cancer of the colon. *Cancer Nursing, 19*(2), 112–117.

Germino, B. B., Mishel, M. H., Belyea, M., Harris, L., Ware, A., & Mohler, J. (1998). Uncertainty in prostate cancer, ethnic and family patterns. *Cancer Practice, 6*(2), 102–113.

Gil, K. M., Mishel, M. H., Belyea, M., Germino, B., Porter, L., & Clayton, M. (2006). Benefits of the uncertainty management intervention for African American and White older breast cancer survivors: 20-month outcomes. *International Journal of Behavioral Medicine, 13*(4), 285–294.

Gil, K. M., Mishel, M. H., Belyea, M., Germino, B., Porter, L. S., LeNey, I. C., … Stewart, J. (2004). Triggers of uncertainty about recurrence and treatment side effects in long-term older breast African American and Caucasian cancer survivors. *Oncology Nursing Forum, 31*(3), 633–639.

Gil, K. M., Mishel, M. H., Germino, B., Porter, L. S., Carlton-LaNey, I., & Belyea, M. (2005). Uncertainty management intervention for older African American and Caucasian long-term breast cancer survivors. *Journal of Psychosocial Oncology, 23*(2–3), 3–21.

Giurgescu, C., Penckofer, S., Maurer, M. C., & Bryant, F. B. (2006). Impact of uncertainty, social support, and prenatal coping on the psychological well-being of high-risk pregnant women. *Nursing Research, 55*(5), 356–365.

Green, J., & Murton, F. (1996). Diagnosis of Duchenne muscular dystrophy: Parents' experiences and satisfaction. *Child: Care, Health & Development, 22*, 113–128.

Hilton, B. A. (1988). The phenomenon of uncertainty in women with breast cancer. *Issues in Mental Health Nursing, 9*, 217–238.

Hilton, B. A. (1989). The relationship of uncertainty, control, commitment, and threat of recurrence to coping strategies used by women diagnosed with breast cancer. *Journal of Behavioral Medicine, 12*(1), 39–54.

Hilton, B. A. (1993). Issues, problems, and challenges for families coping with breast cancer. *Seminars in Oncology Nursing, 9*(2), 88–100.

Hilton, B. A. (1994). The uncertainty stress scale: Its development and psychometric properties. *Canadian Journal of Nursing Research, 26*(3), 15–30.

Horner, S. (1997). Uncertainty in mothers' care for their ill children. *Journal of Advanced Nursing, 26*, 658–663.

Johnson, L. M., Zautra, A. J., & Davis, M. C. (2006). The role of illness uncertainty on coping with fibromyalgia symptoms. *Health Psychology, 25*(6), 696–703.

Jurgens, C. Y. (2006). Somatic awareness, uncertainty, and delay in care-seeking in acute heart failure. *Research in Nursing and Health, 29*(2), 74–86.

Kang, Y. (2005). Effects of uncertainty on perceived health status in patients with atrial fibrillation. *British Association of Critical Care Nurses, Nursing in Critical Care, 10*(4), 184–191.

Kang, Y. (2006). Effect of uncertainty on depression in patients with newly diagnosed atrial fibrillation. *Progress in Cardiology Nursing, 21*(2), 83–88.

Kang, Y. (2011). The relationships between uncertainty and its antecedents in Korean patients with atrial fibrillation. *Journal of Clinical Nursing, 20*, 1880–1886.

Kang, Y., Daly, B. J., & Kim, J. S. (2004). Uncertainty and its antecedents in patients with atrial fibrillation. *Western Journal of Nursing Research, 26*(7), 770–783.

Katz, A. (1996). Gaining a new perspective on life as a consequence of uncertainty in HIV infection. *Journal of the Association of Nurses in AIDS Care, 7*(11), 51–60.

Kazer, M. W., Bailey, D. E., Sanda, M., Colberg, J., & Kelly, K. (2011). An internet intervention for management of uncertainty during active surveillance for prostate cancer. *Oncology Nursing Forum, 38*(5), 561–568.

Kreulen, G. L., & Braden, C. J. (2004). Model test of the relationship between self-helppromoting nursing interventions and self-care and health status outcomes. *Research in Nursing & Health, 27*, 97–101.

Landis, B. J. (1996). Uncertainty, spirituality, well-being, and psychosocial adjustment to chronic illness. *Issues in Mental Health Nursing, 17*, 217–231.

Lazarus, R. S. (1974). Psychological stress and coping in adaptation and illness. *International Journal of Psychiatry in Medicine, 5*, 321–333.

Lee, Y. L. (2006). The relationships between uncertainty and posttraumatic stress in survivors of childhood cancer. *Journal of Nursing Research, 14*(2), 133–142.

Lemaire, G. S. (2004). More than just menstrual cramps: Symptoms and uncertainty among women with endometriosis. *Journal of Obstetric, Gynecologic, and Neonatal Nursing, 33*(1), 71–79.

Lemaire, G. S., & Lenz, E. R. (1995). Perceived uncertainty about menopause in women attending an educational program. *International Journal of Nursing Studies, 32*(1), 39–48.

Light, D. (1979). Uncertainty and control in professional training. *Journal of Health and Social Behavior, 20*, 310–322.

Liu, L., Li, C. Y., Tang, S., Huang, C., & Chiou, A. (2006). Role of continuing supportive cares in increasing social support and reducing perceived uncertainty among women with newly diagnosed breast cancer in Taiwan. *Cancer Nursing, 29*(4), 273–282.

Mandler, G. (1979). Thought processes, consciousness and stress. In V. Hamilton & D. M. Warburton (Eds.), *Human stress and cognition: An information processing approach* (pp. 179–201). New York, NY: Wiley.

Mast, M. E. (1995). Adult uncertainty in illness: A critical review of research. *Scholarly Inquiry for Nursing Practice, 9*(1), 3–24.

Mast, M. E. (1998). Survivors of breast cancer: Illness uncertainty, positive reappraisal, and emotional distress. *Oncology Nursing Forum, 25*(3), 555–562.

McCain, N. L, Munjas, B. A., Munro, C. L., Elswick, R. K., Jr., Robins, J. L., Ferreira-Gonzalez, A., … Cochran K. L. (2003). Effects of stress management on PNI-based outcomes in persons with HIV disease. *Research in Nursing & Health, 26*, 102–117.

McCormick, K. M. (2002). A concept analysis of uncertainty in illness. *Journal of Nursing Scholarship, 34*(2), 127–131.

McCormick, K. M., Naimark, B. J., & Tate, R. B. (2006). Uncertainty, symptom distress, anxiety, and functional status in patients awaiting coronary artery bypass surgery. *Heart & Lung, 35*(1), 34–44.

Mishel, M. H. (1981). The measurement of uncertainty in illness. *Nursing Research, 30*, 258–263.

Mishel, M. H. (1983). Parents' perception of uncertainty concerning their hospitalized child. *Nursing Research, 32*, 324–330.

Mishel, M. H. (1984). Perceived uncertainty and stress in illness. *Research in Nursing and Health, 7*, 163–171.

Mishel, M. H. (1988). Uncertainty in illness. *Image: Journal of Nursing Scholarship, 20*, 225–231.

Mishel, M. H. (1990). Reconceptualization of the uncertainty in illness theory. *Image: Journal of Nursing Scholarship, 22*, 256–262.

Mishel, M. H. (1993). Living with chronic illness: Living with uncertainty. In S. G. Funk, E. M. Tornquist, M. T. Champagne, & R. A. Wiese (Eds.), *Key aspects of caring for the chronically ill: Hospital and home* (pp. 46–58). New York, NY: Springer.

Mishel, M. H. (1997a). Uncertainty in acute illness. *Annual Review of Nursing Research, 15*, 57–80.

Mishel, M. H. (1997b). *The efficacy of the uncertainty management intervention for older White and African American women with breast cancer.* Paper presented at the 11th Annual Conference of the Southern Nursing Research Society, Norfolk, VA.

Mishel, M. H. (1999). Uncertainty in chronic illness. *Annual Review of Nursing Research, 17*, 269–294.

Mishel, M. H., Belyea, M., Germino, B. B., Stewart, J. L., Bailey, D. E., Robertson, C., & Mohler, J. (2002). Helping patients with localized prostate carcinoma manage uncertainty and treatment side effects: Nurse-delivered psychoeducational intervention over the telephone. *Cancer, 94*(6), 1854–1866.

Mishel, M. H., & Braden, C. J. (1987). Uncertainty: A mediator between support and adjustment. *Western Journal of Nursing Research, 9,* 43–57.

Mishel, M. H., & Braden, C. J. (1988). Finding meaning: Antecedents of uncertainty in illness. *Nursing Research, 37,* 98–127.

Mishel, M. H., Germino, B. B., Belyea, M., Stewart, J. L., Bailey, D. E., Mohler, J., & Robertson, C. (2003). Moderators of an uncertainty management intervention, for men with localized prostate cancer. *Nursing Research, 52*(2), 89–97.

Mishel, M. H., Germino, B. B., Gill, K. M., Belyea, M., Laney, I. C., Stewart, J., ... Clayton, M. (2005). Benefits from an uncertainty management intervention for African-American and Caucasian older long-term breast cancer survivors. *Psychooncology, 14,* 962–978.

Mishel, M. H., Hostetter, T., King, B., & Graham, V. (1984). Predictors of psychosocial adjustment in patients newly diagnosed with gynecological cancer. *Cancer Nursing, 7,* 291–299.

Mishel, M. H., & Murdaugh, C. L. (1987). Family adjustment to heart transplantation: Redesigning the dream. *Nursing Research, 36,* 332–336.

Mishel, M. H., Padilla, G., Grant, M., & Sorenson, D. S. (1991). Uncertainty in illness theory: A replication of the mediating effects of mastery and coping. *Nursing Research, 40,* 236–240.

Mishel, M. H., & Sorenson, D. S. (1991). Uncertainty in gynecological cancer: A test of the mediating functions of mastery and coping. *Nursing Research, 40,* 167–171.

Mitchell, M. L., Courtney, M., & Coyer, F. (2003). Understanding uncertainty and minimizing families' anxiety at the time of transfer from intensive care. *Nursing & Health Sciences, 5*(3), 207–217.

Moos, R., & Tsu, V. (1977). The crisis of physical illness: An overview. In R. Moos (Ed.), *Coping with physical illness* (pp. 3–25). New York, NY: Plenum.

Mullins, L. L., Cheney, J. M., Balderson, B., & Hommel, K. A. (2000). The relationship of illness uncertainty, illness intrusiveness, and asthma severity to depression in young adults with long-standing asthma. *International Journal of Rehabilitation and Health, 5*(3), 177–185.

Mullins, L. L., Cheney, J. M., Hartman, V. L., Albin, K., Miles, B., & Roberson, S. (1995). Cognitive and affective features of postpolio syndrome: Illness uncertainty, attributional style, and adaptation. *International Journal of Rehabilitation and Health, 1,* 211–222.

Mullins, L. L., Cote, M. P., Fuemmeler, B. F., Jean, V. M., Beatty, W. W., & Paul, R. H. (2001). Illness intrusiveness, uncertainty, and distress in individuals with multiple sclerosis. *Rehabilitation Psychology, 46*(2), 139–153.

Nelson, J. P. (1996). Struggling to gain meaning: Living with the uncertainty of breast cancer. *Advances in Nursing Science, 18*(3), 59–76.

Neville, K. (1998). The relationships among uncertainty, social support, and psychological distress in adolescents recently diagnosed with cancer. *Journal of Pediatric Oncology Nursing, 15*(1), 37–46.

Neville, K. L. (2003). Uncertainty in illness: An integrative review. *Orthopaedic Nursing, 22*(3), 206–214.

Northouse, L., Mood, D., Templin, T., Mellon, S., & George, T. (2000). Couples' patterns of adjustment to colon cancer. *Social Science and Medicine, 50*(2), 271–284.

Northouse, L., Walker, J., Schafenacker, A., Mood, D., Mellon, S., Galvin, E., ... Freeman-Gibb, L. (2002). A family-based program of care for women with recurrent breast cancer and their family members. *Oncology Nursing Forum, 29*(10), 1411–1419.

Norton, R. (1975). Measurement of ambiguity tolerance. *Journal of Personal Assessment, 39*, 607–619.

Nyhlin, K. T. (1990). Diabetic patients facing long-term complications: Coping with uncertainty. *Journal of Advanced Nursing, 15*, 1021–1029.

Padilla, G., Mishel, M., & Grant, M. (1992). Uncertainty, appraisal and quality of life. *Quality of Life Research, 1*, 155–165.

Parry, C. (2003). Embracing uncertainty: An exploration of the experiences of childhood cancer survivors. *Qualitative Health Research, 13*(2), 227–246.

Pelusi, J. (1997). The lived experience of surviving breast cancer. *Oncology Nursing Forum, 24*(8), 1343–1353.

Penrod, J. (2001). Refinement of the concept of uncertainty. *Journal of Advanced Nursing, 34*(2), 238–245.

Porter, L. S., Clayton, M. E., Belyea, J., Mishel, M., Gil, K. M., & Germino, B. B. (2006). Predicting negative mood state and personal growth in African American and White long-term breast cancer survivors. *Annals of Behavioral Medicine, 31*(3), 195–204.

Prigogine, I., & Stengers, I. (1984). *Order out of chaos: Man's new dialogue with nature.* New York, NY: Bantam Books.

Redeker, N. S. (1992). The relationship between uncertainty and coping after coronary bypass surgery. *Western Journal of Nursing Research, 14*, 48–68.

Righter, B. (1995). Ostomy care. Uncertainty and the role of the credible authority during an ostomy experience. *Journal of Wound and Ostomy Care Nursing, 22*(2), 100–104.

Ritz, L., Nissen, M., Swenson, K., Farrell, J., Sperduto, P., Sladek, M., ... Schroeder, L. M. (2000). Effects of advanced nursing care on quality of life and cost outcomes of women diagnosed with breast cancer. *Oncology Nursing Forum, 27*(6), 923–932.

Rydström, I., Dalheim-Englund, A.-C., Segesten, K., & Rasmussen, B. H. (2004). Relations governed by uncertainty: Part of life of families of a child with asthma. *Journal of Pediatric Nursing, 19*(2), 85–94.

Sammarco, A. (2001). Perceived social support, uncertainty, and quality of life of younger breast cancer survivors. *Cancer Nursing, 24*(3), 212–219.

Sammarco, A., & Konecny, L. M. (2010). Quality of life, social support and uncertainty among Latina and Caucasian breast cancer survivors: A comparative study. *Oncology Nursing Forum, 37*(1), 93–99.

Sanders-Dewey, N., Mullins, L., & Chaney, J. (2001). Coping style, perceived uncertainty in illness, and distress in individuals with Parkinson's disease and their caregivers. *Rehabilitation Psychology, 46*(4), 363–381.

Santacroce, S. (2000). Support from health care providers and parental uncertainty during the diagnosis phase of perinatally acquired HIV infection. *Journal of the Association of Nurses in AIDS Care, 11*(2), 63–75.

Santacroce, S. (2001). Measuring parental uncertainty during the diagnosis phase of serious illness in a child. *Journal of Pediatric Nursing, 16*(1), 3–12.

Santacroce, S. (2002). Uncertainty, anxiety, and symptoms of posttraumatic stress in parents of children recently diagnosed with cancer. *Journal of Pediatric Oncology Nursing, 19*(3), 104–111.

Santacroce, S. J. (2003). Parental uncertainty and posttraumatic stress in serious childhood illness. *Journal of Nursing Scholarship, 35*(1), 45–51.

Santacroce, S. J., & Lee, Y. L. (2006). Uncertainty, posttraumatic stress, and health behavior in young adult childhood cancer survivors. *Nursing Research, 55*(4), 259–266.

Saunders, J. C., & Cookman, C. A. (2005). A clarified conceptual meaning of hepatitis Crelated depression. *Gastroenterology Nursing, 28*(2), 123–129; quiz 120–121.

Sexton, D. L., Calcasola, S. L., Bottomley, S. R., & Funk, M. (1999). Adults' experience with asthma and their reported uncertainty and coping strategies. *Clinical Nurse Specialist, 13*(1), 8–17.

Shalit, B. (1977). Structural ambiguity and limits to coping. *Journal of Human Stress, 3*, 32–45.

Sharkey, T. (1995). The effects of uncertainty in families with children who are chronically ill. *Ho me Healthcare Nurse, 13*(4), 37–42.

Small, S. P., & Graydon, J. E. (1993). Uncertainty in hospitalized patients with chronic obstructive pulmonary disease. *International Journal of Nursing Studies, 30*, 239–246.

Smeltzer, S. C. (1994). The concerns of pregnant women with multiple sclerosis. *Qualitative Health Research, 4*, 497–501.

Sorenson, D. L. S. (1990). Uncertainty in pregnancy. *NAACOG Clinical Issues in Perinatal and Women's Health Nursing, 1*(3), 289–296.

Sterken, D. J. (1996). Uncertainty and coping of fathers of children with cancer. *Journal of Pediatric Oncology Nursing, 13*, 81–90.

Stewart, J. L. (2003). "Getting used to it": Children finding the ordinary and routine in the uncertain context of cancer. *Qualitative Health Research, 13*(3), 394–407.

Stewart, J. L., & Mishel, M. H. (2000). Uncertainty in childhood illness: A synthesis of the parent and child literature. *Scholarly Inquiry for Nursing Practice, 17*, 299–319.

Stewart, J. L., Mishel, M. H., Lynn, M. R., & Terhorst, L. (2010). Test of a conceptual model of uncertainty in children and adolescents with cancer. *Research in Nursing and Health, 33*, 179–191.

Taylor-Piliae, R. E., & Chair, S. Y. (2002). The effect of nursing intervention utilizing music theory or sensory information on Chinese patients' anxiety prior to cardiac catherization: A pilot study. *European Journal of Cardiovascular Nursing, 1*, 203–311.

Taylor-Piliae, R., & Molassiotis, A. (2001). An exploration of the relationships between uncertainty, psychological distress and type of coping strategy among Chinese men after cardiac catheterization. *Journal of Advanced Nursing, 33*(1), 79–88.

Tomlinson, P., Kirschbaum, M., Harbaugh, B., & Anderson, K. (1996). The influence of illness severity and family resources on maternal uncertainty during critical pediatric hospitalization. *American Journal of Critical Care, 5,* 140–146.

Turner, M., Tomlinson, P., & Harbaugh, B. (1990). Parental uncertainty in critical care hospitalization of children. *Maternal-Child Nursing Journal, 19,* 45–62.

Van Riper, M., & Selder, F. E. (1989). Parental responses to birth of a child with Down syndrome. *Loss, Grief and Care: A Journal of Professional Practice, 3*(3–4), 59–76.

Walker, L. O., & Avant, K. C. (1989). *Strategies for theory construction in nursing.* Norwalk, CT: Appleton-Century-Crofts.

Webster, K. K., & Christman, N. J. (1988). Perceived uncertainty and coping post myocardial infarction. *Western Journal of Nursing Research, 10*(4), 384–400.

Weems, J., & Patterson, E. T. (1989). Coping with uncertainty and ambivalence while awaiting a cadaveric renal transplant. *ANNA Journal, 16*(1), 27–32.

Weiss, M. E., Saks, N. P., & Harris, S. (2002). Resolving the uncertainty of preterm symptoms: Women's experiences with the onset of preterm labor. *Journal of Obstetric, Gynecologic, and Neonatal Nursing, 31*(1), 66–76.

Weitz, R. (1989). Uncertainty and the lives of persons with AIDS. *Journal of Health and Social Behavior, 30,* 270–281.

White, R. E., & Frasure-Smith, N. (1995). Uncertainty and psychologic stress after coronary angioplasty and coronary bypass surgery. *Heart & Lung, 24*(1), 19–27.

Wiener, C. L., & Dodd, M. J. (1993). Coping amid uncertainty: An illness trajectory perspective. *Scholarly Inquiry for Nursing Practice, 7*(1), 17–31.

Wineman, N. M. (1990). Adaptation to multiple sclerosis: The role of social support, functional disability, and perceived uncertainty. *Nursing Research, 39,* 294–299.

Wineman, N. M., O'Brien, R. A., Nealon, N. R., & Kaskel, B. (1993). Congruence in uncertainty between individuals with multiple sclerosis and their spouses. *Journal of Neuroscience Nursing, 25,* 356–361.

Wineman, N. M., Schwetz, K. M., Goodkin, D. E., & Rudick, R. A. (1996). Relationships among illness uncertainty, stress, coping, and emotional well-being at entry into a clinical drug trial. *Applied Nursing Research, 9*(2), 53–60.

Wineman, N. M., Schwetz, K. M., Zeller, R., & Cyphert, J. (2003). Longitudinal analysis of illness uncertainty, coping, hopefulness, and mood during participation in a clinical drug trial. *Journal of Neuroscience Nursing, 35*(2), 100–106.

Winters, C. A. (1999). Heart failure: Living with uncertainty. *Progress in Cardiovascular Nursing, 14,* 85–91.

Wonghongkul, T., Dechaprom, N., Phumivichuvate, L., & Losawatkul, S. (2006). Uncertainty appraisal coping and quality of life in breast cancer survivors. *Cancer Nursing, 29*(3), 250–257.

Wonghongkul, T., Moore, S., Musil, C., Schneider, S., & Deimling, G. (2000). The influence of uncertainty in illness, stress appraisal, and hope on coping in survivors of breast cancer. *Cancer Nursing, 23*(6), 422–429.

Wunderlich, R., Perry, A., Lavin, M., & Katz, B. (1999). Patients' perceptions of uncertainty and stress during weaning from mechanical ventilation. *Dimensions of Critical Care Nursing, 18*(1), 8–12.

5

Theory of Meaning

Patricia L. Starck

O ne of the greatest challenges faced by nurses and other health professionals—whether providing care to those with acute, life-threatening illnesses, chronic conditions, or seeking to remain healthy—is to find the key to human motivation. What keeps a person from hanging on versus giving up, from struggling to overcome versus giving in, and from making sacrificial changes now for a better tomorrow? A young man is injured in a diving accident and is suddenly and irrevocably changed with the resulting spinal cord injury. What can the nurse do to promote that fighting spirit to be the best of what can now be? Such were the ponderings that led this author to search for answers.

Motivation and human behavior are usually thought to be the purview of psychology/psychiatry. Sigmund Freud believed that seeking pleasure (and in particular, sexual pleasure) was the primary factor in human behavior. Alfred Adler had a different theory—the chief force was the seeking of power—with the concepts of birth order position, inferiority complex, and so on. The philosophy most resonating with this author was that of Viktor Frankl, who believed that the primary human motivation was to seek meaning and purpose in life (PIL).

Frankl laid the foundational concepts on what has been developed into the Theory of Meaning. Frankl's application was originally with patients with psychiatric or psychological disorders. It has been expanded to help patients with various health problems, including disabilities and catastrophic, life-changing events, as well as to help the average human being cope with the everyday stresses of life. The theory and its application has also evolved past the individual level to groups and to the community/society.

PURPOSE OF THE THEORY AND HOW IT WAS DEVELOPED

In Europe during Frankl's professional era, a precise set of assumptions and philosophy was called a school of thought. Thus, Frankl— as a Viennese psychiatrist and neurologist—was trained in the first school of Viennese psychiatry, known as the Will to Pleasure, espoused by Sigmund Freud, and later, the second school, or the Will to Power, developed by Alfred Adler.

Frankl (1978) acknowledged the worth of Freud and Adler, as well as behaviorists who followed, but based on his own practice and experiences came to believe that humans cannot be seen as beings whose basic concerns are to satisfy drives and gratify instincts or, for that matter, to reconcile id, ego, and superego; nor can the human reality be understood merely as the outcome of conditioning processes or conditioned reflexes. Rather, the human is revealed as a being in search of meaning, and when this search is thwarted, various physical, mental, and spiritual problems become manifest.

Frankl called his concept the Will to Meaning, and it became known as the third school of Viennese psychiatry. He postulated that human beings are motivated to seek answers to such questions as: Why am I here? He went on to develop treatment, which he termed *logotherapy*, the practice of helping people with psychiatric problems find meaning and PIL, no matter what their life circumstances.

There is a common misperception that Frankl's theory emerged as a result of his internment in German concentration camps during World War II. This misperception was a source of great irritation to Frankl as he clarified that in actuality he formulated his ideas about meaning in life when he was a young child, with his first clear understanding at age 5. After his medical education, he planned to write a book about the theory. However, the plan was interrupted when he was seized by the Nazis in Germany and imprisoned (Fabry, 1991). During the concentration camp experience, observing the behavior of prisoners and guards, he validated the premise of the vital importance of humans seeking meaning in life experiences.

He found that in spite of great suffering, survival behaviors were more evident in those who had a strong reason to live than in those who did not. Frankl preserved the theory by recreating a manuscript he had lost when he was imprisoned. During his internment at four different concentration camps over a 2½-year period, he wrote on scraps of paper to keep his mind focused on his reason to survive. After his release at the end of World War II, he published the book that was later titled *Man's Search for Meaning*, under the previous title *From Death Camp to Existentialism*. In the book, he described his experience in prison, detailing the unimaginable sufferings of the imprisoned. He began to develop his concept of human suffering by defining suffering as a challenge. In the experience of suffering, the challenge to the individual is to decide how to respond to unavoidable, deplorable life circumstances. It is an opportunity to show courage and to behave decently in spite of circumstances. He coined the term *logotherapy* from the Greek word, *logos*, denoting meaning. Logotherapy is the practice of the theory, which is intended to assist individuals to find PIL regardless of circumstances.

Starck (1985a) examined Frankl's work in light of Kerlinger's (1973) criteria for a theory that describes, explains, and predicts human behavior. The postulates are the central core of the theory and are generalized statements of truth that serve as essential underpinnings for this body of knowledge. The postulates follow.

- A person's search for meaning is the primary motivation of life. This meaning is unique and specific in that it must and can be fulfilled by the person alone (Frankl, 1984, p. 121).
- A person is free to be responsible and is responsible for the realization of the meaning of life, the *logos* of existence (Frankl, 1961, p. 9).
- A person may find meaning in life even when confronted with a hopeless situation, when facing a fate that cannot be changed (Frankl, 1984, p. 135).
- A person's life offers meaning in every moment and in every situation (Fabry, 1991, p. 130).

The theory of meaning is a framework that lends itself to interdisciplinary endeavors. Frankl's work has been used as the basis for research and practice in many fields, including medicine, psychology, counseling, education, ministry, and nursing. Travelbee (1966, 1969, 1972) was the first nurse to use Frankl's work in practice. She used parables and other stories to help psychiatric patients realize that human suffering comes to all and that we have the means to combat life problems no matter the circumstances.

I had the great privilege of knowing Viktor E. Frankl over a 20-year period beginning when I was a doctoral student seeking ways to promote rehabilitation of patients with spinal cord injuries. I came upon Frankl's work and wrote to him. He responded and encouraged me, saying I would be the first to apply his theory and practice to physically disabled individuals.

I met him in 1979 when I presented my dissertation—including the logotherapeutic nursing intervention I had designed—to the first World Congress of Logotherapy. I was deeply honored when he quoted my work in his publications and presentations. I later received further training in logotherapy from his protégé, Elizabeth Lukas, a logotherapist from Munich, Germany. I visited with Dr. and Mrs. Frankl in their home in Vienna and received several treasured mementos—a photograph of him and me together, his sketches of our two profiles, and a reprint of one of his early publications.

I was pleased to invite him to the University of Texas Health Science Center at Houston in 1985, where he gave a 90-minute lecture to a packed auditorium. We made a videotape of this lecture and another tape in which I interviewed him about human suffering. In this latter tape, we were joined by Jerry Long, a quadriplegic who became a doctorally prepared logotherapist after his injury at age 17. I saw Dr. Frankl at several more World Congresses until health prevented his travel. The only child of Dr. and Mrs. Frankl became a logotherapist and carries on her father's work in Vienna. Frankl's two grandchildren have also developed their careers in ways to enhance his work. In 2011, his grandson, Alexander Vesseley, produced a documentary film, *Viktor and I*.

Dr. Frankl died in 1997, the same week that Princess Diana of England and Mother Teresa of India died. His work goes on as educators, practitioners, and researchers from various disciplines continue to broaden and enrich his theory.

CONCEPTS OF THE THEORY

Three major concepts from Frankl's works are the building blocks of the theory: life purpose, freedom to choose, and human suffering. These concepts are supported by three human dimensions: the physical or soma, the mental or psyche, and the spiritual or noos (Frankl, 1969). The physical and the mental dimensions can become ill but the spiritual dimension cannot. It can only become blocked or frustrated. To explain this three-dimensional assumption, Frankl (1969) described laws of dimensional ontology. He sought to illustrate the simultaneous ontological differences and the anthropological unity of these three dimensions by using geometrical structures as analogies, showing qualitative differences while not destroying the unity of the structure. Dimensional ontology rests on two laws:

1. "One and the same phenomenon projected out of its own dimension into different dimensions lower than its own is depicted in such a way that the individual pictures contradict one another" (p. 23). For example, a cylinder when projected vertically, would be perceived as a rectangle from the vertical view (from the side),

but as a circle when projected as a horizontal view (from above). The meaning ascribed to the shape is relative to one's position in relation to the cylinder view. Therefore, this law articulates complexity emerging from unique perspectives of a single phenomenon.

2. "Different phenomena projected out of their own dimension into one dimension lower than their own are depicted in such a manner that the pictures are ambiguous" (p. 23). This second law articulates the quality of potential sameness occurring when multiple distinct levels of phenomena are viewed in relation to each other. For example, a cylinder, a cone, and a sphere all cast shadows as a circle when projected from above onto a horizontal plane. It would be possible to ascribe the same or different meaning to each of these distinct shapes given a particular perspective.

Frankl's point is that while we have these three dimensions of soma, psyche, and noos, we can be both parts and a whole. From different points of view, different impressions and, therefore, different meanings reveal themselves. He called attention to the fact that a problem in one dimension may show up as a symptom in another. For example, spiritual emptiness may manifest in a physical symptom such as intense headaches. An important understanding when considering dimensional ontology is Frankl's emphasis on the human spirit, the noos, and the "defiant" power of the noos. Fabry (1991) interpreted this conceptualization as, "You *have* a body and a psyche, but you *are* your noos (spirit)" (p. 127). The human spirit can defy the odds and rise above the other dimensions.

Examples of the power of the noos will be provided throughout this chapter as vignettes are shared and stories are told about people who excelled beyond expectations to accomplish extraordinary feats. The noos is essential to the pursuit of life purpose.

Life Purpose

Life purpose is the central concept of the theory of meaning. It is the summary of reasons for one's existence, answering the questions: Who am I? and Why am I here? A sense of life purpose brings satisfaction with one's place in the world. Life purpose is that to which one may feel called and to which one is dedicated. There is a theme to one's life purpose—making a contribution, leaving the world a better place. The major premise of Frankl's theory is that the search for meaning in one's life is an overriding search for purpose. Life purpose flows from the "uniqueness of the person and the singularity of the situation" (Frankl, 1973, p. 63). Every person is "indispensable and irreplaceable" (Frankl, 1973, p. 117).

Fabry (1991) explained meaning from various existential viewpoints. The French existentialists, Sartre and Camus, believed that life itself had no meaning other than the meaning that humans gave to it. In contrast, the German existentialists, including Frankl, maintained that meaning exists and the task is to discover it, and in discovering meaning one also discovers life purpose. Fabry emphasized that our human spirits are the instruments for finding a PIL through tapping the spiritual treasure in each of us.

Frankl asserts that each person must discover his or her own meaning. It cannot be prescribed by another. A professional caregiver working with a person who has recently suffered a loss cannot tell the person how to look for meaning in another dimension of life, but the caregiver can help guide the person to find new avenues of meaning through shifting views of soma, psyche, and noos. "And meaning is something to be found rather than to be given, discovered rather than invented" (Frankl, 1969, p. 62).

Frankl (1984) postulated that meaning in life always changes but never ceases to be. He specified three different ways to find meaning on the path to uncovering life purpose: (1) creating a work or doing a deed that moves beyond self, (2) experiencing something or encountering someone, and (3) choosing our attitude toward our own fate. In the first way, a strong sense of purpose or meaning in life may be seen when a terminally ill person hangs on tenaciously until the achievement of some goal such as that person's child graduating from college. This will to meaning is a strong life force that can defy the odds given by the most expert clinician. Frankl (1984) also emphasized that our past achievements are monuments of meaning in our lives. "All we have done, whatever great thoughts we may have had, and all we have suffered, all this is not lost, though it is past; we have brought it into being. Having been is also a kind of being, and perhaps the surest kind" (p. 104). Fabry (1980) distinguished between "meaning of the moment" in everyday choices we make and "universal meaning" or the bigger picture that we may not completely understand at the time. Meaning of the moment is the everyday situation where one has a chance to act in a meaningful way through action, experiences, and the stand one takes. Ultimate meaning is the trust that there is order in the universe and that humans are part of that order. It is the opposite of seeing the world as chaotic and humans as the victims of whim.

Self-transcendence (Frankl, 1969) is related to life purpose. It is described as getting outside the self for a cause greater than the self. It is creating a work or doing a deed that reaches beyond one's egocentricity toward others, even though it may be difficult to do when life has been cruel (Fabry, 1991). Self-transcendence is contrasted with self-awareness. In self-awareness, the focus is internal, such as guilt, past traumas, or other feelings. By contrast, self-transcendence is distancing from oneself. In the distancing, a different view of the situation comes to light along with a changed meaning of the situation. For example, parents who have lost a child to violence may put energy toward getting new legislation passed that will protect children and prevent the type of loss they have suffered from happening to others. The hardship is deliberately endured so that others may benefit. Self-transcendence should not be confused with self-actualization as defined by Maslow (1968). Frankl (1975) stated that "what is called 'self-actualization' is ultimately an effect, the unintentional by-product of self-transcendence" (p. 78).

A second way to find meaning and enable life purpose is through experiences like loving or encountering another human being. Frankl believed that love goes beyond an individual and is long lasting. "Love is so little directed toward the body of the beloved that it can easily outlast the other's death, can exist in the lover's heart until his own death" (Frankl, 1973, p. 138).

The third way to find meaning on the path of life purpose is by choosing one's own attitude to whatever life presents. Choosing to remain positive, brave, or optimistic in spite of difficult circumstances illustrates this way of finding meaning. PIL can come when a choice is made to deliberately change one's attitude and view the situation in a different way.

Frankl identified two states that describe a lack of meaning: existential frustration and existential vacuum. Existential frustration is searching for meaning in which there is a state of being unsettled, of wanting more from life (Frankl, 1969). Existential vacuum is a sense of utter despair, of hopelessness, that life has no meaning and all is of no use (Frankl, 1969). This is an inner emptiness where one feels trapped in unhappiness. Times of transition may lead to an existential vacuum, such as when a person is dissatisfied with work but is afraid of risking change. Existential vacuum may also occur during times of loss, such as the sudden, unexpected death of a child, when one does not trust values that have formerly been a guide. Fabry (1980) believed that lack of meaning is a major problem in society because people repress their natural desire to find meaning, causing them to feel that life has no purpose, no challenges, and no obligations. This problem is experienced as a crisis among the rich and the poor, the old and the young, the successful and those who have failed. Fabry (1980) identified unhealthy ways that people cope including drugs, workaholism, thrill-seeking, and overeating. This crisis experience may also serve as a stimulus to find a more meaningful existence.

A poignant example of finding meaning and accomplishing life purpose, even at the end of life, is a story that will live in history as one in which individuals transcended self for the good of others. On September 11, 2001, passengers on United Airlines flight #93 found that fate had placed them on a plane hijacked by terrorists intent on a suicide mission to destroy innocent lives and symbols of American democracy. With the aid of cell phone technology, some passengers learned there had already been terrorist attacks occurring through the hijack of other commercial flights that morning and there was no doubt what their fate was to be. Many talked to family members about the things that gave meaning to their lives—the love they had, the expressed wish for the family to go on to complete meaningful lives. Yet, in the face of their own death, they had freedom of choice. They had a chance to transcend their own fears, one last chance to do something good for humanity. In the last moments of their lives, they could and did perform a selfless act—they made sure the plane did not reach its intended target but rather crashed in a nonpopulated area in Pennsylvania. In accomplishing this unexpected life purpose, they gave meaning to their lives and left a legacy of heroism, not only for their loved ones but also for every American citizen and many others around the world. If among this group there were one person whose life had been meaningless, when that person exercised freedom to act and to transcend his/her own needs, by this one act in the final moments, life was flooded with meaning and purpose.

Freedom to Choose

Freedom to choose is the second concept of the theory of meaning. It is the process of selecting among options over which one has control.

In enduring the most intense imaginable hardship, that of the Holocaust, Frankl (1973) pointed out that there is value to be found in a person's attitude toward the limiting factors of life. Being confronted by an unalterable destiny where one can act only by acceptance provides a unique opportunity to choose one's attitude. "The way in which he accepts, the way in which he bears his cross, what courage he manifests in suffering, what dignity he displays in doom and disaster, is the measure of his human fulfillment" (Frankl, 1973, p. 44).

One can be subjected to torture, humiliation, and worse, and yet retain the attitude to face one's fate with courage. It is the attitude of the sufferer that drives the behavior, not the actions of the persecutor. The right to choose one's own attitude may be thought of as spiritual freedom or independence of mind.

> We who lived in concentration camps can remember the men who walked through the huts comforting others, giving away their last piece of bread. They may have been few in number, but they offer sufficient proof that everything can be taken from a man but one thing: the last of the human freedoms—to choose one's attitude in any given set of circumstances, to choose one's own way. (Frankl, 1984, p. 86)

Freedom to be self-determining within the limits of endowment and environment was validated during Frankl's experiences in the concentration camps.

In this living laboratory and on this testing ground, we watched and witnessed some of our comrades behave like swine while others behaved like saints. Man has both potentialities within himself; which one is actualized depends on decisions but not on conditions. (Frankl, 1984, p. 157)

Fabry (1991) offered practical guidelines for modifying attitudes by considering that something positive can be found in all situations. Some sample questions to stimulate one's attitude change are: "What am I still able to do that would benefit someone? Whom do I love and wish to protect in this situation?" (p. 43). By asking these questions, one shifts the attention away from what has been lost and from self to others. Fabry (1991) suggested that one's attitude can begin to change by "acting as if" one has the attribute. For example, if a person wanted to be courageous, then to act "as if" would be to get a change in attitude.

Lukas (1984, 1986) introduced several ideas that are important to Frankl's work. She expanded understanding of freedom to choose by indicating that life events can be classified as either fate or freedom. Fate is when we cannot change the situation, whereas freedom includes what one can do, including choosing what attitude to adopt. When confronting a problem, the person should ask: Where are my areas of freedom? Which possible choices do I have? Which one do I want to actualize?

Human Suffering

Human suffering is the third concept of the theory of meaning. It is a subjective experience that is unique to an individual and varies from simple transitory discomfort to extreme anguish and despair (Starck & McGovern, 1992). Frankl did not define suffering but rather described it as a subjective, all-consuming human experience. He believed that "the meaning of suffering . . . is the deepest possible meaning" (Frankl, 1969, p. 75) and the ultimate meaning of life or human suffering can never be found. He used the following comparison:

> If I point to something with my finger, the dog does not look in the direction in which I point, it looks at my finger and sometimes snaps at it. And what about man? Is not he, too, unable to understand the meaning of something, say the meaning of suffering, and does not he, too, quarrel with his fate and snap at its finger? (Frankl, 1969, p. 145)

Frankl was clear that there is no meaning *in* suffering. For example, there is no meaning in cancer. However, one can find meaning *in spite of* having cancer. Suffering is a part of the human experience. Things happen to us that are undeserved, unexplainable, and unavoidable. We do not need to look for meaning in these events; rather, meaning comes from stances we take toward the suffering, for example, the courageous way a person chooses to live with the cancer. Frankl (1975) described the worst kind of suffering as "despair, suffering without meaning" (p. 137).

Relationships Among the Concepts: The Model

The relationships among the concepts of the theory are depicted in Figure 5.1. This illustration suggests that meaning is a journey toward life purpose with the freedom to choose one's path in spite of inevitable suffering.

USE OF THEORY IN NURSING RESEARCH

Instruments

A number of instruments have been developed that measure concepts related to meaning. These tools have been used in both research and clinical practice. Some are available from: Viktor E. Frankl International Institute for Logotherapy, Box 15211, Abilene, Texas; telephone: 325-692-9597 or 325-670-1451; fax: 325-692-9188; www.logotherapyinstitute.org. Nurses and other professionals are invited to become a member of the institute. A World Congress is held every 2 years where professionals around the globe share their work.

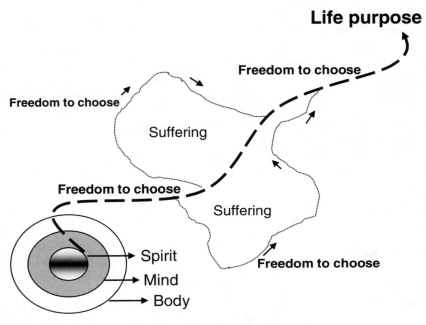

FIGURE 5.1   The Theory of Meaning

Instruments that quantify meaning and that can serve as a clinical guide to planning interventions include the PIL test (Crumbaugh, 1968; Crumbaugh & Maholick, 1976), which measures the degree of purpose one perceives. The Seeking of Noetic Goals (SONG) test (Crumbaugh, 1977) measures motivation to seek meaning, and the Meaning in Suffering Test (MIST) (Starck, 1985b) measures: (1) the extent to which one believes that meaning can be found in suffering and (2) that positive things can emerge from unavoidable suffering. The Life Purpose Questionnaire (LPQ) measures the degree of meaning in life for adults (Hutzell & Peterson, 1986). Another useful instrument is the list of values created by Crumbaugh (1980). This is a list of 20 values from which a person is directed to choose his or her top five values in life.

There are various other instruments available, including the Logotest developed by Elizabeth Lukas, PhD, for use in the practice of logotherapy. Fegg, Kramer, Bausewein, and Borasio (2007) developed and tested a new instrument, the Schedule for Meaning in Life Evaluation (SMiLE) on a large sample of the German population. With this instrument, respondents are asked to list three to seven areas of meaning in their lives, to weigh each in terms of importance, and to rate each for satisfaction. From a total of 3,521 areas, 13 categories of meaning were identified: (1) altruism, (2) animals/nature, (3) family, (4) financial security, (5) friends/acquaintances, (6) health, (7) hedonism, (8) home/garden, (9) leisure time, (10) occupation/work, (11) partnership, (12) psychological well-being, and (13) spirituality/religion. This study also revealed areas of meaning predominant in each age group, which for youth was friends; young adulthood, partnership; middle adulthood, work; retirement, health, and altruism; and advanced age, spirituality/religion and animals/nature.

Fjelland, Barron, and Foxall (2008) conducted a review of 12 instruments to measure (1) search for meaning and (2) meaning in illness. A detailed review of this analysis will help the future researcher select the appropriate instrument.

Nursing Research

Health professionals from various disciplines have contributed to research in the significance of meaning and purpose. Prior to the 1970s, much of the research was in the domain of psychology/psychiatry professionals and related to mental health views. Starck (1979) developed and tested a nursing intervention model for a population of individuals in the community with permanent spinal cord injury. Starck, Ulrich, & Duffy (2009) reported that the most intense suffering was reported by hospitalized psychiatric patients as compared with hospitalized patients with either a medical-surgical or high risk prenatal diagnosis.

In the 1980s and '90s, Steeves and Kahn (1987), Kahn and Steeves (1995), and Steeves (1992, 1996) studied the concept of suffering in various populations including hospice patients and their families and patients undergoing bone marrow transplantations. Steeves, Kahn, and Benoliel (1990) studied how nurses experience and react to a person's suffering. During this same time period, Starck (1992) studied suffering in a nursing home.

Other nursing researchers (Coward, 1991, 1994, 1995, 1996, 1998; Coward & Dickerson, 2003; Coward & Kahn, 2004, 2005; Coward & Lewis, 1993; Coward & Reed, 1996) have studied meaning and PIL in a healthy population as well as patients with breast cancer, AIDS, and at the end-of-life. Coward emphasizes self-transcendence, combining the work of Frankl and others in helping patients overcome spiritual disequilibrium.

Since the turn of the century, research in the role of meaning in health care has greatly expanded—internationally as well as across disciplines. Patient conditions where the role of meaning has been explored include myocardial infarction (MI), cancer, rheumatoid arthritis, addictions, bereavement, battered women, and HIV-positive individuals.

There are several more recent studies addressing life meaning and purpose for populations with chronic diseases. In a 5-year longitudinal study of patients with MI, Baldacchino (2011) documented that by finding meaning in the illness experiences and by clarifying values and PIL, MI patients were motivated to make lifestyle change, particularly in the immediate aftermath of their MI. However, by the third year onward, compliance with lifestyle modification was inconsistent (Baldacchino, 2010). In a study with 156 patients diagnosed with rheumatoid arthritis, Verduin et al. (2008) documented the independent contribution of life purpose to the mental health component of quality of life. In the exploration of the relationship between spirituality, PIL, and well-being in HIV-positive people, Litwinczuk and Groh (2007) found a significant relationship between spirituality and PIL in 46 HIV-positive men and women. The researchers recommended the design of nursing interventions to help HIV-positive people redefine themselves and find meaning in life.

There are several studies of life meaning and purpose with cancer patients. For instance, in longitudinal work with more than 500 cancer survivors, Jim and Anderson (2007) found that loss of life meaning contributed to poor social and physical functioning. In other research where investigators accepted the premise that many newly diagnosed cancer patients experience existential distress, Lee (2008) and Lee, Cohen, Edgar, Laizner, and Gagnon (2006) studied a meaning-making intervention, using a Lifeline exercise. The Lifeline exercise engaged participants in marking important life events in the past, and noting plans to achieve important life goals in the future. Use of the Lifeline exercise resulted in improved self-esteem, optimism, and self-efficacy in this randomized controlled trial.

Life meaning and purpose has also been studied in populations with addictive disorders. In research on Hungarian men and women, meaning in life as measured with the PIL test differentiated nonsmokers from daily smokers. Life meaning had a significant negative impact on smoking intensity for females (Thege, Bachner, Martos, & Kushnir, 2009). In another study of cocaine abusers in treatment, PIL significantly predicted relapse to cocaine and to alcohol use, as well as the number of days of use, 6 months after treatment (Martin, MacKinnon, Johnson, & Rohsenow, 2011). Martin et al. (2011) suggest that increasing one's sense of PIL may be an important component of treatment for cocaine-addicted patients.

Korean researchers (Kang & Kim, 2011) recently reported a study of life purpose and resilience in a group of 110 battered women. Greater life purpose was positively associated with higher resilience, measured as self-efficacy, communication efficiency, and optimism. Findings led the researchers to conclude that practitioners can help battered women to clarify their values and meaning in life and thereby improve their resilience.

Meaning and PIL play a significant role in health outcomes for a broad range of patients. The most often used measure is the PIL test, which was introduced more than 4 decades ago (Crumbaugh, 1968). Nurse researchers are now positioned to develop and test meaning-making interventions, such as the Lifeline exercise (Lee, 2008; Lee et al., 2006) described above. The move to intervention research to examine change in life purpose and health outcomes for people with chronic illness can easily be accommodated with guidance from the theory of meaning.

USE OF THE THEORY IN NURSING PRACTICE

Fabry (1980) has described logotherapy as "guiding people toward understanding themselves as they are and *could be* and their place in the totality of living" (p. xiii). When contrasted with traditional psychotherapy, it is less retrospective and introspective (Frankl, 1984). Other comparisons between psychotherapy and logotherapy are found in Table 5.1.

TABLE 5.1
Contrast of Psychotherapy and Logotherapy

Psychotherapy	Logotherapy
Depth psychology	Height psychology
Sees life in terms of problems	Sees life in terms of solutions
Focuses on obstacles	Focuses on goals
Is reductionistic	Is holistic
Emphasis on uncovering	Emphasis on discovering
Analytical style	Uniqueness and improvisational style
Psychiatrist listens	Logotherapist talks

The goal of logotherapy is to help persons separate themselves from their symptoms, to tap into the resources of their noetic dimension, and to arouse the dynamic power of the human spirit. Helping another find meaning may be described as promoting an unfolding of what is already there. It is helping the other discover his or her values and facilitating awareness of subconscious beliefs and commitments.

Frankl does not advocate techniques in a routine procedural sense but rather encourages creativity based on the situation at hand. Frankl (1969) has described *three* logotherapeutic approaches. These approaches are dereflection, paradoxical intention, and Socratic dialogue. Both dereflection and paradoxical intention "rest on two essential qualities of human existence, namely, man's capacities of self-transcendence and self-detachment" (Frankl, 1969, p. 99).

Dereflection

Dereflection is the act of de-emphasizing or ceasing to focus on a troublesome phenomenon, issue, or problem; it is putting this issue aside. Dereflection strengthens the capacity for self-transcendence.

Obsessions are recognized as hyper reflection or excess attention, described as the "compulsion to self-observation" (Frankl, 1973, p. 253). The urge for better sexual performance is an example. "Sexual performance or experience is strangled to the extent to which it is made either an object of attention or an objective of intention" (Frankl, 1969, p. 101).

Complaining is an example of hyper reflection, as an excessive amount of attention is given to the self. Dereflection helps the person stop fighting an anxiety, a neurosis, or a psychosis, and spares the person the reinforcement of additional suffering. If a person is depressed, dereflection can help achieve distance between the person and the depression, "to see himself—not as a person who is depressed but—as a full human being who has depressions with the capacity to find meaning despite the depressions" (Fabry, 1991, p. 136).

Paradoxical Intention

Paradoxical intention is intentionally acting the opposite to one's desired ends, thereby confronting one's fears and anxieties. Paradoxical intention strengthens the capacity for self-distancing. By distancing from the triggers of problems, these triggers become ineffective. Paradoxical intention is helpful in dealing with the problem of anticipatory anxiety. The object of the person's fear is fear itself. The underlying dynamic is apprehension about the potential effects of the anxiety attacks. And, of course, the fear of the fear increases the fear, producing precisely what the person is afraid of. The person is caught in a restricting cycle. The aim of therapy is to break the cycle, to interfere with the feedback mechanism. In logotherapy, one is asked to replace fear with a paradoxical wish, to wish for the very thing one fears. By this treatment, Frankl said, "the wind is taken out of the sails of the anxiety" (1984, p. 147).

This approach makes use of the specific human capacity for self-detachment. For example, in sleep disturbances when a person worries that he or she will not be able to get to sleep and focuses on trying to go to sleep, sleep will not come. The fear of sleeplessness results in the hyperintention to fall asleep, which inevitably leads to sleeplessness. Paradoxical intention advises the person not to try to sleep, but rather to try to do the opposite, stay awake as long as possible. The person who has been trying to stay awake wakes up to find that he or she has been asleep.

Paradoxical intention can be used to change unwanted behavior patterns. This does not depend upon understanding how and why the behavior started. It simply breaks the cycle of fear. Ascher and Schotte (1999) demonstrated that individuals with public speaking phobia complicated by recursive anxiety—for example, fear of loss of bladder control, vomiting, and so on—showed greater improvement when paradoxical intention was included in treatment.

Based on the finding that 55% of patients with a psychiatric disorder who presented in the emergency department were diagnosed with conversion disorders, Ataoglu, Ozcetin, Icmeli, and Ozbulut (2003) conducted a study and concluded that paradoxical intention therapy provided greater improvement than diazepam therapy.

Socratic Dialogue

Socratic dialogue is a conversation of questions and answers, probing deeply into existential issues such as one's values. It is rhetorical debate to trigger a change in attitude, behavior, or both. Socratic dialogue is self-discovery discourse and seeks to get rid of masks that have been put on to please or to be accepted. The therapist poses questions so that patients become aware of their unconscious decisions, their repressed hopes, and their unadmitted self-knowledge. In Socratic dialogue, experiences of the past are explored as well as fantasies for the future to modulate attitude (Fabry, 1980). Socratic dialogue requires impro-visation and intuition and asks probing questions like the following:

- Was there a time when life had meaning?
- Who do you know who leads a meaningful life? What keeps you from living like this person?
- Who are the people who need you?
- Tell me about an experience that made you see things differently.
- Tell me something you said you couldn't do but you did it.

As an example, Lukas (1984) working with a patient who strongly valued physical ability and who had undergone a leg amputation, asked the question, "Does the value of human existence depend on the use of two legs?" (p. 47).

Fabry (1991) proposed five guideposts to probe areas of meaning. These are self-discovery, choice, uniqueness, responsibility, and self-transcendence. He also identified a number of creative methods and exercises to illustrate choice, where family members act out the role of others in the way they wish the others had responded. The flashlight technique can be useful in self-discovery and in aggressive discussion. The facilitator shines the flashlight on the partner who says some-thing offensive to the other, indicating that the person must rephrase what has been said without hostility or sarcasm, thus helping reshape attitudes and behaviors. Fabry (1991) also has guidelines for groups, wherein the Socratic dialogue becomes a multilogue.

A family who was experiencing problems thought to be caused by one child who had a physical condition requiring most of the moth-er's attention, making her less available to her other children and to her husband, sought logotherapy. The therapist asked the "identified patient" this question in the presence of the entire family—"If you could give your condition to anyone else in the family, who would you give it to?" The mother quickly spoke and said, "I would take it." The therapist specified that the child was the one to answer the ques-tion. After looking at each member of his family, the child responded, "I would keep it myself because I think I am the best one to handle it." This attitude changed the family dynamic; the child was seen as a hero and not a burden to others.

Other Practices Using Logotherapy

Pearce (2005), a parish nurse, declared that Frankl was a forerunner to integrative medicine and holistic nursing, contrasting this with today's fragmented system of healers specializing in healing only a part of the whole. Patients with a complex interaction of physical, psychological, and spiritual suffering often find their way to logotherapy after being disappointed with the existing health care system. Logotherapy provides tools to tap into inner resources to emerge as a stronger and more joyous self.

Winters and Schulenberg (2006) pointed out that diagnosis is a necessary evil in practice. Diagnosis is inherently reductionistic and focuses on defeats. To address this problem, the authors developed a holistic, logotherapeutic model of diagnosis. The diagnostic process is a bio-psychosocial-spiritual one and incorporates an assessment of one's inner strength. For example, the provider might include a positive history of emotional balance and a history of making it through previous difficult times as noetic resources. Logotherapy is aimed at empowering the patient by emphasizing choice, responsibility, and hope.

More recent practice applications of meaning theory, both patient-related and provider-related, have been developed. Wong (2010) presents an interesting approach to meaning therapy including the PURE strategy (purpose, understanding, responsible action, and evaluation) and the ABCDE strategy (accept, believe, commit, discover, and evaluate).

The central ideas of the theory of meaning are proving useful for a range of life-altering illnesses and significant life time points. For instance, there is perhaps no greater challenge than finding meaning when confronting end-of-life. There is a growing recognition that symptoms of psychological distress and existential concerns are ever more prevalent and problematic than pain and other physical concerns when facing imminent death (Breitbart, Gibson, Poppito, & Berg, 2004).

Finding meaning in the traumatic experience of cardiac disease is used by psychotherapists to help patients reconstruct basic assumptions about self and others and to re-establish predictability in their lives (Sheikh & Marotta, 2008). A meaning-centered intervention has been used in treating veterans with chronic combat related posttraumatic stress disorder (Southwick, Gilmartin, McDonough, & Morrissey, 2006).

Not only do patients benefit from a sense of meaning and life purpose, care providers also benefit. Taubman-Ben-Ari and Weintroub (2008) studied physicians and nurses frequently exposed to terminally ill children in Israel. A higher level of exposure to patient death, higher optimism and professional self-esteem, and lower secondary traumatization (being close to someone who experienced trauma), predicted the sense of meaning in life. Fillion and colleagues have studied nurses who work in a palliative care setting. They designed a meaning-centered intervention consisting of group therapy in four sessions plus a closing session (Fillion, Dupuis, Tremblay, De Grace, & Breitbart, 2006). In the intervention, enhancing meaning in palliative care, the focus of each session was (1) search for and sources of meaning, (2) historical perspective and sense of accomplishment as creative values, (3) meaning and suffering through attitudinal change, and (4) affective experiences and humor in experiential values. Each session consisted of didactic content, exercises, and group discussion, plus home assignments. In a follow-up study, the researchers sought to ameliorate stress and improve job satisfaction and quality of life for nurses working in palliative care. The four-session meaning-centered intervention was conducted (Fillion et al., 2009) using a wait list design. Outcome measures included personal and job-related measures. Even though spiritual and emotional quality of life remained unchanged, nurses who received the intervention reported greater job benefits associated with working in the palliative care setting.

CONCLUSION

The theory of meaning can be a useful guide in research and practice. The theory focuses on discovering meaning when facing life challenges that threaten one's purpose in relation to unique circumstances. Nurse researchers and practitioners can draw on the theory to understand ordinary life stresses, as well as life-changing events and human suffering.

REFERENCES

Ascher, L. M., & Schotte, D. E. (1999). Paradoxical intention and recursive anxiety. *Journal of Behavior Therapy and Experimental Psychiatry, 30*, 71–79.

Ataoglu, A., Ozcetin, A., Icmeli, C., & Ozbulut, O. (2003). Paradoxical therapy in conversion reaction. *Journal of Korean medical science, 18*, 581–584.

Baldacchino, D. (2010). Long-term causal meaning of myocardial infarction. *British Journal of Nursing, 19*(12), 774–781.

Baldacchino, D. (2011). Myocardial infarction: A turning point in meaning in life over time. *British Journal of Nursing, 20*(2), 107–114.

Breitbart, W., Gibson, C., Poppito, S. R., & Berg, A. (2004). Psychotherapeutic interventions at the end of life: A focus on meaning and spirituality. *Canadian Journal of Psychiatry, 49*(6), 366–372.

Coward, D. D. (1991). Self-transcendence and emotional well-being in women with advanced breast cancer. *Oncology Nursing Forum, 18*, 857–863.

Coward, D. D. (1994). Meaning and purpose in the lives of persons with AIDS. *Public Health Nursing, 11,* 331–336.

Coward, D. D. (1995). The lived experience of self-transcendence in women with AIDS. *Journal of Obstetric, Gynecologic and Neonatal Nursing, 24,* 314–318.

Coward, D. D. (1996). Self-transcendence and correlates in a health population. *Nursing Research, 45*(2), 116–121.

Coward, D. D. (1998). Facilitation of self-transcendence in a breast cancer support group. *Oncology Nursing Forum, 25*(1), 75–84.

Coward, D. D., & Dickerson, D. (2003). Facilitation of self-transcendence in breast cancer support group: II. *Oncology Nursing Forum, 30*(2), 291–300.

Coward, D. D., & Kahn, D. L. (2004). Resolution of spiritual disequilibrium by women newly diagnosed with breast cancer. *Oncology Nursing Forum, 31*(2), 24–31.

Coward, D. D., & Kahn, D. L. (2005). Transcending breast cancer: Making meaning from diagnosis and treatment. *Journal of Holistic Nursing, 23*(3), 264–283.

Coward, D. D., & Lewis, F. M. (1993). The lived experience of self-transcendence in gay men with AIDS. *Oncology Nursing Forum, 20,* 1363–1368.

Coward, D. D., & Reed, P. G. (1996). Self-transcendence: A resource for healing at the end of life. *Issues in Mental Health Nursing, 17,* 275–288.

Crumbaugh, J. C. (1968). Cross-validation of purpose in life test based on Frankl's concepts. *Journal of Individual Psychology, 24,* 74–81.

Crumbaugh, J. C. (1977). The Seeking of Noetic Goals test (SONG): A complementary scale to the purpose in life test (PIL). *Journal of Clinical Psychology, 33,* 900–907.

Crumbaugh, J. C. (1980). *Logotherapy—new help for problem drinkers.* Chicago, IL: Nelson-Hall.

Crumbaugh, J. C., & Maholick, L. T. (1976). *Purpose in life test.* Abilene, TX: Viktor Frankl Institute for Logotherapy.

Fabry, J. B. (1980). *The pursuit of meaning.* New York, NY: Harper & Row.

Fabry, J. B. (1991). *Guideposts to meaning: Discovering what really matters.* Oakland, CA: New Harbinger.

Fegg, M. J., Kramer, M., Bausewein, C., & Borasio, G. D. (2007). Meaning in life in the Federal Republic of Germany: Results of a representative survey with the schedule for meaning in life evaluation (SMiLE). *Health and Quality of Life Outcomes, 5,* 59. Retrieved from http://www.hqlo.com/contents/5/1/59

Fillion, L., Dupuis, R., Tremblay, I., De Grace, G. R., & Breitbart, W. (2006). Enhancing meaning in palliative care practice: A meaning-centered intervention to promote job satisfaction. *Palliative and Supportive Care, 4,* 333–344.

Fillion, L., Duval, S., Dumont, S., Gagnon, P., Tremblay, I., Bairati, I., & Breitbart, W. S. (2009). Impact of a meaning-centered intervention on job satisfaction and on quality of life among palliative care nurses. *Psycho-Oncology, 18,* 1300–1310.

Fjelland, J. E., Barron, C. R., & Foxall, M. (2008). A review of instruments measuring two aspects of meaning: Search for meaning and meaning in illness. *Journal of Advanced Nursing, 62*(4), 394–406.

Frankl, V. E. (1961). Dynamics, existence, and values. *Journal of Existential Psychiatry, 11*(5), 5–16.

Frankl, V. E. (1969). *The will to meaning.* New York, NY: New American Library.

Frankl, V. E. (1973). *The doctor and the soul.* New York, NY: Vintage.

Frankl, V. E. (1975). *The unconscious God.* New York, NY: Simon & Schuster.

Frankl, V. E. (1978). *The unheard cry for meaning.* New York, NY: Simon & Schuster.

Frankl, V. E. (1984). *Man's search for meaning: An introduction to logotherapy.* Boston, MA: Beacon.

Hutzell, R. R., & Peterson, T. J. (1986). Use of the life purpose questionnaire with an alcoholic population. *International Journal of Addiction, 22*, 51–57.

Jim, H. S., & Andersen, B. L. (2007). Meaning in life mediates the relationship between social and physical functioning and distress in cancer survivors. *British Journal of Health Psychology, 12*, 363–381.

Kahn, D. L., & Steeves, R. H. (1995). The significance of suffering in cancer care. *Seminars in Oncology Nursing, 11*(1), 9–16.

Kang, S. K., & Kim, W. (2011). A study of battered women's purpose of life and resilience in South Korea. *Asian Social Work and Policy Review, 5*, 145–159.

Kerlinger, F. H. (1973). *Foundations of research* (2nd ed.). New York, NY: Holt, Rinehart, and Winston.

Lee, V. (2008). The existential plight of cancer: Meaning making as a concrete approach to the intangible search for meaning. *Support Care Cancer, 16*, 779–785.

Lee, V., Cohen, S. R., Edgar, L., Laizner, A. M., & Gagnon, A. J. (2006). Meaning-making and psychological adjustment to cancer: Development of an intervention and pilot results. *Oncology Nursing Forum, 33*(2), 291–302.

Litwinczuk, K. M., & Groh, C. J. (2007). The relationship between spirituality, purpose in life, and well-being in HIV-positive persons. *Journal of the Association of Nurses in Aids Care, 18*(3), 13–22.

Lukas, E. (1984). *Meaningful living: A logotherapeutic guide to health.* Cambridge, MA: Schenkman.

Lukas, E. (1986). *Meaning in suffering: Comfort in crisis through logotherapy.* Berkeley, CA: Institute of Logotherapy Press.

Martin, R. A., MacKinnon, S., Johnson, J., & Rohsenow, D. (2011). Purpose in life predicts treatment outcome among adult cocaine abusers in treatment. *Journal of Substance Abuse Treatment, 40*, 183–188.

Maslow, A. (1968). *Toward a psychology of being.* New York, NY: Van Nostrand.

Pearce, M. (2005). Appeal and application of logotherapy in parish nursing practice. *The International Forum of Logotherapy: Journal of Search for Meaning, 28*(1), 26–30.

Sheikh, A. I., & Marotta, S. A. (2008). Best practices for counseling in cardiac rehabilitation settings. *Journal of Counseling & Development, 86*, 111–120.

Southwick, S. M., Gilmartin, R., McDonough, P., & Morrissey, P. (2006). Logotherapy as an adjunctive treatment for chronic combat-related PTSD: A meaning-based intervention. *American Journal of Psychotherapy, 60*(2), 161–174.

Starck, P. L. (1979). Spinal cord injured clients' perception of meaning and purpose in life, measurement before and after nursing intervention. *Dissertation Abstracts International, 40*(10), 4741. (UMI No. 8007891)

Starck, P. L. (1985a). Logotherapy comes of age: Birth of a theory. *The International Forum of Logotherapy: Journal of Search for Meaning, 8*(2), 71–75.

Starck, P. L. (1985b). *The meaning in suffering test.* Berkeley, CA: Institute of Logotherapy Press.

Starck, P. L. (1992). Suffering in a nursing home: Losses of the human spirit. *The International Forum of Logotherapy: Journal of Search for Meaning, 15*(2), 76–79.

Starck, P. L., & McGovern, J. P. (1992). The meaning in suffering. In P. L. Starck & J. P. McGovern (Eds.), *The hidden dimension of illness: Human suffering* (pp. 25–42). New York, NY: National League for Nursing Press.

Starck, P. L., Ulrich, E., & Duffy, M. E. (2009). The meaning of suffering experiences. In Batthyany & Levinson (Eds). *Existential Psychotherapy of Meaning: A Handbook of Logotherapy and Existential Analysis.* Phoenix, AZ: Zeis, Tucker & Theisen.

Steeves, R. H. (1992). Patients who have undergone bone marrow transplantation: Their quest for meaning. *Oncology Nursing Forum, 19*, 899–905.

Steeves, R. H. (1996). Loss, grief, and the search for meaning. *Oncology Nursing Society, 23*, 897–903.

Steeves, R. H., & Kahn, D. L. (1987). Experience of meaning in suffering. *Journal of Nursing Scholarship, 19*(3), 114–116.

Steeves, R. H., Kahn, D. L., & Benoliel, J. Q. (1990). Nurses' interpretation of the suffering of their patients. *Western Journal of Nursing Research, 12*(6), 715–731.

Taubman, O., & Weintraub, A. (2008). Meaning in life and personal growth among pediatric physicians and nurses. *Death Studies, 32*, 621–645.

Thege, B. K., Bachner, Y. G., Martos, T., & Kushnir, T. (2009). Meaning in life: Does it play a role in smoking? *Substance Use & Misuse, 44*, 1566–1577.

Travelbee, J. (1966). *Interpersonal aspects of nursing.* Philadelphia, PA: F. A. Davis.

Travelbee, J. (1969). *Intervention in psychiatric nursing: Process in the one-to-one relationship.* Philadelphia, PA: F. A. Davis.

Travelbee, J. (1972). To find meaning in illness. *Nursing, 72*(2), 6–7.

Verduin, P. J. M., de Bock, G. H., Vliet Vlieland, T. P. M., Peeters, A. J., Verhoef, J., & Otten, W. (2008). Purpose in life in patients with rheumatoid arthritis. *Clinical Rheumatology, 27*, 899–908.

Vesseley, A. (2011). Viktor and I. Noetic Films, Inc. Retrieved from http://www.viktorandimovies.com

Winters, M., & Schulenberg, S. (2006). Diagnosis in logotherapy: Overuse and suggestions for appropriate use. *The International Forum of Logotherapy: Journal of Search for Meaning, 29*(1), 16–24.

Wong, P. T. P. (2010). Meaning therapy: An integrative and positive existential psychotherapy. *Journal of Contemporary Psychotherapy, 40*, 85–93.

6

Theory of Self-Transcendence

Pamela G. Reed

A central focus of nursing is facilitating well-being and understanding the capacity for well-being in the context of difficult health-related experiences. The nursing Theory of Self-Transcendence was created from a developmental perspective of human–environment processes of health. The word developmental is used in the theory to emphasize inherent change processes that are ongoing, innovative, and context-related while still acknowledging inevitable changes that may be viewed as random, decremental, or mechanistic. Self-transcendence theory originated from an interest in understanding developmental processes of later adulthood as integral to mental health and well-being. Although the role of development had long been an accepted perspective in work with children and adolescents, little attention was given to its significance for adults and especially older adults. The theory is now applied to individuals across the life span.

PURPOSE OF THE THEORY AND HOW IT WAS DEVELOPED

The purpose of the theory of self-transcendence is to provide a framework for inquiry and practice regarding the promotion of well-being in the midst of difficult life situations, particularly where individuals and families are facing loss or life-limiting illness. According to the intermodern philosophy of nursing science (Reed, 2011), theories are open systems of knowledge development that incorporate various ways of knowing including empirical and practice-based sources. Knowledge from research and practice is organized into theories for creative applications with people who need nursing care. Research and practice using self-transcendence theory can generate new discoveries about the many processes by which people attain well-being. Through inquiry and practice, then, theory becomes a structure and process for building nursing knowledge.

The idea for a theory of self-transcendence was influenced by three major events in the history of science, the history of nursing, and my own professional history. First, the life-span movement of the 1970s in developmental psychology provided philosophic perspective and empirical evidence that the potential for developmental change exists across the life span, beyond childhood and adolescence, into adulthood, and throughout processes of aging and dying (Reed, 1983). Research findings indicated that developmental change was influenced less by chronological age or passage of time and more by normative and non-normative life events and the accruement of life experiences. Second, postulations by the eminent scholar Martha Rogers (1970) about the nature of change in human beings provided further inspiration for development of the theory (Reed, 1997b). Rogerian and life-span principles of development external to the theory influenced the theory's development. Philosophic views include the pandimensionality of human beings and the human potential for healing and well-being. Several nursing theories were also foundational to the theory of self-transcendence.

Third, I was encouraged to formulate this theory by my practice experiences in applying developmental theories in child and adolescent psychiatric–mental health care. Successful approaches to fostering mental health and well-being required an understanding of patients' developmental processes.

Self-transcendence is proposed to facilitate integration of complex and conflicting elements of living, aging, and dying. Health events particularly confront people with increased complexity in terms of new people in their lives, new information, and new feelings and concerns. For example, a chronic or serious illness necessitates relationships with new people such as health care providers and community resources. It confronts the person and family with new information and the challenges of treatments and self-care activities. And illness initiates, if not intensifies patient and family concerns about the future and raises fears about pain, quality of life, economic issues, and about mortality. By expanding one's boundaries and gaining new perspectives, self-transcendence can help the person gain new perspectives and organize these challenges into some meaningful system to sustain well-being and a sense of wholeness.

CONCEPTS OF THE THEORY

The theory of self-transcendence rests on two major assumptions. First, it is assumed that human beings are integral with their environments, as postulated in Rogers's science of unitary human beings. Human beings are "pandimensional" (Rogers, 1980, 1994), coextensive with their environment, and capable of an awareness that extends beyond physical and temporal dimensions (Reed, 1997a). This awareness may be experienced through altered states of consciousness, but more often it is found in everyday practices in reaching deeper within the self and reaching out to others, to nature, to one's God, or other sources of transcendence. Self-transcendence embodies experiences that connect rather than separate a person from self, others, and the environment. It is a concept that enables description and study of the nature of human pandimensionality within everyday and personal contexts of living.

The second assumption is that self-transcendence is a developmental imperative, meaning that it is a human resource that demands expression, much like other developmental processes such as walking in toddlers, abstract reasoning in adolescents, and grieving in those who have suffered a loss. These resources are a part of being human and of realizing one's potential for well-being. As such, the person's participation in self-transcendence is integral to well-being, and nursing has a role in facilitating this process.

Self-Transcendence

Self-transcendence is the major concept of the theory. It refers to the capacity to expand self-boundaries in a variety of ways. Some of these are as follows: intrapersonally (toward greater awareness of one's philosophy, values, and dreams), interpersonally (to relate to others and one's environment), temporally (to integrate one's past and future in a way that has meaning for the present), and transpersonally (to connect with dimensions beyond the typically discernible world). Self-transcendence is a characteristic of developmental maturity in terms of an enhanced awareness of the environment and an orientation toward broadened perspectives about life. It is expressed and measured through life perspectives and behaviors that represent this pandimensional expansion of boundaries.

Neo-Piagetian theories about development in adulthood and later life were influential in formulating the concept of self-transcendence.

Beginning in the 1970s, life-span development researchers discovered postformal patterns of thinking in older adults that extended beyond Piaget's formal operations, once thought to be the final stage of cognitive development. Life-span developmental theories on social–cognitive development extended Piaget's original theory on reasoning, which had identified formal operations (abstract and symbolic reasoning) in youth and young adulthood as the apex of cognitive development. Researchers identified abilities in older adults that indicated that cognitive development continued well into later life beyond the phase of formal operations. Arlin's (1975) problem-finding stage, Riegel's (1976) and Basseches's (1984) dialectic operations, and Koplowitz's (1984) unitary stage are examples of these patterns.

It came to be recognized that this mature reasoning was more contextual, more pragmatic, more spiritual, and more tolerant of ambiguity and the paradoxes inherent in living and dying (e.g., Commons, Demick, & Goldberg, 1996; Sinnott, 1998, 2003). There is greater awareness of the larger social and temporal contexts that extend beyond the self and immediate situation. The person who uses mature forms of reasoning does not seek absolute answers to questions in life but rather seeks meaning of life events as integrated within a moral, social, and historical context. The person has an appreciation of the greater environment and things unseen, as well as an inner knowledge of self. A perspective of relativism from multiple, sometimes conflicting views is balanced by the ability to make a commitment to one's beliefs.

Self-transcendence was conceptualized in reference to these views. I theorized that people facing life-threatening experiences may acquire this expanded awareness of self and environment. With this mature approach to life and death, people reflect goals more in line with Erikson's generativity and ego integrity than with more self-absorbed strivings for identity and intimacy characteristic of earlier developmental phases (Sheldon & Kasser, 2001).

Self-transcendence is expressed through various behaviors and perspectives such as sharing wisdom with others, integrating the physical changes of aging, accepting death as a part of life, having an interest in helping others and learning about the world, letting go of losses, and finding spiritual meaning in life.

Well-Being

A second major concept of the theory is well-being. Well-being is a sense of feeling whole and healthy, in accord with one's own criteria for wholeness and health. It is theorized that self-transcendence, as a basic human pattern of development, is logically linked with positive, health-promoting experiences and is therefore a correlate if not a predictor and resource for well-being. Well-being may be defined in many ways, depending upon the individual or patient population. Indicators of well-being are as diverse as human perceptions of health and wellness. Examples of indicators of well-being include life satisfaction, positive self-concept, hopefulness, happiness, and sense of meaning in life. Well-being is a correlate and an outcome of self-transcendence. Theoretical analyses and empirical studies have consistently supported this foundational conceptualization of self-transcendence as a correlate of and contributor to well-being (Lundman et al., 2010; McCarthy, 2011; Reed, 2009; Teixeira, 2008).

Vulnerability

Another key concept of the theory is vulnerability. Vulnerability involves awareness of personal mortality or the experience of difficult life events. It is theorized that self-transcendence—as a developmental capacity (and perhaps as a survival mechanism)—emerges naturally in health experiences that confront a person with issues of mortality and immortality. Life events that heighten one's sense of mortality, inadequacy, or vulnerability can—if they do not crush the individual's inner self— initiate developmental progress toward a renewed sense of identity and expanded self-boundaries (Corless, Germino, & Pittman, 1994; Erikson, 1986; Frankl, 1963; Marshall, 1980). Examples of these life events include serious or chronic illness, disability, aging, parenting, child rearing, family caregiving, loss of a loved one, career difficulties, and other life crises. Self-transcendence is evoked through such events and may enhance well-being by transforming losses and difficulties into healing experiences (Reed, 1996).

RELATIONSHIPS AMONG THE CONCEPTS: THE MODEL

The model of the theory of self-transcendence is presented in Figure 6.1. Four basic sets of relationships exist among the concepts in the theory. First, there is a relationship between the experience of vulnerability and self-transcendence such that increased levels of vulnerability, as brought on by health events, for example, influence increased levels of self-transcendence. However, this may hold only within certain levels of experienced vulnerability. The relationship between vulnerability and self-transcendence may be nonlinear in that very low and very

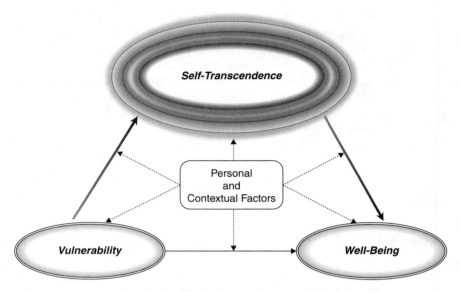

FIGURE 6.1   Self-Transcendence

high levels of vulnerability may not relate to increased levels of self-transcendence or at least not without the influence of other factors in that relationship.

A second relationship exists between self-transcendence and well-being. This relationship is direct and positive. For example, self-transcendence relates positively to sense of well-being and morale but relates negatively to the level of depression, as a "negative" indicator of well-being. This relationship represents more than a coping process; rather it is transcending a current situation to move forward toward a changed life rather than a return to previous perspectives and behaviors (Willis & Grace, 2011).

Third, self-transcendence functions as a mediator of well-being. Research findings indicate that self-transcendence mediates the relationship between vulnerability and well-being. Self-transcendence may mediate the effects of vulnerability (e.g., experienced as illness distress; lack of optimism, hope, or power; uncertainty; or death anxiety) on well-being. Several studies discussed later provide empirical support for the mediator hypothesis. Self-transcendence, then, may be an underlying process that explains how well-being is possible in difficult or life-threatening situations that people endure.

Fourth, personal and contextual factors may also have a role in this healing process. A wide variety of personal and contextual factors and their interactions may influence the process of self-transcendence as it relates to well-being. Examples of these factors are age, gender, cognitive ability, health status, past significant life events, personal beliefs, family support, and sociopolitical environment. These factors can enhance or diminish the strength of the three key variables and their relationships. For example, a recent and significant loss may diminish the potential for vulnerability to generate self-transcendence. Advanced age or education may potentiate the relationship between self-transcendence and well-being. Continued research in other personal and contextual factors is needed to better understand the potential role of these variables in the theory.

In the future, other concepts and relationships may be identified to extend the theory of self-transcendence. The theory was initially constructed to better understand the role of self-transcendence at the end of life. Since then, the findings of the researchers have extended the boundaries of theory beyond later life and end-of-life illness experiences to include other experiences of vulnerability among other age groups. For example, end-of-life health experiences were found to be significant correlates of self-transcendence among younger adults. In another study, middle-aged adults were studied using the variables of parenting and self-acceptance as indicators of self-transcendence. And in a third study, school-age boys were found to employ self-transcendence to overcome victimization by bullies.

Because of my nursing interest in understanding the inherent resources that foster human well-being, I have approached the study of self-transcendence as an independent variable or contributor to well-being and possible predictor of well-being outcomes, rather than as the dependent or outcome variable. Nursing interventions that support the person's inner resource for self-transcendence may focus directly on facilitating self-transcendence. Interventions may also focus on influencing some of the personal and contextual factors that mediate or moderate the relationships between vulnerability and self-transcendence and between self-transcendence and well-being (Figure 6.1).

Self-transcendence is a concept relevant to the discipline of nursing. Themes of self-transcendence are evident in other nursing theories (Reed, 1996). For example, in Watson's (1985/1999) theory of human caring, transcendence is integral to understand the essence of patients and nurses and their inner strivings toward greater self-awareness and inner healing. In Parse's (1992) theory of human becoming, cotranscending is a major theme underlying the philosophical assumptions of her theory and mobilizing transcendence is an exemplary nursing practice. Newman's (1994) theory of health as expanding consciousness postulates a transcendence of time and space as one reaches beyond illness to develop an awareness of one's patterns, self-identity, and higher level of consciousness. Although all of these theorists present unique views of transcendence, they generally share the idea of expanded awareness beyond the immediate or constricted views of oneself and the world to transform life experiences into healing (Reed, 1996).

Self-transcendence is also congruent with philosophic views of nursing. Newman's (1992) unitary–transformative paradigm presents human beings as embedded in an ongoing developmental process of changing complexity and organization, a process integrally related to well-being. Furthermore, self-transcendence is an example of Reed's (1997a) nursing process, which is a self-organizing process inherent among human systems that is related to well-being.

Other disciplines, particularly transpersonal psychology and psychiatry, have addressed the concept of self-transcendence. Cloninger, Svrakic, and Svrakic (1997) conceptualized self-transcendence as a factor in the organization of the personality and in development of psychopathology. Cloninger (1997) measured self-transcendence as one of three dimensions in his instrument, the temperament and character inventory (TCI). Psychologists Frankl (1963) and Maslow (1969) are frequently cited for their emphasis on the self-transcendent capacity of human beings. However, psychologists' conceptualizations of self-transcendence diverge from nursing in their emphasis on self-transcendence as involving an elevation or a separation of self from the environment, whereas nursing regards self-transcendence as awareness of one's wholeness in person–environment connections when fragmentation threatens one's well-being (Reed, 1997b).

USE OF THE THEORY IN NURSING RESEARCH

An increasing number of studies have provided empirical support for self-transcendence theory and in so doing, will lead to extensions, modifications, or refinements of the theory since all theories undergo change as they are used in research. In general, the results to date indicate that self-transcendence is a resource that accompanies serious life experiences that intensify one's sense of vulnerability or mortality. Specifically, self-transcendence functions as a mediator between experiences of vulnerability and well-being outcomes. Findings also support the theorized direct relationship between self-transcendence and many indicators of well-being across groups of study participants facing a wide variety of health experiences.

The Self-Transcendence Scale

Reed's (2009) *Self-Transcendence Scale* (STS) has been used in much of the research that most directly relates to the theory. The STS is a 15-item, one-dimensional scale. It is originated from a 36-item instrument, the Developmental Resources of Later Adulthood (DRLA) scale (Reed, 1986, 1989), which measured the level of developmentally based psychosocial resources in a person. The DRLA was constructed from an extensive review of theoretical and empirical literatures on adult development and aging, selected nursing conceptual models and life-span theories, and clinical encounters with older adults.

A self-transcendence factor, which explained nearly half of the variance in the instrument and had good internal consistency, was identified within the scale. The STS was developed around this empirically based factor. The STS was subsequently used in research to measure intrapersonal, interpersonal, temporal, and transpersonal experiences that reflect expanded boundaries of the self in developmentally mature adults. The STS has demonstrated reliability and construct validity and is brief and easy to administer as a questionnaire or in an interview format. Many researchers and graduate students have used the instrument in studying self-transcendence as it relates to various health experiences and outcomes. Most recently, a group of Norwegian researchers examined the factor structure of the STS in a sample of 202 older adults across 44 nursing homes (Haugan, Rannestad, Garåsen, Hammervold, & Espnes, 2011). They found that a two-factor solution that was both statistically and clinically meaningful in this sample. This solution involved an interpersonal dimension and an intrapersonal dimension that included transpersonal and temporal indicators of self-transcendence. Their findings supported the theory by providing empirical evidence of various dimensions by which individuals expand their boundaries to achieve a sense of sell-being.

Initial Research

The initial research used to build the theory of self-transcendence focused on well elders and elders hospitalized for psychiatric treatment of depression (Reed, 1986, 1989). Elders were selected as a group potentially facing end-of-life issues. Correlational and longitudinal studies were designed to examine the nature and significance of the relationship between self-transcendence and mental health outcomes. It was found consistently that self-transcendence was a correlate and predictor of mental health in these elders. Correlations were significant and of moderate magnitude. Reed's (1986) longitudinal study provided empirical evidence for a potential link between self-transcendence and subsequent occurrence of depression among mentally healthy adults; this link approached statistical significance and was in the expected direction among clinically depressed adults.

Self-transcendence was next examined for its relevance to mental health among the oldest-old, adults 80 to 100 years of age (Reed, 1991). Quantitative and qualitative data generated further support for the theory. Significant inverse correlations of moderate magnitude were found between self-transcendence and both depression and overall mental health symptomatology. In addition, four conceptual clusters representing different aspects of self-transcendence were generated from a content analysis: generativity, introjectivity, temporal integration, and body transcendence. Elders who scored high on depression reflected weak patterns in these four areas, particularly in body-transcendence, inner-directed activities, and positive integration of present and future. These qualitative findings provided further support for the theory, which posited the salience of self-transcendence as a correlate of well-being in later adulthood or other critical times of life.

Basic and Practice-Based Research by Coward

Coward, who as a doctoral student studied with Reed, continued research into self-transcendence with a focus on middle-aged adults confronting their mortality through serious illness, advanced cancer, and AIDS. Coward (1990, 1995) initially studied the lived experience of self-transcendence in women with advanced breast cancer. Results from her phenomenological study were consistent with findings from quantitative studies. Self-transcendent perspectives were salient in this group, which had a heightened awareness of personal mortality; self-transcendence was expressed in terms of reaching out beyond self to help others, to permit others to help them, and to accept the present, unchangeable events in time.

This research validated Reed's (1989) quantitative measure of self-transcendence. In subsequent phenomenological research, Coward and Lewis (1993) explored self-transcendence in women and men with

AIDS. Despite increased fear and sadness at the prospect of death, all participants indicated self-transcendent perspectives, which in turn helped them find meaning and achieve emotional well-being.

Findings from a study of 107 women with Stages III and IV breast cancer, in which structural equation modeling was used to analyze responses, indicated that self-transcendence had a significant and direct positive effect on emotional well-being by mediating the effect of illness distress on well-being (Coward, 1991).

Coward (1996) also studied healthy adults, who ranged in age from 19 to 85 years. She was interested in extending the theory of self-transcendence by examining its salience in a group of adults who were not as actively confronted with end-of-life issues as other seriously ill populations. Self-transcendence was again found to be a significant and strong correlate of well-being indicators, namely coherence, self-esteem, hope, and other variables assessing emotional well-being. Coward concluded that while her research supported the hypothesized relationship between self-transcendence and mental health variables, the findings, as generated from a sample of healthy adults, did not necessarily support the theoretical link between awareness of end-of-life issues and self-transcendence. Coward cited Frankl (1969) in proposing that self-transcendence is an essential human characteristic that may surface at any time in the life span.

Although Coward's interpretation of the results may expand the boundaries of the theory in terms of populations where self-transcendence may be salient, her results do not necessarily dispute the idea that some awareness of human mortality is integral to self-transcendence. Awareness of mortality is a basic characteristic of the human condition among both healthy and ill adults. This awareness may emerge slowly from the accumulation of life experiences as well as suddenly by a health crisis event.

Intervention research by Coward and Kahn (2004, 2005) focused on the experiences and functions of self-transcendence in women newly diagnosed with breast cancer. Self-transcendent practices and perspectives were particularly effective in helping women to resolve spiritual disequilibrium often experienced after diagnosis of breast cancer (Coward & Kahn, 2004). In their 2005 study, the investigators compared a traditional community cancer support group with a self-transcendence theory-based group on outcomes regarding the experiences of self-transcendence and physical and emotional well-being. Women in the treatment group were able to attain a better sense of community with their support group. However, the most striking finding was that women in both groups had self-transcendent experiences as described in Reed's theory, which sustained them through the diagnosis and treatment of their illness. They expressed themes of outward, inward, and temporal expansion of self-boundaries such as reaching out for support and information, finding inner strength to endure, and constructing meaning out of past experiences and future hopes. The authors interpreted this finding as support for the idea that the capacity for transcending an adverse event is a universal trait that motivates expansion of one's conceptual boundaries in multiple and beneficial ways.

In summary, Coward's program of research has provided empirical evidence to support and possibly extend the theory of self-transcendence. Her findings from various studies have consistently indicated that self-transcendence is a resource that accompanies serious illness and is significantly related to indicators of well-being. This was found with women facing the end of life through advanced breast cancer and AIDS and through men's experience with AIDS. Her research with a healthy population provided further support for the theory of self-transcendence while raising new questions about the significance of awareness of personal mortality in the emergence of self-transcendence.

Research by Colleagues and Reed

In an attempt to examine the theory in a group of adults that was healthy and younger than the elders typically studied, Ellermann and Reed (2001) reported on their study of self-transcendence in middle-aged adults. Theorizing as Coward did several years earlier that self-transcendence was a life-span phenomenon and not confined to later life, they sought evidence that extended applications of the theory of self-transcendence. They identified parenting, self-acceptance, and spirituality as expressions of self-transcendence in middle-aged adults in particular and related these experiences to mental health. The results indicated a strong inverse relationship between self-transcendence and level of depression in this group, particularly among women.

In comparing their findings to those from other studies, Ellermann and Reed (2001) found that self-transcendence was higher among groups of older participants although still salient among the middle-aged participants. Gender differences were identified, including the finding that self-transcendence was more predominant among women than men. Their research not only supported the theory of self-transcendence but also introduced questions about the role of human experiences such as parenting and spirituality in the theory; that is, do they function as indicators, correlates, or antecedents of self-transcendence?

Decker and Reed (2005) studied self-transcendence and moral reasoning within the context of several contextual and developmental factors to better understand end-of-life treatment preferences among older adults. Self-transcendence was found to be significantly and positively related to level of integrated moral reasoning, which is reasoning that includes both the autonomous and social domains of moral decision making. This was expected based on life-span developmental theory on adult thinking processes. Self-transcendence did not relate significantly to desired level of aggressiveness of end-of-life treatment, although investigators argued that more research is needed into the role of self-transcendence and end-of-life decisions. The results help explain why reasoning about end-of-life treatment options reflects a complex and integrated approach among some elders.

Runquist and Reed (2007) reported on findings from Runquist's master's thesis research in which self-transcendence along with the variables of spiritual perspective, fatigue, and health status were measured to identify significant correlates of well-being in 61 homeless men and women. Self-transcendence coupled with physical health factors was theorized to be statistically independent correlates (resources) for well-being in this sample. A strong positive relationship between self-transcendence and well-being was found, as theorized. In addition, two variables, self-transcendence and health status, together explained a significant 60% of the variance in well-being, with self-transcendence having the greater correlation with well-being. These findings suggest that an effective clinical approach with homeless persons does not necessarily require extensive clinical applications to enhance well-being. The investigators concluded that attention to the spiritual side of living, in addition to physical health, may be equally important in fostering well-being among homeless persons.

Research by Other Investigators

Other research conducted over the past 15 years has provided support for the theory of self-transcendence. In most of the quantitative studies reported here, researchers measured self-transcendence with Reed's (2009) STC. In the case of qualitative studies, researchers worked from a conceptualization of self-transcendence congruent with Reed's definition unless or until the findings indicated something different. Research has focused on various populations including older adults with chronic illness and adults with life-threatening illness.

Chronic Illness and Aging

Several researchers in addition to Reed have studied self-transcendence in older adults. These studies include older adults who have chronic, serious, or mental illness, and older adults who are relatively healthy.

Walton and colleagues (1991) reported one of the earliest studies. They explored self-transcendence as measured by a 58-item scale based on Peck's (1968) developmental stages of old age. They identified a significant inverse relationship between self-transcendence and loneliness among 107 healthy older adults.

Billard (2001) examined the role of self-transcendence in the well-being of aging Catholic sisters for her doctoral research. Specifically, she combined Reed's (1987) *Spiritual Perspective Scale* with Reed's (1991) STC to measure the concept of spiritual transcendence and its relationship to the variable of emotional intelligence in a sample of 377 elder Catholic sisters. She found that spiritual transcendence, along with selected personality and demographic factors, contributed significantly to explaining emotional intelligence. Fostering spiritual transcendence was recommended as a resource for helping aging sisters who transform their own lives and the lives of others in positive ways.

In suicide research by Buchanan, Farran, and Clark (1995), the findings supported the hypothesis that self-transcendence was integral to older adults coping with the changes in later life. Other important factors in coping were loss of spouse and friends, loss of work, and state of finances. In studying 35 elders hospitalized for depression, the researchers found that desire for death and self-transcendence (as measured by the STS) were significantly and inversely related. All other relationships between self-transcendence and suicide ideation were in the expected direction but were not significant, likely due to the small sample size.

Klaas (1998) studied self-transcendence and depression in 77 depressed and nondepressed elders. Her results in both groups supported the theory of self-transcendence. Significant negative correlations were found between depression and self-transcendence. In addition, self-transcendence was significantly and positively correlated with meaning in life in this group. Last, the depressed group of elders scored significantly lower on the STS as well as on meaning in life. Scores on the STS and purpose in life test were significantly and positively related, supporting the construct validity of the STS.

In research by Upchurch (1999), a significant positive relationship was found between self-transcendence and activities of daily living among 88 chronically ill elders. She proposed a theoretical model in which self-transcendence, as a developmental strength and part of human essence, may partly explain why some elders continued to remain independent while others did not, regardless of health status.

Walker (2002) measured self-transcendence and mastery of stress in testing his theory of transformative aging. His study was based upon the idea that stressful events can bring about transformative change that enables the person to deal with the losses and challenges that accompany aging. Self-transcendence was conceptualized as a process of transforming among middle-aged adults and older adults. Results of the study lent support to the hypothesized relationships derived from his theory; self-transcendence was significantly and positively related to mastery of stress and significantly inversely related to stress of aging. His findings have implications for engaging the resource of self-transcendence to assist middle-aged and older adults in mastering stress and existential anxiety over the aging process. Similarly, in a study of older women living with rheumatoid arthritis, Neill (2002) found that transcendence of self-boundaries and personal transformation represented a process of living successfully with a chronic illness.

In a correlational study of oldest-old adults, a group of Swedish researchers studied self-transcendence and similar variables as related to mental and physical health outcomes in later life (Nygren et al., 2005). They found significant, positive relationships of moderate magnitude between self-transcendence and several variables in both the men's and women's groups including resilience, sense of coherence, and purpose in life. Self-transcendence was also positively related to indicators of mental health but significantly so only in the women's group. The results overall indicated that oldest-old adults were capable of experiencing levels of self-transcendence and other positive factors comparable to those in younger adults. The investigators concluded that the impact of aging on inner strength and other spiritually related and psychological variables may differ between men and women and suggested further research. More knowledge about gender differences would help refine the theory of self-transcendence.

Elderly nursing home residents were studied for their perceptions on what personal qualities allowed them to rise above the difficulties faced in their advanced age (Bickerstaff, Grasser, & McCabe, 2003). Results from this qualitative study were consistent with patterns of self-transcendence identified earlier by Reed (1991) in her study of community-dwelling oldest-old adults: generativity, introjectivity, temporal integration, body-transcendence, and one not previously identified, "relationship with self/others/higher being." Many participants exhibited more than one pattern of self-transcendence. The researchers concluded that caregivers of older adults in long-term care facilities and at home should look beyond custodial care to incorporate activities that build upon the residents' capacity for self-transcendence that can help them cope with the losses of later life.

In a study of factors related to self-care in older African Americans, Upchurch and Mueller (2005) found that self-transcendence was significantly and positively related to the ability to carry out instrumental activities of daily living (IADLs). They also found a significant interaction effect between self-transcendence and education, which related positively to IADLs among the least-educated elders. The investigators recommended that caregivers consider interventions designed to enhance self-transcendence to help caregivers support self-care abilities of older adults.

Serious and Life-Threatening Illness in Adults

Several researchers in addition to Coward have studied self-transcendence in people who have life-threatening illnesses. Stevens (1999) examined the relationships between self-transcendence and depression in young adults with AIDS and found the two variables to be significantly and inversely related, consistent with the theory of self-transcendence.

Wright (2003) studied the relationship between quality of life and self-transcendence in liver transplant recipients. She found a significant positive relationship between self-transcendence and quality of life. Self-transcendence was also significantly and inversely related to fatigue in this sample. Women scored significantly higher on self-transcendence than men. They concluded that self-transcendence along with illness distress, fatigue, and age is an important factor related to quality of life. Bean and Wagner (2006) also studied persons ($n = 471$) who were liver transplant recipients. The researchers proposed and found that self-transcendence becomes salient following the experience of liver transplant and was related significantly to higher quality of life and potentially functioned as a mediator to decrease the effects of illness distress on quality of life.

In a phenomenological study of eight women who had completed breast cancer therapy, Pelusi (1997) found that surviving breast cancer very much involved self-transcendence. In this population, self-transcendence was expressed as setting life priorities, finding meaning in life, and looking within self. Similar findings occurred in a study by Kinney (1996), who reported on her own journey through breast cancer. A process of listening to and trusting one's inner voice facilitated transcendence. Self-transcendence in turn was central to reconstruction of self.

Self-transcendence and quality of life were studied in 46 HIV-positive adults by Mellors, Riley, and Erlen (1997). Data analysis revealed a significant moderate positive relationship between self-transcendence and quality of life for the group, particularly for those who were the most seriously ill. The dimensions of quality of life that related most significantly to self-transcendence were health and functioning and psychological/spiritual dimensions.

Chin-A-Loy and Fernsler (1998) examined self-transcendence among 24 men, aged 61 to 84, attending a prostate cancer support group. The participants scored fairly high on the STS, averaging 50 of a possible 15 to 60. The high level of self-transcendence in this group indicated that group members had developed ways to expand beyond the limitations posed by their cancer, despite or perhaps because of aging and living with prostate cancer. Results from other research also attest to the capacity for seriously ill individuals to transcend their illness. In a study of persons with AIDS, researchers found evidence that they were able to transcend the suffering associated with their illness (Mellors, Erlen, Coontz, & Lucke, 2001). The participants demonstrated three dominant patterns indicative of self-transcendence: creating a meaningful life pattern, achieving a sense of connectedness, and engaging in self-care.

A group of investigators (Ramer, Johnson, Chan, & Barrett, 2006) interested in quality of life among persons with HIV/AIDS studied 420 mostly Hispanic, male patients to determine the relationships of self-transcendence and spirituality to demographic, cultural, and clinical factors. Among the findings was a significant positive relationship between self-transcendence and level of energy in the patients. In addition, researchers found that levels of acculturation and self-transcendence were significantly related, suggesting that the meaning of self-transcendence may be influenced by cultural factors. Their study not only provided support for the relevance of self-transcendence among these patients but also suggested that acculturation may moderate the relationship between self-transcendence and health outcome variables in people with HIV/AIDS.

In a group of 93 women receiving radiation treatment for breast cancer, Matthews and Cook (2009) found that self-transcendence alone partially mediated the relationship between optimism and emotional well-being and was an important factor in emotional health among people facing life-threatening illness. Sarenmalm, Thorén-Jönsson, Gaston-Hohansson, and Öhlén (2009) found that women use self-transcendence to adjust to the recurrence of breast cancer. Several authors emphasize the need for more research into factors that foster or increase self-transcendence in women with breast cancer.

Farren's (2010) study of 104 breast cancer survivors produced findings that self-transcendence was a significant mediator in two relationships—between power (knowing participation) and quality of life and between uncertainty and quality of life. Uncertainty reduces quality of life by reducing self-transcendence. Farren used Reed's theory to describe self-transcendence as a profound awareness of one's wholeness while having awareness of fluctuations in one's human–environmental field patterns.

Williams (2012) conducted a phenomenological study of eight men and women who had received a stem cell translation the previous year. Analyses showed that self-transcendence is brought about by the intense suffering, as lived through the physical effects of the treatment, facing death, and eventually drawing strength from within themselves and from spiritual support. The findings suggested that effects of vulnerability on well-being were mediated by self-transcendence.

Research on Nurses and Other Caregivers

Self-transcendence has also been studied as it occurs in family caregivers, nurses, and others providing care to patients. This area of research has been increasing in recent years.

Enyert and Burman (1999) conducted a qualitative study of self-transcendence in caregivers of terminally ill persons. They found that caregivers' self-transcendent behaviors, such as being with and doing for their loved one as death approached, provided personal growth and other positive consequences for them. They found new meaning, a new view of life and were able to reach out to help others besides their family member.

Poole (1999) found that self-transcendence was an important phase in being a caregiver. Using the grounded theory method, Poole studied 19 family caregivers in the process of being a caregiver for frail older adults at home. Three phases of caregiving were identified by which the caregiver became able to work with health care personnel as a partner instead of perpetuating conflict in the relationship. The three phases were connecting, discovering self, and transcending self.

Acton and Wright (2000) and Acton (2002) addressed self-transcendence in family caregivers of adults with dementia. Based on the literature they found it to be a relevant and potentially therapeutic experience for family caregivers and identified strategies to facilitate self-transcendence in family caregivers. However, when Acton (2002) conducted a naturalistic field study of family caregivers, she found that caregivers of adults with dementia had little opportunity to nurture self-transcendence; instead they experienced social isolation, ambivalence, emotional fragility, and burden of caring for their family member. She concluded that some of these negative experiences associated with caregiving may inhibit development of self-transcendence in caregivers and interfere with their continued growth and well-being.

Reese and Murray (1996) examined the role of self-transcendence in great-grandmothering in a qualitative study of African American and White groups of great-grandmothers. From interviews of 16 great-grandmothers, they identified five domains of self-transcendence: connectedness, religion, being wise, values, and stories. These domains reflect dimensions in the definition of self-transcendence in Reed's theory. The authors considered great-grandparents vital in facilitating self-transcendence and good relationships among family members.

As part of her study of spiritual growth in nurses, Kilpatrick (2002) studied the relationships among self-transcendence, spiritual perspective, and spiritual well-being in female nursing students and faculty. She found positive correlations among those variables in students and faculty. Nursing students and faculty differed significantly on level of self-transcendence and spiritual well-being, suggesting that self-transcendence may increase with development.

McGee (2004) reported on her research into self-transcendence in nursing. She employed the method of interpretive phenomenology to examine self-transcendence and its impact on nurses' practice. Among the results from the moving stories of nurses, McGee found self-transcendence to be an important mechanism of healing for nurses who have experienced difficult and traumatic personal life experiences. Her work expands the theory of self-transcendence by revealing the role of self-transcendence in healing the *nurse* and in enriching the practice of nurses for the mutual benefit of both patient and nurse.

Along a similar line of thinking, Hunnibell, Reed, Quinn-Griffin, & Fitzpatrick (2008) conducted dissertation research based on self-transcendence theory. She studied self-transcendence as related to burnout syndrome in hospice and oncology nurses. Both groups of nurses face death and life-threatening illness through their work with patients. However, she hypothesized that because of the philosophy of their health care setting and opportunities to process loss, hospice nurses would demonstrate higher levels of self-transcendence and lower levels of burnout than oncology nurses. Her findings also provided empirical support for the hypothesis and for an inverse relationship between self-transcendence and three types of burnout. Hunnibell concluded that self-transcendence is a resource for nurses and may protect them against burnout.

Palmer and her colleagues (2010) found significantly positive relationships between work engagement (measured as vigor, dedication, and absorption) and self-transcendence among 84 acute care staff registered nurses. Through self-transcendence, the nurses had increased self-awareness and inner strength and made sense of challenging work situations.

This review of research on self-transcendence provides consistent evidence of the significance of this variable on the well-being of nurses and other caregivers. Nurses and caregivers experience vulnerability and related health experiences through the challenges of their work as well as in their personal lives. It is important not to overlook the importance of research to gain a better understanding of self-transcendence as a resource for well-being in caregivers.

USE OF THE THEORY IN NURSING PRACTICE

Research findings have shown that self-transcendence is integral to well-being across a diversity of health experiences that confront a person with end-of-life issues. Nursing practices that facilitate self-transcendence result in healing outcomes during these health events, as in, for example, diminished depression over time among clinically depressed elders, increased hopefulness and self-care among chronically ill elders, sense of well-being among persons with advanced breast cancer or with HIV/AIDS, and decreased suicidal ideation among hospitalized depressed elders. Although these particular health events have been the focus of self-transcendence research, many if not most health events confront a person with vulnerability and mortality and, therefore, are potential contexts for promoting healing and well-being through self-transcendence.

Encouraged by these results, nurses continue to identify other health experiences in which they can promote well-being by facilitating self-transcendence, for example, in bereavement (Joffrion & Douglas, 1994), family caregiving (Acton & Wright, 2000), and in maintenance of sobriety and well-being (McGee, 2000).

Advanced practice nurses increasingly provide spiritual care to specialty populations; this care extends beyond that typically provided by primary care practitioners (McCormick, Holder, Wetsel, & Cawthon, 2001). This care includes an integrative approach to spiritual care that includes facilitating self-transcendence. Wasner, Longaker, Fegg, and Borasio (2005) studied the effects of spiritual care intervention training on 48 palliative care professionals' self-transcendence, spiritual well-being, and attitude toward work with dying patients. Spiritual well-being but not religion was related to self-transcendence. So, the phrase self-transcendence brings in ideas of the spiritual, and the two concepts are often found to be related. However, self-transcendence is typically measured as a human experience that encompasses the psychosocial, physical, and emotional as well as spiritual.

Theory-Informed Strategies for Practice

Research findings indicate that a variety of strategies derived from self-transcendence theory have been successful in promoting well-being or in diminishing negative outcomes in practice settings. These strategies expand boundaries intrapersonally, interpersonally, and transpersonally.

Intrapersonal Strategies

Intrapersonal strategies help the person expand inward and make room to integrate loss in all its diverse experiences. Meditation, prayer, visualization, life review, structured reminiscence, self-reflection, and journaling are the techniques of self-transcendence that nurses can guide and facilitate (Acton & Wright, 2000; McGee, 2000; Stinson & Kirk, 2006). These approaches help a person look inward to clarify and expand knowledge about self and find or create meaning and purpose in the experience. Encouraging patients to keep a journal, for example, helps them become more aware of their process of transformation and transcendence. Recognition of the process and the pattern of their own healing is empowering for patients.

Diener (2003) conducted a randomized, clinical trial to examine the effectiveness of personal narrative as an intervention for enhancing self-transcendence in women with HIV, multiple sclerosis, and systemic lupus erythematosus. The STS scores increased significantly in the intervention groups, suggesting that the intervention was successful in helping the women address issues related to having a life-threatening or life-altering illness.

The nurse may also encourage cognitive strategies that help patients integrate a health event into their lives. Acquiring information about the illness, using positive self-talk, and engaging in meaningful and challenging activities are all techniques that can help a person integrate and grow from the illness experience (Coward & Reed, 1996).

Interpersonal Strategies

Interpersonal strategies for facilitating self-transcendence focus on connecting the person to others through formal or informal means, including face-to-face, telephone, or through the Internet. Maintaining meaningful relationships and strengthening affiliations with civic groups and with a supporting faith community are also strategies that the nurse can facilitate (McCormick et al., 2001). Nurse visits, peer counseling, informal networks, and formal support groups are examples of interpersonal strategies that the nurse may arrange for the person (Acton & Wright, 2000).

Support groups are often cited as an effective way to connect people facing a difficult life situation. Groups that bring together people of similar health experiences can facilitate self-transcendence by connecting the person to others who can share the loss and exchange information and wisdom about coping with the experience and by providing an opportunity to reach beyond the self to help another. Joffrion and Douglas (1994) reported that nurses can facilitate self-transcendence during bereavement by helping the person participate in church or civic groups, develop or resume a hobby, share personal experiences of grief with others, and support others who have experienced loss.

In pre-experimental and quasiexperimental studies, Coward (1998, 2003) developed and refined a series of support group sessions to facilitate self-transcendence. These sessions provided a variety of activities designed to support self-transcendence in women facing breast cancer: orientation and information sessions, sharing cancer stories, problem solving, assertive communication training, relaxation training, values clarification, ongoing educational components, constructive thinking and self-instructional training, feelings management, and pleasant activity planning. The self-transcendence–based sessions resulted in expanded perspectives and views—and in an improved sense of well-being at the end of treatment—although this did not hold 1 year later. Ongoing group support based on self-transcendence theory may be helpful to women, depending on their available resources.

Group psychotherapy is another intervention strategy for enhancing self-transcendence. Young and Reed (1995) found that this intervention approach was effective in generating a variety of outcomes for a group of elders, for example, intrapersonally in terms of achieving self-enrichment, self-esteem, and self-affirmation; interpersonally in terms of bonding with and helping others, enabling self-disclosure, and overcoming self-absorption; and temporally in terms of gaining acceptance of one's past and feeling empowered about the future.

Similarly, Stinson and Kirk (2006) reported research in which they tested the effect of group reminiscing on depression (measured by the Geriatric Depression Scale) and self-transcendence (measured by the STS) in a group of older women living in an assisted living facility. Given previous findings that consistently supported the relationship between self-transcendence and depression, it was logical to examine interventions that may increase self-transcendence as well as decrease depression. Results indicated a nonsignificant decrease in depression and an increase in self-transcendence after 6 weeks of reminiscence group sessions. Findings also indicated a significant inverse relationship between depression and self-transcendence as theorized.

Altruistic activities facilitate self-transcendence. They provide a context for learning new things and expanding awareness about oneself and one's world (Coward & Reed, 1996). Altruism also enhances a person's inner sense of worth and purpose. McGee (2000) explained that practicing humility and providing service to others are tools of self-transcendence that can empower individuals to maintain a healthy lifestyle. Connections between people, whether to receive or provide support, are key strategies for enhancing self-transcendence. Chan and Chan (2011) tested interventions designed to expand boundaries toward others through participation in volunteer work and social activities. These activities promoted acceptance and finding meaning in spousal death by facilitating the passing of time among bereaved Hong Kong Chinese older adults.

In a study by Willis and Griffith (2010) of school-age boys victimized by bullying, altruistic views and practices were found to facilitate healing. The boys reached out to others in helping and seeking help, having an interest in learning and engaging in fun hobbies, and feeling empathy toward others. The authors suggested that it is very important for practitioners to plan activities and interactions that can foster self-transcendence.

Transpersonal Strategies

Transpersonal strategies of self-transcendence are designed to help the person connect with a power or purpose greater than self. The nurse's role in this process is often one of creating an environment in which transpersonal exploration can occur. For example, to foster self-transcendence in family caregivers of adults with dementia, Acton and Wright (2000) identify the importance of helping arrange for in-home assistance or day care so the family members have the time and energy to engage in activities that promote transpersonal awareness. Religious activities and prayer in particular are frequently identified as significant to the well-being of persons facing life crises. McGee (2000) explained the need for the nurse to provide an environment in which patients can look beyond themselves toward a higher power for help and be inspired to help others. In addition, several of the strategies that foster intrapersonal growth also can foster a sense of transpersonal connection, such as meditation, visualization, and journaling.

Spiritual perspective or spiritual well-being in particular—rather than religion per se—has been found to relate to self-transcendence by several researchers over the years, including Haase and colleagues (1992), Thomas, Burton, Quinn Griffin, and Fitzpatrick (2010), and Sharpnack and colleagues (2010, 2011) in their two studies on the Amish community's use of spiritual and alternative health care practices to foster well-being.

Schumann (1999) found that self-transcendence enhanced well-being in ventilated patients. Spiritual connections enabled patients to use temporal perspectives of past and future to empower themselves; they synchronized their lives with the realities of being on a ventilator and anticipating extubation and were then better able to manage this life-threatening health experience.

Artistic modalities such as art-making activities, creative bonding practice, memorial quilt making, and watching a therapeutic music video were based on self-transcendence theory. These artistic modalities expand personal boundaries and facilitate transcendence, which in turn increase well-being (Burns, Robb, & Haase, 2009; Chen & Walsh, 2009; Kausch & Amer, 2007; Walsh, Radcliffe, Castillo, Kumar, & Broschard, 2007). Other researchers found that poetry writing was an expressive therapy for facilitating self-transcendence in caregivers facing difficult life situation, and subsequently leading to positive outcomes of self-affirmation, sense of achievement, catharsis, and acceptance among dementia caregivers (Kidd, Zauszniewski, & Morris, 2011).

CONCLUSION

Professional nurses are defined in large part by their ability to engage human capacities for healing and well-being. Self-transcendence was presented as a resource for well-being. It represents "both a human capacity and a human struggle that can be facilitated by nursing" (Reed, 1996, p. 3). A goal in developing the theory was to gain better understanding of the dynamics of self-transcendence as it relates to health and well-being. This knowledge, in addition to that acquired through personal and ethical knowing and practice experience, can be used by nurses to foster well-being through strategies of self-transcendence.

There is consistency among the elements internal to the theory—the concepts, their definitions, and proposed relationships. Positive relationships were identified between vulnerability and self-transcendence and between self-transcendence and well-being. However, new twists in the stated relationships may yet be discovered. A number of researchers have studied self-transcendence as an outcome or a process of well-being in its own right, disregarding the third key relationship identified in the theory between self-transcendence and well-being. In other research, self-transcendence functions as a resource, correlate, or facilitator of specific indicators of well-being. In addition, research findings provide evidence to support the role of mediators and moderators in the process of self-transcendence as proposed in the theory.

The theory now reaches beyond the initial focus on elders to include children, adolescents, and adults of all ages who experience vulnerability. The theory is being studied across cultures around the world. Research findings are broadening the scope of the theory to include other normative life transitions and developmental events among youth and children, whose processes of self-transcendence have yet to be explored indepth. The scholarship of advanced practice nurses, graduate students, and researchers can continue to offer new insights into personal, contextual, and cultural factors that influence the process of self-transcendence.

The theory is significant in that it is a theory for the present. Self-transcendence reflects a nursing perspective of human beings and proposes a mechanism by which human beings generate well-being in times of vulnerability. This process has been supported by research. Findings consistently indicate that self-transcendence is associated with a wide variety of well-being indicators, from successful aging and inner strength to specific human experiences such as decreased fatigue or increased self-care activities of daily living. Nursing, through its theories and practices that inspire human transcendence, can make a significant contribution to sustaining human beings within the context of their everyday experiences. Authors emphasize application of self-transcendent theory in developing therapeutic modalities for practice.

Self-transcendence is emerging as a foundational process in promoting well-being. Self-transcendence may very well be a developmental imperative for all ages of individuals, and for those who are well or ill. As such, nursing must be there to generate the knowledge and provide the expert support that facilitates this cost-effective and holistic process of well-being.

REFERENCES

Acton, G. J. (2002). Self-transcendent views and behaviors: Exploring growth in caregivers of adults with dementia. *Journal of Gerontological Nursing, 28*(12), 22–30.

Acton, G. J., & Wright, K. B. (2000). Self-transcendence and family caregivers of adults with dementia. *Journal of Holistic Nursing, 18*, 143–158.

Arlin, P. K. (1975). Cognitive development in adulthood: A fifth stage? *Developmental Psychology, 11*, 602–606.

Basseches, M. (1984). *Dialectical thinking and adult development*. Norwood, NJ: Ablex.

Bean, K. B., & Wagner, K. (2006). Self-transcendence, illness distress, and quality of life among liver transplant recipients. *The Journal of Theory Construction & Testing, 10*(2), 47–53.

Bickerstaff, K. A., Grasser, C. M., & McCabe, B. (2003). How elderly nursing home residents transcend losses of later life. *Holistic Nursing Practice, 17*(3), 159–165.

Billard, A. (2001). *The impact of spiritual transcendence on the well-being of aging Catholic sisters*. Unpublished doctoral dissertation, Loyola College, Baltimore, MD.

Buchanan, D., Farran, C., & Clark, D. (1995). Suicidal thought and self-transcendence in older adults. *Journal of Psychosocial Nursing, 33*(10), 31–34.

Burns, D. S., Robb, S. L., & Haase, J. E. (2009). Exploring the feasibility of a therapeutic music video intervention in adolescents and young adults during stem cell transplantation. *Cancer Nursing, 32*(5), 8–16.

Chan, W. C., & Chan, C. L. W. (2011). Acceptance of spousal death: The factor of time in bereaved older adults' search for meaning. *Death Studies, 35*, 147–162.

Chen, S., & Walsh, S. M. (2009). Effect of a creative-bonding intervention on Taiwanese nursing students' self-transcendence and attitudes toward elders. *Research in Nursing & Health, 32*, 204–216.

Chin-A-Loy, S. S., & Fernsler, J. I. (1998). Self-transcendence in older men attending a prostate cancer support group. *Cancer Nursing, 21*, 358–363.

Cloninger, C. R., Svrakic, N. M., & Svrakic, D. M. (1997). Role of personality self-organization in development of mental order and disorder. *Development and Psychopathology, 9,* 881–906.

Commons, M., Demick, J., & Goldberg, C. (1996). *Clinical approaches to adult development.* Norwood, NJ: Ablex.

Corless, I. B., Germino, B. B., & Pittman, M. (1994). *Dying, death, and bereavement: Theoretical perspectives and other ways of knowing.* Boston, MA: Jones and Bartlett.

Coward, D. (1990). The lived experience of self-transcendence in women with advanced breast cancer. *Nursing Science Quarterly, 3,* 162–169.

Coward, D. (1991). Self-transcendence and emotional well-being in women with advanced breast cancer. *Oncology Nursing Forum, 18,* 857–863.

Coward, D. (1995). Lived experience of self-transcendence in women with AIDS. *Journal of Obstetric, Gynecologic, and Neonatal Nursing, 24,* 314–318.

Coward, D. (1996). Self-transcendence and correlates in a healthy population. *Nursing Research, 45,* 116–122.

Coward, D. (1998). Facilitation of self-transcendence in a breast cancer support group. *Oncology Nursing Forum, 25,* 75–84.

Coward, D. D. (2003). Facilitation of self-transcendence in a breast cancer support group: Part II. *Oncology Nursing Forum, 30*(2), 291–300.

Coward, D. D., & Kahn, D. L. (2004). Resolution of spiritual disequilibrium by women newly diagnosed with breast cancer. *Oncology Nursing Forum, 31*(2), E1–E8.

Coward, D. D., & Kahn, D. L. (2005). Transcending breast cancer: Making meaning from diagnosis and treatment. *Journal of Holistic Nursing, 23*(3), 264–283.

Coward, D. D., & Lewis, F. M. (1993). The lived experience of self-transcendence in gay men with AIDS. *Oncology Nursing Forum, 20,* 1363–1369.

Coward, D. D., & Reed, P. G. (1996). Self-transcendence: A resource for healing at the end of life. *Issues in Mental Health Nursing, 17,* 275–288.

Decker, I. M., & Reed, P. G. (2005). Developmental and contextual correlates of elders' anticipated end-of-life treatment decisions. *Death Studies, 29,* 827–846.

Diener, J. E. S. (2003). *Personal narrative as an intervention to enhance self-transcendence in women with chronic illness.* Unpublished doctoral dissertation. University of Missouri, St. Louis.

Ellermann, C. R., & Reed, P. G. (2001). Self-transcendence and depression in middle-aged adults. *Western Journal of Nursing Research, 23,* 698–713.

Enyert, G., & Burman, M. E. (1999). A qualitative study of self-transcendence in caregivers of terminally ill patients. *American Journal of Hospice and Palliative Care, 16*(2), 455–462.

Erikson, E. H. (1986). *Vital involvement in old age.* New York, NY: Norton.

Farren, A. T. (2010). Power, uncertainty, self-transcendence, and quality of life in breast cancer survivors. *Nursing Science Quarterly, 23*(1), 63–71.

Frankl, V. E. (1963). *Man's search for meaning.* New York, NY: Pocket Books.

Frankl, V. E. (1969). *The will to meaning.* New York, NY: New American Library.

Haase, J. E., Britt, T., Coward, D. D., Leidy, N. K., & Penn, P. E. (1992). Simultaneous concept analysis of spiritual perspective, hope, acceptance and self-transcendence. *Image: Journal of Nursing Scholarship, 24,* 141–147.

Haugan, G., Rannestad, R., Garåsen, H., Hammervold, R., & Espnes, G. A. (2011). The self-transcendence scale: An investigation of the factor structure among nursing home patients. *Journal of Holistic Nursing,* Advance online publication, 1–6.

Hunnibell, L. S., Reed, P. G., Quinn-Griffin, M. Q., & Fitzpatrick, J. J. (2008). Self-transcendence and burnout in hospice and oncology nurses. *Journal of Hospice and Palliative Nursing, 10*(3), 172–179.

Joffrion, L. P., & Douglas, D. (1994). Grief resolution: Facilitating self-transcendence in the bereaved. *Journal of Psychosocial Nursing, 32*(3), 13–19.

Kausch, K. D., & Amer, K. (2007). Self-transcendence and depression among AIDS memorial quilt panel makers. *Journal of Psychosocial Nursing, 45*(6), 45–53.

Kidd, L. I., Zauszniewski, J. A., & Morris, D. L. (2011). Benefits of a poetry writing intervention for family caregivers of elders with dementia. *Issues in Mental Health Nursing, 32,* 598–604.

Kilpatrick, J. A. W. (2002). *Spiritual perspective, self-transcendence, and spiritual wellbeing in female nursing students and female nursing faculty.* Unpublished doctoral dissertation, Widener University, Wilmington, DE.

Kinney, C. K. (1996). Transcending breast cancer: Reconstructing one's self. *Issues in Mental Health Nursing, 17*(3), 201–216.

Klaas, D. (1998). Testing two elements of spirituality in depressed and non-depressed elders. *The International Journal of Psychiatric Nursing Research, 4,* 452–462.

Koplowitz, H. (1984). A projection beyond Piaget's formal operational stage: A general systems stage and a unitary stage. In M. L. Commons, F. A. Richards, & C. Armon (Eds.), *Beyond formal operations: Late adolescence and adult cognitive development* (pp. 272–296). New York, NY: Praeger.

Lundman, B., Aléx, L., Jonsén, E., Norberg, A., Nygren, B., Santamäki, R., & Strandberg, G. (2010). Inner strength—A theoretical analysis of salutogenic concepts. *International Journal of Nursing Studies, 47*(2), 251–260.

Marshall, V. M. (1980). *Last chapter: A sociology of aging and dying.* Monterey, CA: Brooks-Cole.

Maslow, A. H. (1969). Various meanings of transcendence. *Journal of Transpersonal Psychology, 1,* 56–66.

Matthews, E. E., & Cook, P. F. (2009). Relationships among optimism, well-being, self-transcendence, coping, and social support in women during treatment for breast cancer. *Psycho-Oncology, 18,* 716–726.

McCarthy, V. L. (2011). A new look at successful aging: Exploring a mid-range nursing theory among older adults in a low-income retirement community. *The Journal of Theory Construction & Testing, 15*(1), 17–23.

McCormick, D. P., Holder, B., Wetsel, M. A., & Cawthon, T. W. (2001). Spirituality and HIV disease: An integrated perspective. *Journal of the Association of Nurses in AIDS Care, 12*(3), 58–65.

McGee, E. M. (2000). Alcoholics anonymous and nursing. *Journal of Holistic Nursing, 18*(1), 11–26.

McGee, E. M. (2004). *I'm better for having known you: An exploration of self-transcendence in nurses.* Unpublished doctoral dissertation, Boston College, Boston.

Mellors, M. P., Erlen, J. A., Coontz, P. D., & Lucke, K. T. (2001). Transcending the suffering of AIDS. *Journal of Community Health Nursing, 18*(4), 235–246.

Mellors, M. P., Riley, T. A., & Erlen, J. A. (1997). HIV, self-transcendence, and quality of life. *Journal of the Association of Nurses in AIDS Care, 2,* 59–69.

Neill, J. (2002). Transcendence and transformation in the life patterns of women living with rheumatoid arthritis. *Advances in Nursing Science, 24*(4), 27–47.

Newman, M. (1992). Prevailing paradigms in nursing. *Nursing Outlook, 40,* 10–13.

Newman, M. (1994). *Health as expanding consciousness* (2nd ed.). New York, NY: National League for Nursing.

Nygren, B., Aléx, L., Jonsén, E., Gustafson, Y., Norberg, A., & Lundman, B. (2005). Resilience, sense of coherence, purpose in life and self-transcendence in relation to perceived physical and mental health among the oldest old. *Aging & Mental Health, 9*(4), 354–362.

Palmer, B., Quinn Griffin, M. T., Reed, P., & Fitzpatrick, J. J. (2010). Self-transcendence and work engagement in acute care staff registered nurses. *Critical Care Nursing Quarterly, 33*(2), 138–147.

Parse, R. (1992). Human becoming: Parse's theory of nursing. *Nursing Science Quarterly, 5,* 35–42.

Peck, R. C. (1968). Psychological development in the second half of life. In B. L. Neugarten (Ed.), *Middle age and aging* (pp. 88–92). Chicago, IL: University of Chicago Press.

Pelusi, J. (1997). The lived experience of surviving breast cancer. *Oncology Nursing Forum, 24*(8), 1343–1353.

Poole, D. K. (1999). *Partnering with a formal program: Expanding the boundaries of family caregiving for frail older adults.* Unpublished doctoral dissertation, Medical College of Georgia, Augusta.

Ramer, L., Johnson, D., Chan, L., & Barrett, M. T. (2006). The effect of HIV/AIDS disease progression on spirituality and self-transcendence in a multi-cultural population. *Journal of Transcultural Nursing, 17*(3), 280–289.

Reed, P. G. (1983). Implications of the life-span developmental framework for well-being in adulthood and aging. *Advances in Nursing Science, 6,* 18–25.

Reed, P. G. (1986). Developmental resources and depression in the elderly: A longitudinal study. *Nursing Research, 35,* 368–374.

Reed, P. G. (1987). Spirituality and well-being in terminally ill hospitalized adults. *Research in Nursing and Health, 10*(5), 335–344.

Reed, P. G. (1989). Mental health of older adults. *Western Journal of Nursing Research, 11*(2), 143–163.

Reed, P. G. (1991). Self-transcendence and mental health in oldest-old adults. *Nursing Research, 40,* 7–11.

Reed, P. G. (1996). Transcendence: Formulating nursing perspectives. *Nursing Science Quarterly, 9*(1), 2–4.

Reed, P. G. (1997a). Nursing: The ontology of the discipline. *Nursing Science Quarterly, 10*(2), 76–79.

Reed, P. G. (1997b). The place of transcendence in nursing's science of unitary human beings: Theory and research. In M. Madrid (Ed.), *Patterns of Rogerian knowing* (pp. 187–196). New York, NY: National League for Nursing.

Reed, P. G. (2009). Demystifying self-transcendence for mental health nursing practice and research. *Archives of Psychiatric Nursing, 23*(5), 397–400.

Reed, P. G. (2011). The spiral path of nursing knowledge. In P. G. Reed & N. B. C. Shearer (Eds.), *Nursing knowledge and theory innovation: Advancing the science of nursing practice* (pp. 1–35). New York, NY: Springer.

Reese, C. G., & Murray, R. B. (1996). Transcendence: The meaning of great-grandmothering. *Archives of Psychiatric Nursing, 10*(4), 245–251.

Riegel, K. F. (1976). The dialectics of human development. *American Psychologist, 31*, 631–647.

Rogers, M. E. (1970). *Introduction to the theoretical basis of nursing*. Philadelphia, PA: F. A. Davis.

Rogers, M. E. (1980). A science of unitary man. In J. P. Riehl & C. Roy (Eds.), *Conceptual modes for nursing practice* (2nd ed., pp. 329–337). New York, NY: Appleton-Century-Crofts.

Rogers, M. E. (1994). The science of unitary human beings: Current perspectives. *Nursing Science Quarterly, 7*(1), 33–35.

Runquist, J. J., & Reed, P. G. (2007). Self-transcendence and well-being in homeless adults. *Journal of Holistic Nursing, 25*(1), 5–13; discussion, 14–15.

Sarenmalm, E. K., Thorén-Jönsson, A., Gaston-Hohansson, F., & Öhlén, J. (2009). Making sense of living under the shadow of death: Adjusting to a recurrent breast cancer illness. *Qualitative Health Research, 19*(8), 1116–1130.

Schumann, R. R. (1999). *Intensive care patients' perceptions of the experience of mechanical ventilation*. Unpublished doctoral dissertation, Texas Women's University, Denton.

Sharpnack, P. A., Quinn Griffin, M. T., Benders, A. M., & Fitzpatrick, J. J. (2010). Spiritual and alternative healthcare practices of the Amish. *Holistic Nursing Practice, 24*, 64–72.

Sharpnack, P. A., Quinn Griffin, M. T., Benders, A. M., & Fitzpatrick, J. J. (2011). Self-transcendence and spiritual well-being in the Amish. *Journal of Holistic Nursing, 29*(2), 91–97.

Sheldon, K. M., & Kasser, T. (2001). Getting older, getting better? Personal strivings and psychological maturity across the life span. *Developmental Psychology, 37*, 491–501.

Sinnott, J. D. (1998). *The development of logic in adulthood: Postformal thought and its applications*. New York, NY: Plenum.

Sinnott, J. D. (2003). Postformal thought and adult development: Living in balance. In J. Demick & C. Andreoletti (Eds.), *Handbook of adult development* (pp. 221–238). New York, NY: Kluwer Academic/Plenum.

Stevens, D. D. (1999). *Spirituality, self-transcendence and depression in young adults with AIDS*. Unpublished doctoral dissertation. University of Miami, Coral Gables, FL.

Stinson, C. K., & Kirk, E. (2006). Structured reminiscence: An intervention to decrease depression and increase self-transcendence in older women. *Journal of Clinical Nursing, 15*(2), 208–218.

Teixeira, M. E. (2008). Self-transcendence: A concept analysis for nursing praxis. *Holistic Nursing Practice, 22*(1), 25–31.

Thomas, J. C., Burton, M., Quinn Griffin, M. T., & Fitzpatrick, J. J. (2010). Self-transcendence, spiritual well-being, and spiritual practices of women with breast cancer. *Journal of Holistic Nursing, 28*(2), 115–122.

Upchurch, S. (1999). Self-transcendence and activities of daily living: The woman with the pink slippers. *Journal of Holistic Nursing, 17*, 251–266.

Upchurch, S., & Mueller, W. H. (2005). Spiritual influences on ability to engage in self-care activities among older African Americans. *International Journal of Aging and Human Development, 60*(1), 77–94.

Walker, C. A. (2002). Transformative aging: How mature adults respond to growing older. *The Journal of Theory Construction & Testing, 6*(2), 109–116.

Walsh, S. M., Radcliffe, S., Castillo, L. C., Kumar, A. M., & Broschard, D. M. (2007). A pilot study to test the effect of art-making classes for family caregivers of patients with cancer. *Oncology Nursing Forum, 34*(1), online exclusive, 1–8.

Walton, C. G., Shultz, C., Beck, C. M., & Walls, R. C. (1991). Psychological correlates of loneliness in the older adult. *Archives of Psychiatric Nursing, 5*(3), 165–170.

Wasner, M., Longaker, C., Fegg, J. J., & Borasio, G. D. (2005). Effects of spiritual care training for palliative care professionals. *Palliative Medicine, 19*, 99–104.

Watson, J. (1985/1999). *Nursing: Human science and human care.* Sudbury, MA: Jones & Bartlett. (Original work published 1985.)

Williams, B. J. (2012). Self-transcendence in stem cell transplantation recipients: A phenomenologic inquiry. *Oncology Nursing Forum, 39*(4), E41–E48.

Willis, D. G., & Grace, P. J. (2011). The applied philosopher-scientist: Intersections among phenomenological research, nursing science, and theory as a basis for practice aimed at facilitating boys' healing from being bullied. *Advances in Nursing Science, 34*(1), 19–28.

Willis, D. G., & Griffith, C. A. (2010). Healing patterns revealed in middle school boys' experiences of being bullied using Rogers' Science of Unitary Human Beings. *Journal of Child and Adolescent Psychiatric Nursing, 23*(3), 125–132.

Wright, K. B. (2003). *Quality of life, self-transcendence, illness distress, and fatigue in liver transplant recipients.* Unpublished doctoral dissertation, University of Texas at Austin.

Young, C., & Reed, P. G. (1995). Elders' perceptions of the effectiveness of group psychotherapy in fostering self-transcendence. *Archives of Psychiatric Nursing, 9*, 338–347.

7

Theory of Symptom Management

Janice Humphreys, Susan Janson, DorAnne Donesky,
Kathleen Dracup, Kathryn A. Lee, Kathleen Puntillo,
Julia A. Faucett, Bradley Aouizerat, Christine Miaskowski,
Christina Baggott, Virginia Carrieri-Kohlman, Mary
Barger, Linda Franck, Christine Kennedy; the University
of California, San Francisco (UCSF) School of Nursing
Symptom Management Faculty Group

A symptom is defined as a subjective experience reflecting changes in the biopsychosocial functioning, sensations, or cognition of an individual. In contrast, a sign is defined as any abnormality indicative of disease that is detectable by the individual or others (Dodd et al., 2001). Signs and symptoms are important aspects of health and illness that disrupt physical, mental, and social functioning. An acute or unrelenting symptom is often what brings the patient into the health care system, particularly after self-care management strategies have failed. The presence of a symptom or a cluster of symptoms may be the first indication to the patient or provider of a developing illness. Symptoms can also be brought on by prescribed pharmacologic or medical therapy. Whether the goal is to eliminate the symptom or to minimize the distress of the symptom experience, the theory of symptom management provides useful information. This middle range theory serves to guide symptom assessment and treatment in nursing practice and to suggest questions and hypotheses for nursing research.

PURPOSE OF THE THEORY AND HOW IT WAS DEVELOPED

The faculty at the University of California, San Francisco (UCSF) School of Nursing first introduced the symptom management model in 1994 (Larson et al., 1994). That original model provided a framework to allow faculty involved in symptom research and clinical practice to improve collaboration and move forward in a more organized way of thinking about the symptom experience, management strategies, and outcomes of symptom management. The conceptualization at that time was based on models that had been developed by nurses, such as Orem's self-care model (1971, 1980, 1985) and Sorofman, Tripp-Reimer, Lauer, and Martin's (1990) model of symptoms of self-care, and other related models from anthropology, sociology, and psychology. The UCSF faculty concluded that none of these frameworks adequately addressed the patient's role in self-care *and* the "patient's experience, his or her tested management strategies, or the desired outcomes" (Larson et al., 1994, p. 273). With further testing of the model and its components and ongoing discussion among the UCSF faculty and students, the UCSF symptom management model was revised in 2001 (Dodd et al., 2001). Selected published research studies were used to build an evidence-based foundation and to compare and contrast the concepts across symptoms. In the 2008 revision, the concept labels and nature of the relationships among the concepts were slightly altered. In addition, the influence of person, environment, and health and illness domains were made explicit by situating the entire model within these spheres. With this chapter, we have updated the growing body of research that uses the Symptom Management Theory (SMT) as a theoretical basis. As depicted in Figure 7.1, the three components of symptom experience, management strategies, and status outcomes continue to form the conceptual basis of the SMT for research and practice. The SMT addresses specific phenomena but does not necessarily limit application to one narrow group. The SMT also proposes explicit and testable relationships among three concepts, provides a structure for understanding the connections among these concepts, and provides a framework for considering interventions and outcomes. As will be shown later in this chapter, the SMT continues to provide a strong basis for research and has also begun to inform practice and education in nursing.

CONCEPTS OF THE THEORY

The three essential concepts of the SMT are symptom experience, symptom management strategies, and symptom status outcomes. These concepts are nested within three domains of nursing science (person, environment, and heath/illness) to serve as a reminder of the contextual considerations for nursing research. For instance, a

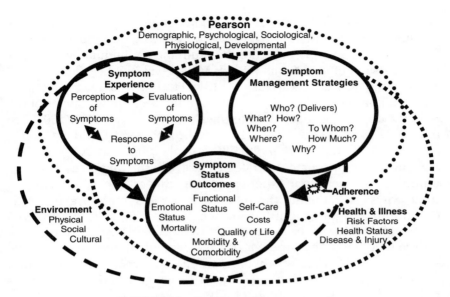

FIGURE 7.1 Symptom Management

Source: Reprinted with permission from Dodd, M., Janson, S., Facione, N., Faucett, J., Froelicher, E. S., Humphreys, J., ... Taylor, D. (2001). Advancing the science of symptom management. *Journal of Advanced Nursing*, *33*, 668–676.

woman's symptom experience will vary by age and reproductive status as well as by her genetic risk factors (person domain), her cultural beliefs about the meaning of a symptom or whether she is assessed in the laboratory, clinic, home, or job (environmental domain), and her current state of health or diagnosis (health/illness domain).

Symptom experience is a simultaneous perception, evaluation, and response to a change in one's usual feeling. The change can be in frequency (how often) or severity (how bad). Further, frequency or severity may not change, but distress associated with the symptom could be altered by an intervention strategy. For example, a woman may suddenly feel hot and diaphoretic. In response to her awareness of these symptoms, she begins to evaluate and consider potential responses that may include taking no action. This symptom perception and response differs depending on whether it occurs during an important meeting or during the night while asleep. If it continues with sufficient frequency and severity over time and is perceived as distressing and interfering with her life, her response is likely to include seeking help and more effective strategies to eliminate or minimize the symptom that is conceptualized within symptom management strategies of the theory.

The symptom experience may include not just one but several synergistic symptoms. Some of the investigators who developed the SMT have explored this phenomenon by studying individuals who experience clusters of symptoms (Dodd, Miaskowski, & Lee, 2004; Dodd, Miaskowski, & Paul, 2001; Voss, Portillo, Holzemer, & Dodd, 2007). In fact, this approach is one of the more rapidly developing aspects of the SMT (Dodd, Cho, Cooper, & Miaskowski, 2010; E. Kim et al., 2009; Lee et al., 2009; Miaskowski, 2006c; Miaskowski, Aouizerat, Dodd, & Cooper, 2007; Miaskowski, Paul et al., 2011; Voss et al., 2007; Xiao, 2010).

Symptom management strategies are efforts to avert, delay, or minimize the symptom experience. The strategy can be effective in three ways: (1) reducing the frequency of the symptom experience, (2) minimizing the severity of the symptom, or (3) relieving the distress associated with the symptom (Portenoy et al., 1994). A framework for the study and development of management strategies include the specifications of who, how, where, when, and what the intervention strategy entails. To continue again with the woman who suddenly feels hot and diaphoretic—to cool her body temperature down to relieve the symptom at one moment in time—she might either remove some clothing or begin to fan herself. Her circumstances (environment), personal characteristics (person), and health status (health/illness) continue to influence her symptom management strategies as do the frequency and severity of the symptoms, among other factors, over time.

Increasing attention is being given to self-management strategies used by patients (Landers, McCarthy, & Savage, 2011; Zimmerman et al., 2011). An outcome of this effort is to shift more of the responsibility of managing symptoms to the individual, particularly in the setting of a chronic illness. Patients essentially become their own primary caregivers and manage their symptoms themselves on a day-to-day basis. The location where an intervention strategy is tested or used, such as in the laboratory or home, can impact or modulate the symptom. For example, an intervention for insomnia may have a different effect when tested in the home compared with a sleep laboratory. The "what" is viewed as the strategy itself; one strategy might be a medical therapy that also needs provider input (e.g., adjusting a daily diuretic dosage to manage symptoms of dyspnea and orthopnea), whereas another may involve a complementary therapy or relaxation technique that the patient or family can carry out on a daily basis. Yet another may involve alteration of the hospital room, home, or work environment. Patients and providers may also attempt more than one strategy and use a combination of interventions that have a greater effect on the symptom or cluster of symptoms. Tailoring the management strategy to the person or the family has been shown to be important in bringing about behavior change (Committee on Quality of Health Care in America, 2001; Leeman, Skelly, Burns, Carlson, & Soward, 2008; Skelly, Carlson, Leeman, Soward, & Burns, 2009) and symptom reduction.

The dose (i.e., how much) and the timing (i.e., when) aspects of interventions or strategies are also important to modulate symptoms in nursing practice and research. The dose is an important consideration, particularly when implementing a behavioral intervention. Dose could include actual time spent exercising, number of times a stress reduction session was attended, or amount of time spent in an education session. The dose of time spent by the health care provider or family member administering the intervention is also critical to consider in terms of how much time and support is actually provided to the person experiencing the symptom. One example of dose related to environmental management may be the degree of job improvement or disability accommodation that a workplace provides (Faucett & McCarthy, 2003). Donesky-Cuenco, Janson, Neuhaus, Neilands, and Carrieri-Kohlman (2007) found that when reporting dose and timing, the use of intuitively understood units of measurement improved comparisons across interventions and programs of research. In their study, "minutes per session" and "number of sessions per week" were units of exercise measurement that were easily understood; in contrast, cumulative minutes during a 6-month study were less useful as a measurement unit of comparison.

Symptom status outcomes are clear and measurable outcomes to assess following the implementation of a strategy. Outcomes include the obvious change in symptom status, whereby the symptom is less frequent, less intense, or less distressing. This improvement in symptoms can lead to better physical and mental functioning, improved quality of life, shorter hospital stay, quicker return to work, and greater productivity, all with less cost to the individual, family, health care system, or employer.

RELATIONSHIPS AMONG THE CONCEPTS: THE MODEL

The SMT has three major concepts: symptom experience, symptom management strategies, and symptom status outcomes. The bidirectional arrows within the model of SMT are meant to indicate a simultaneous interaction among all three concepts. The symptom experience is conceptualized as influencing and being influenced by both symptom management strategies and symptom status outcomes. As individuals become aware of symptoms, initiate strategies, and assess symptom outcomes, their symptom perception is affected. This interaction can take place in a matter of moments as is often the case in common symptom self-care management (e.g., minor colds, rashes, stomach upset). However, when symptoms are more pronounced and/or distressing, other sources of symptom management strategies may be sought and symptom status outcomes may be assessed in a more formal fashion. This iterative process continues until symptoms resolve and/or are stabilized. However, the process of managing symptoms goes amiss when adherence (i.e., whether the intended recipient of the strategy actually receives or uses the strategy prescribed) becomes a problem. This breakdown is illustrated by the broken arrow between the symptom management strategies and symptoms status outcomes components of the SMT. Within the SMT, nonadherence occurs when interventions are too demanding, are not applied, or are applied inconsistently. In addition, factors situated in the person, environment, and health/illness domains may contribute to nonadherence in managing symptoms.

USE OF THE THEORY IN NURSING RESEARCH

The SMT has evolved as more research studies have contributed to the understanding and development of relationships among the three concepts of the theory. Likewise, the study of symptom experiences and responses—both with individual and clusters of symptoms— has continued to flourish using the SMT as a conceptual guide. The works of Carrieri-Kohlman, Janson-Bjerklie, and colleagues provide an illustration of the systematic development of knowledge for clinical practice that has been possible with the SMT. Their initial research sought to explore patient symptom experience and responses to dyspnea (Carrieri & Janson-Bjerklie, 1986; Carrieri, Kieckhefer, Janson-Bjerklie, & Souza, 1991; Carrieri-Kohlman, Demir-Deviren, Cuenco, Eiser, & Stulbarg, 2000; Carrieri-Kohlman, Gormley, Douglas, Paul, & Stulbarg, 1996; Carrieri-Kohlman et al., 2001; Janson-Bjerklie, Carrieri, & Hudes, 1986; Janson-Bjerklie, Ferketich, Benner, & Becker, 1992). Their research uncovered the diverse symptom experience of individuals and the variety of terms patients used to describe their experience. They produced some of the earliest evidence for the affective dimension of dyspnea and have continued to explore dyspnea-related distress in the clinical setting (Carrieri-Kohlman et al., 2010).

Subsequent testing of the effect of management strategies on symptom experience and other multivariate outcomes, such as exercise performance, depression, self-efficacy for managing dyspnea, health-related quality of life, adherence, and health care utilization, have provided an understanding of how patients manage their symptoms and how those symptoms and their management affect functional status (Carrieri-Kohlman et al., 2005; Davis, Carrieri-Kohlman, Janson, Gold, & Stulbarg, 2006; Donesky et al., 2011; Nguyen & Carrieri-Kohlman, 2005). More recently, the dyspnea self-management program developed from the work of Carrieri-Kohlman et al. has been transferred to an internet platform to improve accessibility of self-management support outside the traditional time and space of a clinic (Nguyen et al., 2011, 2008). Adoption of alternative modalities of exercise, such as yoga, has also shown promise as a dyspnea management strategy (Donesky-Cuenco, Nguyen, Paul, & Carrieri-Kohlman, 2009).

Similarly, application of this research trajectory to asthma revealed the distinct role of symptoms in monitoring asthma control. Increasing chronic asthma symptoms or the sudden onset of acute symptoms signals the loss of asthma control and requires actions to preserve life, yet many adults delay seeking urgent medical care when asthma worsens (Janson & Becker, 1998). Interventions designed to increase self-management skills for responding to acute episodes and controlling chronic asthma have produced improved adherence to anti-inflammatory therapy and improved control of asthma (Janson et al., 2003). A refinement of the self-management intervention tailored to the severity of asthma, inhaler technique, and skin test allergy profile of individual participants was further tested in a randomized controlled trial (Janson, McGrath, Covington, Cheng, & Boushey, 2009). Self-management skills training significantly improved adherence to inhaled corticosteroid therapy, nighttime asthma symptoms, and perception of asthma control in the intervention group compared with the attention control group. Building on the importance of symptom recognition as a warning sign of worsening asthma, a cluster randomized controlled trial was also conducted to test the effect of providing asthmatic adults with monthly written interpretations of their graphed peak flow data based on zones of reduction to match with their symptom reports (Janson, McGrath, Covington, Baron, & Lazarus, 2010). This feedback intervention resulted in significant improvement in self-management during winter (physical environment)—typically a period of vulnerability related to colds and flu—as evidenced by significantly fewer episodes of worsening symptoms, fewer courses of oral steroids, and fewer urgent care visits in the intervention group compared with the control group. All these studies show the effects of informed self-monitoring on asthma symptoms—a marker of loss of asthma control. Moreover, the results provide a growing body of evidence to support the SMT.

The SMT has seen increasing use in other areas since the 2008 revision. A search of both research and practice-focused literature from 2007 until the present produced 40 additional publications that explicitly address the theory and 64 additional publications that cite the SMT in support of the study of symptoms and/or symptom clusters. Among these documents, 35 reported on research that used the theory as the conceptual basis. Two articles discussed the model as part of a focused review of the literature on acute coronary syndromes (Arslanian-Engoren & Engoren, 2010) and symptom clusters (Xiao, 2010). Another article used the symptom management model as a basis for developing a tailored intervention (Skelly, Leeman, Carlson, Soward, & Burns, 2008; Skelly et al., 2009) that was subsequently tested. Linder (2010) conducted a theoretical analysis and Brant, Beck, and Miaskowski (2010) compared the SMT with another and suggested directions for new theory development. In addition to these publications, 10 nationally funded research grants (Alsten, 2008, 2009; Dracup, 2006; Lee, 2004; Miaskowski, 2003, 2006a, 2006b, 2007, 2009a; Puntillo, 2010) and 2 training grants supporting faculty development or pre- and postdoctoral scholars (Lee, 2011; Miaskowski, 2009b) were found that explicitly use the SMT. One additional foundation grant directly supported international collaboration addressing symptoms and the development of a more global analysis (Dracup, 2011).

Research Studies Using the SMT

Research has varied in the extent of use of the SMT as a conceptual basis but has continued to develop over time. In fact, the body of knowledge grounded in the SMT in areas of patients with cancer, dyspnea, and diabetes mellitus has now progressed to the point where researchers have described patients' symptom experiences, developed symptom management strategies, and conducted tests of their effectiveness. Moreover, the research methods used to test all or part of the SMT have diversified and become even more sophisticated. Regardless, findings remain remarkably similar and supportive of the theory across diverse study populations using varied methods. In particular, the patients' varied symptom experiences, diverse management strategies, and the influence of person, environment, and health and illness domains were confirmed in every study where they were included.

Symptom Experience

The most researched aspect of the SMT is the symptom experience. Five studies sought to describe the symptom experience of cancer patients before (Merriman et al., 2011; Van Onselen et al., 2010) and while undergoing various treatments (Dodd et al., 2010; Miaskowski, Lee et al., 2011; Miaskowski, Paul et al., 2011). Fletcher, Dodd, Schumacher, and Miaskowski (2008) found that symptoms were also a common problem for caregivers of patients undergoing treatment for cancer. Likewise, Yuan et al. (2011) found that shift work contributed to fatigue in nurses in Taiwan. Finally, Johnson, Moore, and Fortner (2007) used the symptom management model as a basis for quality improvement programs intended to improve symptom assessment in cancer patients. Given the number and pervasiveness of symptoms in this population (according to patient report data), it was disappointing to find that symptoms were documented in health records far less frequently. The authors conclude that more work is needed to assess seamlessly and routinely multiple symptoms in patients.

Nieveen, Zimmerman, Barnason, and Yates (2008) used the symptom experience concept as the basis for development of the Cardiac Symptom Survey. Arslanian-Engoren and Engoren (2010) used the symptom experience as a framework for reviewing the available research on acute coronary syndromes.

Symptom Experience Within the Domains

More common were studies that describe the symptom experience and also sought to explore the relationship between this concept and one or more of the three domains. Doorenbos, Given, Given, and Verbitsky (2006) conducted a secondary data analysis from their three prospective, descriptive longitudinal studies to determine whether end-of-life symptom experiences changed with proximity to death or differed by gender, cancer site, or age. Nosek et al. (2010) found that the environmental factors influenced women's menopausal symptom experience. Kim and Lee (2009) compared the sleep and fatigue experiences of women before and at two time points after a hysterectomy according to procedure and contextual factors. Three different studies examined the relationship between symptoms and one or more domains in HIV-positive patients. Lee et al. (2009) found that on an average, patients reported nine symptoms, with more than 50% reporting fatigue, drowsiness, difficulty sleeping, and pain. Corless et al. (2008) and Voss et al. (2007) found that fatigue severity was related to the health/illness domain;

however, in the study by Voss, demographic and environmental variables influenced patients' symptom experiences more than the health/illness domain. Barnason et al. (2008) examined the relationship between fatigue and early recovery over time among older adults after coronary artery bypass graft surgery. Byma, Given, Given, and You (2009) found that mastery, conceptualized within the person domain, influenced the resolution of pain, but not fatigue severity in patients with solid tumors. Bay and Bergman (2006) examined the symptom experience of individuals with mild-to-moderate traumatic brain injury and found that postinjury symptoms varied by age and gender. Borge, Wahl, and Moum (2010) were among the several researchers who studied symptom experience of people with chronic obstructive pulmonary disease (COPD). They found that individuals with COPD suffered a wide array of symptoms that were greatly affected by personal, environmental, and health/illness factors. They concluded that the health care providers who work with people with COPD need to expand their focus beyond single-item measure of symptoms. Similar to studies with Western samples, Korean immigrants with COPD or asthma report dyspnea as the most frequent and distressing symptom. Possibly due to cultural differences, the Korean immigrants identified "problems with urination" and "numbness and tingling" as frequent, distressing symptoms (Park, Stotts, Douglas, Donesky-Cuenco, & Carrieri-Kohlman, 2011) and were less likely to report sadness, feeling irritable, or nervousness compared with the Western samples.

Aouizerat is working in collaboration with nurse researchers to identify genetic predictors of symptoms (e.g., sleep disturbance, fatigue, pain, dyspnea, nausea, and vomiting) that play a role in interindividual variation in symptom experience that are either disease specific (e.g., cancer, HIV disease) or general determinants of symptoms that operate across chronic diseases (Baggott, 2012; Bentsen, Rustoen, & Miaskowski, 2011; Lee, 2003, 2006; Miaskowski, Cooper et al., 2006; Miaskowski, Aouizerat, Dodd, & Cooper, 2007). The role of genetics in human disease occupies the person domain of the SMT. However, Aouizerat is quick to note that genetics can occupy both the environment and health/illness domains as well.

Symptom Experience of Children and Families

There are also an increasing number of studies exploring the symptom experience of children. Gedaly-Duff et al. (2006) studied children with leukemia and their parents. They found that both children and their parents report a variety of symptoms and that the children could differentiate between different causes of fatigue. Van Cleve et al. (2004) also studied children with leukemia over time and reported that pain was frequent and at multiple sites. Rodgers et al. (2008) studied gastrointestinal symptoms in children after stem cell transplantation and also noted ongoing symptoms throughout the course of the prospective study. Most recently, Baggott et al. (2011) found that children undergoing chemotherapy suffered from a variety of symptoms and that these symptoms could be grouped into relatively stable clusters according to symptom occurrence and severity. However, all these researchers note the SMT as a framework for research into pediatric symptom assessment and management needs further development.

Symptom Management Strategies

Six recent studies focused on symptom management strategies (Faucett, Meyers, Miles, Janowitz, & Fathallah, 2007; Landers et al., 2011; Suwanno, Petpichetchian, Riegel, & Issaramalai, 2009; Webel & Holzemer, 2009; Wells et al., 2007; Zimmerman et al., 2011). Their findings documented that patients and others use a variety of approaches to manage their symptoms. Using qualitative methods, Landers, McCarthy, and Savage (2011) found that even 2 years after sphincter-saving surgery for rectal cancer, patients struggled to manage an array of symptoms with varying success. Zimmerman et al. (2011) found gender-based differences in their test of the effectiveness of a symptom management intervention with women reporting fewer symptoms and better outcomes postcoronary artery bypass surgery compared with men. Suwanno et al. (2009) noted that person, health/illness, and environment domains influenced symptom management strategies in heart failure patients. They further suggest that continuity-care programs promoting self-management ability should be developed and implemented in both hospital-based and home-based settings to improve health status. Faucett et al. (2007) tested a symptom management strategy to reduce the musculoskeletal pain and fatigue associated with strenuous fieldwork in the agricultural industry. In a cross-over trial with groups of agricultural workers on piece rate, significant reductions in work-related pain and fatigue were obtained with the addition of four brief rest breaks (20 minutes total) to the usual shift pattern, while leaving productivity relatively unchanged. The success of this intervention was most clearly demonstrated when the managers and workers agreed to retain the intervention after the research was completed. Finally, Webel and Holzemer (2009) found that urban, HIV-infected women were very interested in participating in a community-based, peer-led intervention and that the program facilitated symptom management. A randomized clinical trial to change the environment of the bedroom improved the sleep of parents and, in fact, worked best for parents with low socioeconomic status (Lee & Gay, 2011). The totality of research on symptom management provides strong evidence that providers need to foster open communication with patients if they are to learn patients' self-care strategies and increase the likelihood that patients are aware of approaches that have been shown to be most beneficial.

In a significant increase from the past, ten recent studies were found that included measures of all the three key concepts: symptom experience, symptom management strategies, and symptom status outcomes (Eller et al., 2005; Fuller, Welch, Backer, & Rawl, 2005; Hearson, 2006; Janson et al., 2003, 2009, 2010; Tsai, Holzemer, & Leu, 2005). Henoch et al. (2008) used qualitative methods to uncover the full range of symptom experiences, management strategies, and symptom outcomes for lung cancer patients with dyspnea. They concluded that the dyspnea experience and management strategies were complex and influenced the lives of patients in both immediate and long-term reactions. Of particular note was their finding that patients' symptom experience also included an existential impact involving hope, hopelessness, and thoughts of death, an area of the symptom experience that has not previously been reported.

Fall-Dickson et al. (2008) sought to describe stomatitis-related pain in women with breast cancer undergoing autologous hematopoietic stem cell transplant. They found that 47% had varying degrees of oral pain with a subset reporting continuous moderate-to-severe oral pain despite pain management algorithms. Chou, Dodd, Abrams, and Padilla (2007) explored the cancer symptom experience, self-care strategies, and quality of life among Chinese Americans during outpatient chemotherapy. Their participants reported experiencing approximately 14 symptoms weekly. Participants also averaged two self-care strategies per symptom that were of low-to-moderate effectiveness. For 20% of the participants, this included Chinese medicine strategies. Utne et al. (2010) conducted a longitudinal study of cancer patients in Norway. They also found that participants experienced multiple symptoms and that those who reported both depression and anxiety had poorer quality of life.

Three studies reported on interventions to reduce symptoms in patients with different types of cancer. Lee, Dodd, Dibble, and Abrams (2008) focused on nausea as a symptom experience, exercise as a strategy for its management, and nausea intensity as a symptom outcome. Even moderate exercise was shown to reduce nausea intensity in this sample of women undergoing treatment for cancer, suggesting that although symptoms may be common among cancer patients, effective management strategies can be found. Ruegg, Curran, and Lamb (2009) conducted a randomized controlled trial to determine whether differences exist in perceived pain during preprocedure anesthetic injection for bone marrow biopsy between buffered and unbuffered lidocaine and whether pain levels change over time. Skrutkowski et al. (2008) at the McGill University examined the impact of care delivered by a "pivot" nurse (who accompanies patients and families from diagnosis of cancer onward) on symptoms in patients with lung or breast cancer. Although the researchers found no significant differences in symptom distress, fatigue, quality of life, or health care usage between groups, they concluded that both groups had frequent contact with nurses who were experienced in oncology care. They hypothesized that in less urban settings (environment), the treatment group might show greater benefits.

Skelly and colleagues (Leeman et al., 2008; Skelly et al., 2008, 2009) used the SMT to develop a conceptual model of symptom-focused diabetes care for African Americans. They subsequently conducted a randomized controlled trial of their nursing intervention to improve health outcomes among older African American women with type 2 diabetes. They also reported on the success of a pilot test of a tailored diabetes self-care intervention with older, rural African American women. Both of these tests demonstrated the success of well-conceptualized and tailored interventions to reduce symptoms and improve outcomes. Moreover, the totality of this work provides a useful guide for the systematic study of symptomatic individuals using the SMT.

An intriguing and rapidly growing area of interest is the study of symptom clusters. Although the original SMT focused on how a single symptom can be studied—as has been noted in earlier sections of this chapter—the symptom experience is likely to involve more than one symptom. Dodd et al. (2004) define symptom clusters as two or more symptoms that are both related to one another and occur concurrently. Commonly occurring clusters are symptoms such as nausea, vomiting and poor appetite; pain, depression and disturbed sleep; or wheezing, chest tightness, and shortness of breath. Although there is a developing body of research that addresses symptom clusters (Dodd et al., 2010; E. Kim et al., 2009; Voss et al., 2007; Xiao, 2010), there are still considerable methodological issues that must be resolved (Miaskowski, 2006c; Miaskowski, Aouizerate, Dodd, & Cooper, 2007). However, the concept of a symptom cluster is consistent with the SMT. Miaskowski (2006c) suggests that research into symptom clusters may provide new insights into the underlying mechanisms. "If common biological mechanisms are found for specific symptom clusters, this knowledge may lead to the development of novel symptoms management strategies" (p. 793). In asthma, symptom clusters occur commonly: chest tightness, shortness of breath, wheeze, and cough often occur together when asthma flares. These symptoms have been measured together on separate visual analog or numerical rating scales (Janson, Hardie, Fahy, & Boushey, 2001; Janson et al., 2003).

USE OF THE THEORY IN NURSING PRACTICE

Reports of the use of the SMT in practice are found less frequently in the literature. Jablonski and Wyatt (2005) applied the model to end-of-life care as a means of expanding understanding of the needs of dying patients and environmental barriers that prevent them from getting necessary care. Ahlberg, Ekman, and Gaston-Johansson (2005) used the SMT to illustrate a framework for dealing with cancer-related fatigue. Maag, Buccheri, Capella, and Jennings (2006) synthesized the SMT with other theories to form a conceptual framework for a clinical nurse leader education program. They include the theory to ensure that the clinical nurse leader graduate will effectively evaluate patient symptoms and develop and implement effective management strategies, thus achieving optimal outcomes. Finally, as previously noted, Johnson et al. (2007) and others (Carpenter et al., 2008) have noted that symptom assessments can be computerized, but unless such systems are seamlessly integrated into electronic health records, symptoms are unlikely to be assessed.

An asthma clinic was established at the UCSF in June 2008 that provides evidence-based care and self-management training to adults with persistent asthma. The major objectives of the clinic are to provide expert consultation and care and prevent asthma exacerbations, by optimizing asthma control. Self-monitoring of symptoms and indicators of asthma control, and optimal use of inhaled medications by patients are key components of the care provided by a nurse practitioner, a respiratory therapist, and a pulmonologist. Research by the team formed the blueprint provided in this ongoing practice (Cisnero, 2009).

A multidisciplinary symptom management and quality-of-life pulmonary clinic opened at the UCSF in 2012 to serve the needs of patients with chronic lung disease who experience high symptom burden and frequent readmissions, and/or who desire a palliative care focus. The team includes a pulmonologist, nurse practitioner, palliative care physician, social worker, pharmacist, physical therapist, respiratory therapist, and chaplain. This team is adapting the internet-based dyspnea self-management program developed by Carrieri-Kohlman and colleagues as a support tool for their clinic. In addition, coordination with the UCSF Medical Center discharge planning services, integration of a pulmonary rehabilitation program within the clinic, and affiliation with the UCSF pulmonary clinical services will provide seamless continuity of care for patients across the illness trajectory. Pilot funding has been obtained for a program of clinical research designed to document methodology and outcomes related to the symptom management clinic.

CONCLUSION

The body of knowledge acquired from research using the SMT is growing. Across multiple studies with diverse samples and methods, the results are remarkably similar. Patients experience a wide range of symptoms and use a variety of terms and phrases to describe these sensations. They largely attempt to manage these symptoms themselves using strategies that have evidence-based support and strategies of questionable value. Providers are seen as an important source for information about symptoms, but so are family, friends, employers, the media, and the Internet including chat rooms. There is clear evidence that providers must establish and maintain good patient–provider communication if they are to understand their patient's symptom perception, accept symptom experience, and implement management strategies. It is also essential for providers to consider the strengths and limitations imposed on patients within the person, environment, and health/illness dimensions. When symptoms are not adequately addressed, patients continue to suffer reduced quality of life and altered functional status at high costs to the individual, family, and society.

However, the SMT may also be in need of reconsideration and possible revision. The temporal dimension of time is largely missing from the model. This is increasingly apparent as more sophisticated studies use longitudinal designs. The need to consider that changes in symptoms over time is also important to understand patient adherence to prescribed strategies and to determine when management strategies are best received and best measured for the highest possible benefit.

Recent technologic advances (e.g., electronic symptom diaries) have facilitated the collection of patient-reported outcomes in real time. Likewise, researchers can now collect patients' daily reports of their self-care intervention utilization. The comparison of symptom severity with symptom management patterns over time may lead to important discoveries regarding the efficacy of the symptom interventions. Henly, Kallas, Klatt, and Swenson (2003) attempted to address this limitation by synthesizing a new theory that includes four temporal dimensions of symptoms. However in doing so, they have created a far more linear framework that fails to consider the multidimensional nature of symptoms. Nonetheless, their efforts may provide some insight into future versions of the SMT.

Donesky has also noted that adherence—currently situated in the SMT between symptom management strategies and symptom status outcomes—may need reconsideration. In research with patients with COPD, Donesky and Carrieri-Kohlman found a bidirectional relationship between adherence and all three concepts of the SMT, as well as the person, environment, and health/illness dimensions of nursing science (Donesky-Cuenco et al., 2007). For example, a person who is less short of breath or who has cognitively restructured their experience of shortness of breath will walk more; and walking more will decrease the shortness of breath experience over the long term. These researchers further note that not only does adherence influence the relationship between intervention and outcome but also the characteristics of the intervention will influence adherence (e.g., desirability of the intervention will influence whether a person adheres). They have concluded that placement of adherence solely at the intervention–outcome link may be too restrictive.

Ongoing discussion with the UCSF faculty and trainees in our T32 Nurse Research Training in Symptom Management has noted that the current two-dimensional depiction of the SMT model may not do it justice. It has often been suggested that the ideal figure would involve a holographic, three-dimensional representation that depicts the three suspended concepts of the SMT within three revolving spheres representing the person, environment, and health/illness dimensions. Such a modification could also be used to represent visually the multiple perspectives of patient's symptom experience much better. Rarely are patients' symptom reports told solely from the perspective of the patient. Collection of family caregivers' perspectives of the symptom experience is ubiquitous in pediatrics and commonplace in the care of most adults with chronic conditions. The family caregivers' perspective is not always congruent with that of the patient, adding complexity to the evaluation of symptoms. Revision of the SMT to make it clearer, more parsimonious, and more representative of "real life" may also increase its usefulness to researchers and clinicians.

In almost two decades since the SMT was originally introduced, it has gained acceptance as a valuable theory for organizing knowledge for research and clinical practice, especially in the symptom experience domain within the person, environment, and health/illness dimensions of nursing science. The management strategies domain of the theory provides guidance in evaluating self-management strategies in addition to clinician-prescribed strategies, and the symptom status outcomes domain underscores the importance of measuring the symptom as an outcome (its frequency, severity, and distress) following an intervention as well as distinguishing other important outcomes related to the symptom experience. The SMT has brought together researchers and clinicians from diverse backgrounds and populations around the shared interest in managing symptoms, with the result that knowledge is expanding in the areas of symptom clusters and extrapolating knowledge gained in one symptom area to similarities of assessment, management, and evaluation strategies with other symptoms. Research related to the SMT supports its current value and encourages continuing efforts to refine the theory for ongoing research and application to clinical practice.

REFERENCES

Ahlberg, K., Ekman, T., & Gaston-Johansson, F. (2005). Fatigue, psychological distress, coping resources, and functional status during radiotherapy for uterine cancer. *Oncology Nursing Forum, 32*(3), 633–640.

Alsten, C. (2008). *Evaluation of a sleep enhancement program for experienced nurses.* Bethesda, MD: National Heart, Lung, and Blood Institute. 1R43HL090110.

Alsten, C. (2009). *Evaluation of a sleep enhancement program for novice shiftworkers.* Bethesda, MD: National Institute of Nursing Research. 1R43NR010688.

Arslanian-Engoren, C., & Engoren, M. (2010). Physiological and anatomical bases for sex differences in pain and nausea as presenting symptoms of acute coronary syndromes. *Heart & Lung, 39*(5), 386–393.

Baggott, C. (2012). *Evaluation of candidate genes for chemotherapy-induced nausea and vomiting* (Mentored Research Scholar Grant ed.). New York, NY: American Cancer Society. MRSG-12-01-PCSM.

Baggott, C., Cooper, B. A., Marina, N., Matthay, K. K., & Miaskowski, C. (2011). Symptom cluster analyses based on symptom occurrence and severity ratings among pediatric oncology patients during myelosuppressive chemotherapy. *Cancer Nursing, 35*(1), 19–28.

Barnason, S., Zimmerman, L., Nieveen, J., Schulz, P., Miller, C., Hertzog, M., & Rasmussen, D. (2008). Relationships between fatigue and early postoperative recovery outcomes over time in elderly patients undergoing coronary artery bypass graft surgery. *Heart & Lung: The Journal of Critical Care, 37*(4), 245–256.

Bay, E., & Bergman, K. (2006). Symptom experience and emotional distress after traumatic brain injury. *Care Management Journals: Journal of Case Management; The Journal of Long Term Home Health Care, 7*(1), 3–9.

Bentsen, S. B., Rustoen, T., & Miaskowski, C. (2011). Prevalence and characteristics of pain in patients with chronic obstructive pulmonary disease compared to the Norwegian general population. *The Journal of Pain: Official Journal of the American Pain Society, 12*(5), 539–545.

Borge, C. R., Wahl, A. K., & Moum, T. (2010). Association of breathlessness with multiple symptoms in chronic obstructive pulmonary disease. *Journal of Advanced Nursing, 66*(12), 2688–2700.

Brant, J. M., Beck, S., & Miaskowski, C. (2010). Building dynamic models and theories to advance the science of symptom management research. *Journal of Advanced Nursing, 66*(1), 228–240.

Byma, E. A., Given, B. A., Given, C. W., & You, M. (2009). The effects of mastery on pain and fatigue resolution. *Oncology Nursing Forum, 36*(5), 544–552.

Carpenter, J. S., Rawl, S., Porter, J., Schmidt, K., Tornatta, J., Ojewole, F., ... Giesler, R. B. (2008). Oncology outpatient and provider responses to a computerized symptom assessment system. *Oncology Nursing Forum, 35*(4), 661–669.

Carrieri, V. K., & Janson-Bjerklie, S. (1986). Strategies patients use to manage the sensation of dyspnea. *Western Journal of Nursing Research, 8*(3), 284–305.

Carrieri, V. K., Kieckhefer, G., Janson-Bjerklie, S., & Souza, J. (1991). The sensation of pulmonary dyspnea in school-age children. *Nursing Research, 40*(2), 81–85.

Carrieri-Kohlman, V., Demir-Deviren, S., Cuenco, D., Eiser, S., & Stulbarg, M. S. (2000). Effect of exercise dose on affective response to dyspnea in COPD. *American Journal of Respiratory and Critical Care Medicine (Suppl), 161,* A705.

Carrieri-Kohlman, V., Donesky-Cuenco, D., Park, S. K., Mackin, L., Nguyen, H. Q., & Paul, S. M. (2010). Additional evidence for the affective dimension of dyspnea in patients with COPD. *Research in Nursing & Health, 33*(1), 4–19.

Carrieri-Kohlman, V., Gormley, J. M., Douglas, M. K., Paul, S. M., & Stulbarg, M. S. (1996). Differentiation between dyspnea and its affective components. *Western Journal of Nursing Research, 18*(6), 626–642.

Carrieri-Kohlman, V., Gormley, J. M., Eiser, S., Demir-Deviren, S., Nguyen, H., Paul, S. M., & Stulbarg, M. S. (2001). Dyspnea and the affective response during exercise training in obstructive pulmonary disease. *Nursing Research, 50*(3), 136–146.

Carrieri-Kohlman, V., Nguyen, H. Q., Donesky-Cuenco, D., Demir-Deviren, S., Neuhaus, J., & Stulbarg, M. S. (2005). Impact of brief or extended exercise training on the benefit of a dyspnea self-management program in COPD. *Journal of Cardiopulmonary Rehabilitation, 25*(5), 275–284.

Chou, F. Y., Dodd, M., Abrams, D., & Padilla, G. (2007). Symptoms, self-care, and quality of life of Chinese American patients with cancer. *Oncology Nursing Forum, 34*(6), 1162–1167.

Cisnero, L. (2009). Research breathes life into new asthma clinic. *UCSF Science of Caring, 21*(1), 14–17.

Committee on Quality of Health Care in America. (2001). *Crossing the quality chasm.* Washington, DC: National Academy Press.

Corless, I. B., Voss, J. G., Nicholas, P. K., Bunch, E. H., Bain, C. A., Coleman, C., … Valencia, C. P. (2008). Fatigue in HIV/AIDS patients with comorbidities. *Applied Nursing Research: ANR, 21*(3), 116–122.

Davis, A. H., Carrieri-Kohlman, V., Janson, S. L., Gold, W. M., & Stulbarg, M. S. (2006). Effects of treatment on two types of self-efficacy in people with chronic obstructive pulmonary disease. *Journal of Pain and Symptom Management, 32*(1), 60–70.

Dodd, M., Janson, S., Facione, N., Faucett, J., Froelicher, E. S., Humphreys, J., … Taylor, D. (2001). Advancing the science of symptom management. *Journal of Advanced Nursing, 33*(5), 668–676.

Dodd, M. J., Cho, M. H., Cooper, B. A., & Miaskowski, C. (2010). The effect of symptom clusters on functional status and quality of life in women with breast cancer. *European Journal of Oncology Nursing: The Official Journal of European Oncology Nursing Society, 14*(2), 101–110.

Dodd, M. J., Miaskowski, C., & Lee, K. A. (2004). Occurrence of symptom clusters. *Journal of the National Cancer Institute. Monographs,* (32), 76–78.

Dodd, M. J., Miaskowski, C., & Paul, S. M. (2001). Symptom clusters and their effect on the functional status of patients with cancer. *Oncology Nursing Forum, 28*(3), 465–470.

Donesky, D., Janson, S. L., Nguyen, H. Q., Neuhaus, J., Neilands, T. B., & Carrieri-Kohlman, V. (2011). Determinants of frequency, duration, and continuity of home walking in patients with COPD. *Geriatric Nursing, 32*(3), 178–187.

Donesky-Cuenco, D., Janson, S., Neuhaus, J., Neilands, T. B., & Carrieri-Kohlman, V. (2007). Adherence to a home-walking prescription in patients with chronic obstructive pulmonary disease. *Heart & Lung: The Journal of Critical Care, 36*(5), 348–363.

Donesky-Cuenco, D., Nguyen, H. Q., Paul, S., & Carrieri-Kohlman, V. (2009). Yoga therapy decreases dyspnea-related distress and improves functional performance in people with chronic obstructive pulmonary disease: A pilot study. *Journal of Alternative and Complementary Medicine, 15*(3), 225–234.

Doorenbos, A. Z., Given, C. W., Given, B., & Verbitsky, N. (2006). Symptom experience in the last year of life among individuals with cancer. *Journal of Pain and Symptom Management, 32*(5), 403–412.

Dracup, K. (2006). *Improving self-care behavior and outcomes in rural patients with heart failure.* Bethesda, MD: National Heart, Lung, and Blood Institute. R01HL083176.

Dracup, K. (2011). Collaborative research grant with Queensland University of Technology (QUT) in Brisbane, Australia. New York, NY: Atlantic Philanthropies.

Eller, L. S., Corless, I., Bunch, E. H., Kemppainen, J., Holzemer, W., Nokes, K., ... Nicholas, P. (2005). Self-care strategies for depressive symptoms in people with HIV disease. *Journal of Advanced Nursing, 51*(2), 119–130.

Fall-Dickson, J. M., Mock, V., Berk, R. A., Grimm, P. M., Davidson, N., & Gaston-Johansson, F. (2008). Stomatitis-related pain in women with breast cancer undergoing autologous hematopoietic stem cell transplant. *Cancer Nursing, 31*(6), 452–461.

Faucett, J., & McCarthy, D. (2003). Chronic pain in the workplace. *The Nursing Clinics of North America, 38*(3), 509–523.

Faucett, J., Meyers, J., Miles, J., Janowitz, I., & Fathallah, F. (2007). Rest break interventions in stoop labor tasks. *Applied Ergonomics, 38*(2), 219–226.

Fletcher, B. A. S., Dodd, M. J., Schumacher, K. L., & Miaskowski, C. (2008). Symptom experience of family caregivers of patients with cancer. *Oncology Nursing Forum, 35*(2), E23–E44; E23.

Fuller, E., Welch, J. L., Backer, J. H., & Rawl, S. M. (2005). Symptom experience of chronically constipated women with pelvic floor disorders. *Clinical Nurse Specialist, 19*, 34–40.

Gedaly-Duff, V., Lee, K. A., Nail, L., Nicholson, H. S., & Johnson, K. P. (2006). Pain, sleep disturbance, and fatigue in children with leukemia and their parents: A pilot study. *Oncology Nursing Forum, 33*(3), 641–646.

Hearson, B. (2006). Sleep disturbance in family caregivers: Application of the revised symptom management model. *Journal of Palliative Care, 22*(3), 216.

Henly, S. J., Kallas, K. D., Klatt, C. M., & Swenson, K. K. (2003). The notion of time in symptom experiences. *Nursing Research, 52*(6), 410–417.

Henoch, I., Bergman, B., & Danielson, E. (2008). Dyspnea experience and management strategies in patients with lung cancer. *Psycho-Oncology, 17*(7), 709–715.

Jablonski, A., & Wyatt, G. K. (2005). A model for identifying barriers to effective symptom management at the end of life. *Journal of Hospice & Palliative Nursing, 7*(1), 23–36.

Janson, S., & Becker, G. (1998). Reasons for delay in seeking treatment for acute asthma: The patient's perspective. *The Journal of Asthma: Official Journal of the Association for the Care of Asthma, 35*(5), 427–435.

Janson, S., Hardie, G., Fahy, J., & Boushey, H. (2001). Use of biological markers of airway inflammation to detect the efficacy of nurse-delivered asthma education. *Heart & Lung: The Journal of Critical Care, 30*(1), 39–46.

Janson, S. L., Fahy, J. V., Covington, J. K., Paul, S. M., Gold, W. M., & Boushey, H. A. (2003). Effects of individual self-management education on clinical, biological, and adherence outcomes in asthma. *The American Journal of Medicine, 115*(8), 620–626.

Janson, S. L., McGrath, K. W., Covington, J. K., Baron, R. B., & Lazarus, S. C. (2010). Objective airway monitoring improves asthma control in the cold and flu season: A cluster randomized trial. *Chest, 138*(5), 1148–1155.

Janson, S. L., McGrath, K. W., Covington, J. K., Cheng, S. C., & Boushey, H. A. (2009). Individualized asthma self-management improves medication adherence and markers of asthma control. *The Journal of Allergy and Clinical Immunology, 123*(4), 840–846.

Janson-Bjerklie, S., Carrieri, V. K., & Hudes, M. (1986). The sensations of pulmonary dyspnea. *Nursing Research, 35*(3), 154–159.

Janson-Bjerklie, S., Ferketich, S., Benner, P., & Becker, G. (1992). Clinical markers of asthma severity and risk: Importance of subjective as well as objective factors. *Heart & Lung: The Journal of Critical Care, 21*(3), 265–272.

Johnson, G. D., Moore, K., & Fortner, B. (2007). Baseline evaluation of the AIM higher initiative: Establishing the mark from which to measure. *Oncology Nursing Forum, 34*(3), 729–734.

Kim, E., Jahan, T., Aouizerat, B. E., Dodd, M. J., Cooper, B. A., Paul, S. M., ... Miaskowski, C. (2009). Changes in symptom clusters in patients undergoing radiation therapy. *Supportive Care in Cancer: Official Journal of the Multinational Association of Supportive Care in Cancer, 17*(11), 1383–1391.

Kim, K. H., & Lee, K. A. (2009). Sleep and fatigue symptoms in women before and 6 weeks after hysterectomy. *Journal of Obstetric, Gynecologic, and Neonatal Nursing: JOGNN/NAACOG, 38*(3), 344–352.

Landers, M., McCarthy, G., & Savage, E. (2011). Bowel symptom experiences and management following sphincter saving surgery for rectal cancer: A qualitative perspective. *European Journal of Oncology Nursing: The Official Journal of European Oncology Nursing Society, 16*(3), 293–300.

Larson, P. J., Carrieri-Kohlman, V., Dodd, M. J., Douglas, M., Faucett, J., Froelicher, E. S., ... Underwood, P. R. (1994). A model for symptom management. *Journal of Nursing Scholarship, 26*(4), 272–276.

Lee, J., Dodd, M. J., Dibble, S. L., & Abrams, D. I. (2008). Nausea at the end of adjuvant cancer treatment in relation to exercise during treatment in patients with breast cancer. *Oncology Nursing Forum, 35*(5), 830–835.

Lee, K. A. (2003). *Biomarkers of insomnia and fatigue in HIV/AIDS.* Bethesda, MD: National Institute of Mental Health. 5R01MH074358.

Lee, K. A. (2004). *Biomarkers of insomnia and fatigue in HIV/AIDS.* Bethesda, MD: National Institute of Mental Health. 1R01MH074358.

Lee, K. A. (2006). *Nursing research training in symptom management.* Bethesda, MD: National Institute of Nursing Research. 2T32NR07088-11.

Lee, K. A. (2011). *Nursing research training in symptom management.* Bethesda, MD: National Institute of Nursing Research. 2T32NR07088-16.

Lee, K. A., Gay, C., Portillo, C. J., Coggins, T., Davis, H., Pullinger, C. R., & Aouizerat, B. E. (2009). Symptom experience in HIV-infected adults: A function of demographic and clinical characteristics. *Journal of Pain and Symptom Management, 38*(6), 882–893.

Lee, K. A., & Gay, D. L. (2011). Can modifications to the bedroom environment improve the sleep of new parents? *Research in Nursing & Health, 34*, 7–19.

Leeman, J., Skelly, A. H., Burns, D., Carlson, J., & Soward, A. (2008). Tailoring a diabetes self-care intervention for use with older, rural African American women. *Diabetes Educator, 34*(2), 310–317.

Linder, L. (2010). Analysis of the UCSF symptom management theory: Implications for pediatric oncology nursing. *Journal of Pediatric Oncology Nursing: Official Journal of the Association of Pediatric Oncology Nurses, 27*(6), 316–324.

Maag, M. M., Buccheri, R., Capella, E., & Jennings, D. L. (2006). A conceptual framework for a clinical nurse leader program. *Journal of Professional Nursing: Official Journal of the American Association of Colleges of Nursing, 22*(6), 367–372.

Merriman, J. D., Dodd, M., Lee, K., Paul, S. M., Cooper, B. A., Aouizerat, B. E., ... Miaskowski, C. (2011). Differences in self-reported attentional fatigue between patients with breast and prostate cancer at the initiation of radiation therapy. *Cancer Nursing, 34*(5), 345–353.

Miaskowski, C. (2003). *Symptom management after breast cancer surgery.* Bethesda, MD: National Cancer Institute. 5R01CA118658.

Miaskowski, C. (2006a). *Improving cancer pain management through self care.* Bethesda, MD: National Cancer Institute. 6R01CA116423.

Miaskowski, C. (2006b). *Long-term arm morbidity following breast cancer treatment.* Bethesda, MD: National Cancer Institute. 5R01CA118658.

Miaskowski, C. (2006c). Symptom clusters: Establishing the link between clinical practice and symptom management research. *Supportive Care in Cancer: Official Journal of the Multinational Association of Supportive Care in Cancer, 14*(8), 792–794.

Miaskowski, C. (2007). *Symptom clusters in pediatric oncology patients.* Bethesda, MD: National Institute of Nursing Research. 5R21NR010600.

Miaskowski, C. (2009a). *Symptom clusters in oncology patients receiving chemotherapy.* Bethesda, MD: National Cancer Institute. 7R01CA134900.

Miaskowski, C. (2009b). *Symptom management faculty scholars program.* Bethesda, MD: National Institute of Nursing Research. 1P30NR11934.

Miaskowski, C., Aouizerat, B. E., Dodd, M., & Cooper, B. (2007). Conceptual issues in symptom clusters research and their implications for quality-of-life assessment in patients with cancer. *Journal of the National Cancer Institute Monographs,* (37), 39–46.

Miaskowski, C., Cooper, B. A., Paul, S. M., Dodd, M., Lee, K., Aouizerat, B. E., ... Bank, A. (2006). Subgroups of patients with cancer with different symptom experiences and quality-of-life outcomes: A cluster analysis. *Oncology Nursing Forum, 33*(5), E79–E89.

Miaskowski, C., Lee, K., Dunn, L., Dodd, M., Aouizerat, B. E., West, C., ... Swift, P. (2011). Sleep-wake circadian activity rhythm parameters and fatigue in oncology patients before the initiation of radiation therapy. *Cancer Nursing, 34*(4), 255–268.

Miaskowski, C., Paul, S. M., Cooper, B. A., Lee, K., Dodd, M., West, C., ... Wara, W. (2011). Predictors of the trajectories of self-reported sleep disturbance in men with prostate cancer during and following radiation therapy. *Sleep, 34*(2), 171–179.

Nguyen, H. Q., & Carrieri-Kohlman, V. (2005). Dyspnea self-management in patients with chronic obstructive pulmonary disease: Moderating effects of depressed mood. *Psychosomatics, 46*(5), 402–410.

Nguyen, H. Q., Donesky-Cuenco, D., Wolpin, S., Benditt, J. O., Paul, S., & Carrieri-Kohlman, V. (2011). A randomized controlled trial of an internet-based dyspnea self-management program in patients with COPD. *American Journal of Respiratory and Critical Care Medicine, 183,* A5818.

Nguyen, H. Q., Donesky-Cuenco, D., Wolpin, S., Reinke, L. F., Benditt, J. O., Paul, S. M., & Carrieri-Kohlman, V. (2008). Randomized controlled trial of an internet-based versus face-to-face dyspnea self-management program for patients with chronic obstructive pulmonary disease: Pilot study. *Journal of Medical Internet Research, 10*(2), e9.

Nieveen, J. L., Zimmerman, L. M., Barnason, S. A., & Yates, B. C. (2008). Development and content validity testing of the cardiac symptom survey in patients after coronary artery bypass grafting. *Heart & Lung: The Journal of Acute and Critical Care, 37*(1), 17–27.

Nosek, M., Kennedy, H. P., Beyene, Y., Taylor, D., Gilliss, C., & Lee, K. (2010). The effects of perceived stress and attitudes toward menopause and aging on symptoms of menopause. *Journal of Midwifery & Women's Health, 55,* 328–334.

Orem, D. E. (1971). *Nursing: Concepts of practice.* New York, NY: McGraw-Hill.

Orem, D. E. (1980). *Nursing: Concepts of practice* (2nd ed.). New York, NY: McGraw-Hill.

Orem, D. E. (1985). *Nursing: Concepts of practice* (3rd ed.). New York, NY: McGraw-Hill.

Park, S. K., Stotts, N. A., Douglas, M. K., Donesky-Cuenco, D., & Carrieri-Kohlman, V. (2011). Symptoms and functional performance in Korean immigrants with asthma or chronic obstructive pulmonary disease. *Heart & Lung: The Journal of Critical Care, 41*(3), 226–237.

Portenoy, R. K., Thaler, H. T., Kornblith, A. B., Lepore, J. M., Friedlander-Klar, H., Kiyasu, E., & Norton, L. (1994). The memorial symptom assessment scale: An instrument for the evaluation of symptom prevalence, characteristics and distress. *European Journal of Cancer, 30A*(9), 1326–1336.

Puntillo, K. (2010). *Palliation of thirst in intensive care unit patients.* Bethesda, MD: National Institute of Nursing Research. 5R01NR011825.

Rodgers, C., Wills-Alcoser, P., Monroe, R., McDonald, L., Trevino, M., & Hockenberry, M. (2008). Growth patterns and gastrointestinal symptoms in pediatric patients after hematopoietic stem cell transplantation. *Oncology Nursing Forum, 35*(3), 443–448.

Ruegg, T. A., Curran, C. R., & Lamb, T. (2009). Use of buffered lidocaine in bone marrow biopsies: A randomized, controlled trial. *Oncology Nursing Forum, 36*(1), 52–60.

Skelly, A. H., Carlson, J., Leeman, J., Soward, A., & Burns, D. (2009). Controlled trial of nursing interventions to improve health outcomes of older African American women with type 2 diabetes. *Nursing Research, 58*(6), 410–418.

Skelly, A. H., Leeman, J., Carlson, J., Soward, A. C., & Burns, D. (2008). Conceptual model of symptom-focused diabetes care for African Americans. *Journal of Nursing Scholarship, 40*(3), 261–267.

Skrutkowski, M., Saucier, A., Eades, M., Swidzinski, M., Ritchie, J., Marchionni, C., & Ladouceur, M. (2008). Impact of a pivot nurse in oncology on patients with lung or breast cancer: Symptom distress, fatigue, quality of life, and use of healthcare resources. *Oncology Nursing Forum, 35*(6), 948–954.

Sorofman, B., Tripp-Reimer, T., Lauer, G. M., & Martin, M. E. (1990). Symptom self-care. *Holistic Nursing Practice, 4*(2), 45–55.

Suwanno, J., Petpichetchian, W., Riegel, B., & Issaramalai, S. (2009). A model predicting health status of patients with heart failure. *Journal of Cardiovascular Nursing, 24*(2), 118–126.

Tsai, Y. F., Holzemer, W. L., & Leu, H. S. (2005). An evaluation of the effects of a manual on management of HIV/AIDS symptoms. *International Journal of STD & AIDS, 16*(9), 625–629.

Utne, I., Miaskowski, C., Bjordal, K., Paul, S. M., & Rustoen, T. (2010). The relationships between mood disturbances and pain, hope, and quality of life in hospitalized cancer patients with pain on regularly scheduled opioid analgesic. *Journal of Palliative Medicine, 13*(3), 311–318.

Van Cleve, L., Bossert, E., Beecroft, P., Adlard, K., Alvarez, O., & Savedra, M. C. (2004). The pain experience of children with leukemia during the first year after diagnosis. *Nursing Research, 53*(1), 1–10.

Van Onselen, C., Dunn, L. B., Lee, K., Dodd, M., Koetters, T., West, C., ... Miaskowski, C. (2010). Relationship between mood disturbance and sleep quality in oncology outpatients at the initiation of radiation therapy. *European Journal of Oncology Nursing, 14*(5), 373–379.

Voss, J., Portillo, C. J., Holzemer, W. L., & Dodd, M. J. (2007). Symptom cluster of fatigue and depression in HIV/AIDS. *Journal of Prevention & Intervention in the Community, 33*(1–2), 19–34.

Webel, A. R., & Holzemer, W. L. (2009). Positive self-management program for women living with HIV: A descriptive analysis. *JANAC-Journal of the Association of Nurses in Aids Care, 20*(6), 458–467.

Wells, M., Sarna, L., Cooley, M. E., Brown, J. K., Chernecky, C., Williams, R. D., ... Danao, L. L. (2007). Use of complementary and alternative medicine therapies to control symptoms in women living with lung cancer. *Cancer Nursing, 30*(1), 45–55.

Xiao, C. (2010). The state of science in the study of cancer symptom clusters. *European Journal of Oncology Nursing, 14*(5), 417–34.

Yuan, S. C., Chou, M. C., Chen, C. J., Lin, Y. J., Chen, M., Liu, H., & Kuo, H. (2011). Influences of shift work on fatigue among nurses. *Journal of Nursing Management, 19*(3), 339–345.

Zimmerman, L., Barnason, S., Hertzog, M., Young, L., Niemen, J., Schulz, P., & Tu, C. (2011). Gender differences in recovery outcomes after an early recovery symptom management intervention. *Heart & Lung, 40*(5), 429–439.

8

The Theory of Unpleasant Symptoms

Elizabeth R. Lenz and Linda C. Pugh

Symptom management has become increasingly central to nursing practice and continues to emerge as an important focus of nursing science. The National Institute of Nursing Research (NINR) has identified symptom management as one of the key investment areas in its strategic plan (NINR, 2011), noting that "a better understanding of symptoms and symptom clusters ... will improve clinical management of illness and lead to more productive lives" (p. 14). As nurses assume more of the responsibility for managing care of patients with both acute and chronic illnesses, their interest in improving the management of symptoms has stimulated additional basic and translational research. One of the most important, yet challenging, developments has been the burgeoning empirical literature revealing the complexity and pervasiveness of symptom clusters. With the notable exception of the Symptom Management Model, developed and updated by faculty and students at the University of California, San Francisco (Dodd et al., 2001; Humphreys et al., 2008), and the relatively few theoretical models addressing symptom clusters (e.g., Barsevick, Whitmore, Nail, Beck, & Dudley, 2006; Kim, McGuire, Tulman, & Barsevick, 2005), much of the theoretical work that has been carried out to elucidate the experience of symptoms and to guide research and management has been symptom or disease specific. In this chapter, we describe the middle range Theory of Unpleasant Symptoms (TOUS): its components, the process by which it was developed, examples and theoretical implications of its application in nursing research and practice, and plans for future development. Notable features of this theory are that it is applicable to multiple symptoms that can occur in conjunction with many different illnesses; it highlights the multidimensionality of symptoms; and it includes the reality that multiple symptoms often occur together.

PURPOSE OF THE THEORY AND HOW IT WAS DEVELOPED

TOUS was designed to integrate existing knowledge about a variety of symptoms. It was based on the premise that there are commonalities across different symptoms experienced by a variety of clinical population in varied situations. A framework that highlights common elements and dimensions has potential to be useful in both nursing practice and research. The purpose of the theory is to improve understanding of symptom experience in various contexts and to provide information useful for designing effective interventions to prevent, ameliorate, or manage unpleasant symptoms and their negative effects. Because it is more general than a situation-specific theory describing or explaining a specific symptom, illness, or experience, the TOUS lacks some of the detail that may be useful in working with a particular symptom in a given clinical population. On the other hand, by highlighting dimensions and considerations that are common to many symptoms and illnesses, investigators and clinicians are encouraged to think about aspects that are not readily apparent and to consider symptoms both alone and in combination. It serves as a useful heuristic tool by providing an organizing schema that encourages thought about the interplay among the many aspects of the symptom experience.

A model such as the TOUS provides a framework within which multiple researchers can work simultaneously, ultimately combining the results of their many programs of research. The TOUS provides common definitions and dimensions for examining symptoms, ultimately enhancing the probability that the results from multiple studies can be combined to produce convincing evidence on which to base practice.

Because the symptom experience, by definition, occurs at the level of individual perception, the theory is applicable at the level of the individual. However, the TOUS does not consider the individual in isolation. Rather, it positions the individual within the context of his or her family, social and organizational networks, and community by taking into account situational factors in the environment that may influence the symptom experience. It embodies an inclusive perspective that is not limited to the physical domain of human experience, but also acknowledges the important influence of psychological factors and situational or environmental factors, as well as their interplay on the experience of symptoms. It also defines the outcome of the symptom experience in terms of performance, a notion that considers its impact on the individual's interactions with others and his or her short- and long-term physical, cognitive, and social functioning.

The TOUS was developed by four nurse researchers who shared interest in the nature and experience of different symptoms (specifically fatigue and dyspnea) and in the processes of concept and theory development. Audrey Gift, Renee Milligan, Linda Pugh, and Elizabeth Lenz had collaborated in dyads or triads on various empirical studies and theoretical articles. They shared geographic proximity, which facilitated collaboration, and, by virtue of their common association with one PhD program in nursing, they also shared exposure to the same philosophical and meta-theoretical perspectives regarding the development and substance of nursing science. They had access to an eminent philosopher of science colleague, Frederick Suppe, who played an important role in shaping their understanding of middle range theory and who assisted in the theory development process.

This is a theory that was developed inductively from specific to general and from concrete observation in the practice environment to theoretical ideas. That is, it had its beginnings at relatively narrow scope of a single symptom and is grounded in the reality of practice. Three of the theory developers—all with extensive clinical experience—had conducted dissertation research regarding a specific symptom: Gift studied dyspnea, and Milligan and Pugh studied fatigue. When their initial studies about individual symptoms were carried out, they had no intention of developing a theory. The opportunity to do so evolved over time, as they began to realize that their work on individual symptoms represented concept development activity. It became apparent— as they continued to identify and discuss the elements that were common across the experience of dyspnea and fatigue in both ill and healthy populations—that their thinking was moving to the level of middle range theory.

The initial collaboration took place between Pugh and Milligan, each of whom was studying the symptom of fatigue during a different phase of the perinatal experience. Pugh (1990) studied correlates of fatigue during labor and delivery. Milligan (1989) had conducted qualitative and quantitative research about fatigue during the postpartum period and was also carrying out concept development and measurement studies (Milligan, Lenz, Parks, Pugh, & Kitzman, 1996). Pugh and Milligan (1993)—who were also engaged in clinical practice in labor and delivery and postpartum environments—combined their findings about the concept to develop a framework for the study of fatigue during childbearing. Milligan's inductive analysis of fatigue during the postpartum period included clinical observations, interviews with postpartum mothers, and data from a quantitative measure of fatigue. Her work pointed out the importance of differentiating fatigue from related concepts, such as depression, and the desirability of differentiating different types of fatigue. From Pugh's deductive work—which was based on existing models of fatigue—came the identification of physiological, psychological, and situational factors that influence fatigue during labor, and the recognition that fatigue is a multidimensional phenomenon. Pugh and Milligan (1995) recognized commonalities in their conceptualizations of and findings about fatigue at different stages in the childbearing process, developing a framework that they then tested in a longitudinal study of pregnant women. Examples of the commonalities include the cumulative nature of the symptom experience and the importance of energy depletion. The framework that emerged from this collaboration incorporated a nursing diagnosis–based definition of fatigue and the results of empirical studies of fatigue from other disciplines, as well as theoretical models developed within nursing to explain fatigue in childbearing situations.

The second collaboration took place when Pugh began to discuss the model of fatigue with Gift (Gift, 1990; Gift & Cahill, 1990), who had conducted multiple studies of dyspnea in patients with chronic obstructive pulmonary disease (COPD) and asthma. They realized that their conceptualizations were similar and discovered a number of commonalities between two symptoms. They developed a model combining elements of their previous work that was meant to be equally applicable to dyspnea and fatigue (Gift & Pugh, 1993).

Gift had carried out Wilsonian concept development activities, which clarified the nature and measurement of dyspnea as a subjective phenomenon. She used pain as an analog to develop a model depicting dyspnea with physiological and psychological components and as variable in intensity, duration, and the degree of distress experienced. Her conceptualization bore similarities to Pugh and Milligan's framework for studying fatigue; for example, the respective symptom having both acute and chronic manifestations, being influenced by the same categories of factors, and affecting performance or functional ability.

Having developed the multiple-concept dyspnea/fatigue model, which was also potentially applicable to pain, the investigators went on to reason that they could develop a more generic theory that was at an even higher level of abstraction and could be extended to encompass additional symptoms. Lenz had expertise in model and theory development, was familiar with the work of all three researchers, and had offered ongoing critique of their work. Collaboratively they decided to develop a middle range theory and began to meet regularly. Discussions revolved around resolving differences in the models for individual symptoms and agreeing on the elements of a more inclusive theory. The resulting TOUS was introduced and described briefly in an article advocating the development of middle range theories to guide nursing practice (Lenz, Suppe, Gift, Pugh, & Milligan, 1995). The call for papers about middle range nursing theory by *Advances in Nursing Science* (*ANS*) served as an important stimulus to this theory development activity.

The TOUS generated considerable interest in the nursing academic community, as indicated by correspondence received by the authors, much of which came from graduate students who sought clinically relevant theories on which to base their research. Its publication and more general exposure also pointed out some weaknesses of the theory and some aspects that were unclear. As a result, the authors continued to work on refining it, and an updated, improved version was subsequently published (Lenz, Pugh, Mulligan, Gift, & Suppe, 1997). Again, the prospect of an opportunity to publish the refinements in *ANS* served to stimulate the revision.

In considering the process by which the TOUS was developed, several observations are pertinent. First, it was not preplanned but occurred spontaneously, stimulated by shared interests and the opportunity for frequent communication. Proximity that allowed face-to-face meetings, a common background in philosophy and interest in theory development acquired during doctoral study, a tradition of scholarly and collegial interchange, and the ability to take the time required to debate difficult conceptual issues facilitated the collaborative efforts at all stages. Such elements have been identified as important in building communities of scholars (Parse, 2005; Roy, 2005). Second, forward movement on the development of the theory has tended to occur in spurts of activity, undertaken in response to external stimuli, primarily publication opportunities, and explicit critiques. This seems to underscore the importance of nursing journal editors' willingness to publish the results of theoretical work and empirical research findings. It also reaffirms the value of scholarly dialogue and debate of ideas. Third, the development of the theory occurred in an inductive fashion, which contributed to its practice relevance. At every step, concept analysis and clarification were grounded in nursing practice and in practice-related research. The theory was not conceived from armchair musings but was based on real-world observations and attempts to study and solve problems encountered in practice. With time, the salience of symptoms and their management, and corresponding interest in and use of the theory, has mushroomed.

CONCEPTS OF THE THEORY

The TOUS has three major concepts: the symptom(s), influencing factors, and performance outcomes. The overall structure of the theory, which is portrayed in Figure 8.1, asserts that three interrelated categories of factors (physiological, psychological, and situational) influence predisposition to and manifestation of a given symptom or multiple symptoms and the nature of the symptom experience. The symptom experience, in turn, affects the individual's performance, which encompasses cognitive, physical, and social functioning. The performance outcomes can feed back to influence the symptom experience itself, as well as to modify the influencing factors. Literature supporting the structure of the theory was cited in the published descriptions of the original theory (Lenz et al., 1995) and the updated version (Lenz et al., 1997) and is also incorporated below in the description of the theory components.

Symptoms

Symptoms were the starting point for conceptualizing the theory, hence should be considered to be the central concept. Thus far, the

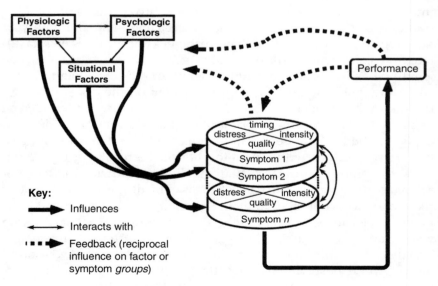

FIGURE 8.1   Unpleasant Symptoms
Source: Reprinted with permission from Lenz, E. R., Pugh, L.C., Milligan, R. A., Gift, A. G., & Suppe, F. (1997). The middle-range theory of unpleasant symptoms: An update. *Advances in Nursing Science, 19*(3), 17.

TOUS has focused on subjectively perceived symptoms rather than objectively observable signs. However, Kim et al. (2005) argued in their discussion of "symptom clusters" that the term—by definition including multiple symptoms and often signs, and by extension including theories that address them—should be broad enough to include both self-reported symptoms and objective, observed signs. For purposes of the TOUS, symptoms are defined subjectively as "the perceived indicators of change in normal functioning as experienced by patients" (Rhodes & Watson, 1987, p. 242). Most but not all symptoms are experienced as unpleasant sensations. The perception-based definition assumes awareness by the individual and that the nature of a symptom can only be truly known and described by the individual experiencing it. The implication of this stance is that measurement of the theory's component concepts must be subjective. The extent to which objectively observable signs can be explained by the theory warrants systematic attention. Such exploration hypothetically would expand the applicability of the theory, particularly in light of the reality that many expressions of the symptom experience are nonverbal and very easily observed by others. Examples include the grimace of an individual experiencing pain, the shrill cry of an infant receiving an injection or the observable act of vomiting.

The TOUS asserts that symptoms can occur either in isolation—one at a time—or in combination and potentially in interaction with other symptoms. Although the term is not used in the TOUS and the model does not depict clusters in the usual way, the TOUS has been recognized to be one of the few generic theories of the symptom experience to address and visually depict multiple symptoms experienced simultaneously (Brant, Beck, & Miaskowski, 2009; Jurgens et al., 2009). Currently, the concept of symptom cluster is being given considerable attention in the literature regarding cancer and other chronic illnesses (Armstrong, Cohen, Eriksen, & H. Kim et al., 2005; Hickey, 2004; Barsevick, Dudley, & Beck, 2006; Chen et al., 2011; Chow & Merrick, 2010; Dodd, Miaskowski, & Lee, 2004; Fox & Lyon, 2006; Jurgens et al., 2009; Lang et al., 2006; Miaskowski, Dodd, & Lee, 2004; Motl et al., 2009; Motl, Suh, & Weikert, 2010; Motl, Weikert, Suh, & Dlugonski, 2010).

In some situations, one symptom may precede and possibly give rise to another. For example, extreme fatigue may precipitate episodes of nausea and vertigo. When more than one symptom is experienced at the same time, or even cumulatively as total symptom burden (a related concept (Abbott, Baranson, & Zimmerman, 2010; Farrell & Savage, 2010), the net effect can be stunning, often more powerful than a sum of the separate symptoms would suggest (Motl, McAuely, Wynn et al., 2010; Wilmoth, Coleman, Smith, & Davis, 2004). For example, when pain is accompanied by one or more other symptoms, such as fatigue and nausea, it tends to be perceived as considerably worse than when it occurs alone, suggesting that a synergistic, possibly multiplicative, relationship may exist. On the other hand, Motl, Weikert, Sueh, & Diugonski (2010) found that a cluster of three symptoms and a cluster of five symptoms related to comparable strength with physical activity in persons with relapsing–remitting multiple sclerosis, suggesting that the addition of two more symptoms to the cluster of fatigue, that is, depression and pain, made little difference in the magnitude of the cluster's effect on the performance outcome. Different levels of pain can also moderate the relationship of fatigue with psychological variables. For example, Francoeur (2005) found several interactions among symptoms in a study of 268 cancer patients with recurrent disease, including the interaction of pain with fever, fatigue, and weight loss in predicting depressive affect.

In the TOUS, symptoms are conceptualized as manifesting multiple variable and measurable dimensions. It is asserted that all symptoms vary in intensity or severity, degree of associated distress, timing, and quality. These dimensions are also related to one another (Jurgens et al., 2009). Intensity is the dimension that quantifies the degree, strength, or severity of the symptom and is the most frequently measured aspect of the symptom experience. It is part of the routine assessment of postsurgical patients to ask them to express the intensity or severity of their pain in numeric terms or on a visual analog scale. Intensity is often the simplest characteristic for patients to rate. In pediatric practice, nonnumeric measures of pain are used to capture children's ratings of its intensity (e.g., the faces pain scale).

The distress dimension reflects an affective aspect of the symptom experience in that it refers to the degree to which the individual experiencing the symptom is bothered by it. Kugler et al. (2008) defined symptom distress as the emotional burden caused by the symptom. Because of differences in pain threshold levels and cultural expectations, for example, individuals exposed to the same intensity of pain-inducing stimuli can experience very different levels of distress. Generally the degree of distress experienced with a symptom is related to its intensity; however, it can also be influenced by other considerations. Distress can be affected by the degree of focused attention that the individual directs toward the symptom. Symptom management strategies designed to lessen distress include diverting attention from the symptom. For example, the breathing techniques during childbirth help divert attention from pain, or introduction of another stimulus can compete with pain for the individual's attention. One of the most important influences on the degree of distress that is associated with a given symptom is the meaning that the individual attaches to the symptom. For example, a woman who has been treated for infertility may perceive nausea associated with pregnancy as a very welcome symptom and not be bothered by it, whereas a cancer patient could perceive considerable distress associated with chemotherapy-induced nausea of the same severity because of its potentially negative connotations. Armstrong (2003), in her concept analysis-based model of the symptom experience, included meaning as a dimension that is separate from, and additional to, distress (Armstrong, Cohen, Eriksen, & Hickey, 2004). She determined that meaning is an important dimension to consider when the emotional consequences of the symptom experience are being examined.

The time dimension includes the way symptoms vary in duration, frequency, and pattern of occurrence. Duration is the length of time that a symptom continues; thus, it highlights the importance of the patient's experiential history. It is common to differentiate acute from chronic symptom experiences because they tend to be different in nature and to be treated differently. They also may hold very different meaning for the individual experiencing them. Chronic symptoms may be particularly distress producing; moreover, the approaches to managing a symptom often change with duration. Strategies that are appropriate for acute pain, for example, are not necessarily useful in treating chronic pain. The dimension of time also takes into account the frequency or rapidity with which symptoms occur and also the pattern with which they vary over time or recur. For example, symptoms that are intermittent can vary in regularity and periodicity. Likewise, persistent symptoms can vary in intensity over time (Chen, Li, Shieh, Yin, & Chiou, 2010). Nausea that occurs every morning for 3 hours during the first trimester of pregnancy can be described, and hence measured, along several time-related dimensions. The importance of time as a dimension of the symptom experience was emphasized by Henley, Kallas, Klatt, and Swenson (2003) in their Symptom Experience in Time model, which underscores the importance of examining intraindividual change over time. They also expanded the notion of the time dimension, arguing that the analysis of time-related symptom patterns should take into consideration perceived, biological/social, and clock/calendar conceptions of time. They described the impact of time on the meaning the individual attaches to the symptom by virtue of its effect on the individual's self-evaluation of the symptom experience and emotional response to it. In the TOUS, this would suggest considering the impact of symptom timing on the extent of distress in the symptom experience, demonstrating the relatedness of the four-variable symptom dimensions identified in the theory.

The final dimension of the symptom experience incorporated in the TOUS is the quality of the symptom. This dimension refers to the nature of the symptom or the way in which it is manifested or experienced, that is, what it feels like to have the symptom. By including this dimension, the TOUS acknowledges that in addition to reflecting characteristics that are common across all symptoms, each symptom has unique characteristics. The descriptors that best characterize each symptom are highly specific. For example, pain is often characterized by the nature of the sensation, such as stinging, burning, stabbing, pounding, and so forth, and by its location. Changes in the nature of the pain may signal changes in disease progression; hence, they are incorporated in many of the widely used symptom-specific measures. Dyspnea can be characterized by the way the shortness of breath feels to the individual, for example, tight versus suffocating. These descriptors are important because they differ systematically from one disease state or stage of progression to another and may provide valuable clues to assessment and effective symptom management.

Describing and measuring the quality of specific symptoms (and symptom clusters) depends on the patient's ability to articulate what he or she is experiencing. Individuals differ in the descriptors that they use and also in their ability to communicate. Qualitative research with a variety of patient populations is often valuable in describing the quality of the symptom experience (Wilmoth, Hatmaker-Flannigan, LaLoggia, & Nixon, 2011). Qualitative methods are frequently appropriate in the early phases of a study to identify descriptors, which are then used as the basis for the subsequent development of quantitative measures (Lang et al., 2006; Waltz, Strickland, & Lenz, 2010). They are also useful in helping to analyze whether two different terms that are often used interchangeably actually name the same concept or two different concepts (Milligan et al., 1996). The measurement of the symptom(s) would be more descriptive when all four characteristics are included. However, measuring one, two, or three characteristics is valid and informative for health care providers in managing the symptom(s).

Influencing Factors

Three categories of factors that influence the symptom experience (and can, in turn, be influenced by it and by one another) are identified in the TOUS: physiological factors, psychological factors, and situational factors. The specific factors that are most relevant in influencing a given symptom may be different from those that are most influential

for another. The combination and/or interaction of multiple influencing factors can impact the symptom experience differently from any
given influencing factor alone. For example, the combination of a late-
stage illness (physiological), depressive mood (psychological), and lack
of social support (situational) is likely to result in a more intense and
distressing symptom experience than one or even two of these factors
alone.

Physiological Factors

Physiological factors include anatomical/structural, physiological,
genetic, illness-related, and treatment-related variables. Examples of
variables in this category include the presence of structural anoma-
lies, existence of pathology or disease states including comorbidities,
stage and duration of illness, inflammation due to infection or trauma,
fluctuations in hormonal or energy levels, adequacy of hydration and
nutrition, level of consciousness, genetic makeup, race/ethnicity, age,
developmental stage, and type and duration of treatment. All may
influence the occurrence of a symptom and how it is experienced. The
interplay among different physiologic influencing factors can be quite
complex, as is pointed out in the many studies of symptom clusters.
For example, see the study of symptom clusters in heart failure by
Jurgens et al. (2009) and the concept analysis of symptom clusters in
cancer populations by Kim et al. (2005). Breastfeeding mothers' experiences of fatigue are influenced by many physiologic factors, including the duration of labor, type of delivery, level of hydration, time
since delivery, hormonal changes, maternal age, presence of infection, and the amount and quality of sleep (Pugh & Milligan, 1998).
Lifestyle behaviors such as exercise, diet, and smoking can impact
the symptom experience. In addition, treatments often give rise to
unpleasant symptoms; the classic examples are cancer chemotherapy
and radiation. Many medications used to treat illnesses or to prevent
complications (e.g., immunosuppressant drugs following transplant
surgery) produce side effects that are experienced as unpleasant
symptoms (Francoeur, 2005; Kiser, Greer, Wilomtoh, Dmochowski, &
Naumann, 2010; Kugler et al., 2009; Lester & Bernhard, 2009; Wilmoth
et al., 2004).

Symptoms are often the indicators that pathology exists and is
either worsening or improving, but the relationship is not necessarily straightforward or simple. Jurgens et al. (2009) pointed out
complications that advanced age may impose on individuals' perceptions and interpretations of the symptom experience. They provided the example that heart failure patients experiencing dyspnea

associated with that diagnosis may be unable to differentiate it from dyspnea associated with comorbid conditions. As a result, they may ignore symptom changes indicating worsening of heart failure and delay seeking advice or initiating self-help measures, ultimately leading to further deterioration in their condition. This example demonstrates that there is a reciprocal relationship between physiologic factors and symptoms and that age, one of the physiological factors, can moderate that relationship.

Psychological Factors

Psychological factors represent one of the more complex components of the model. They include both affective and cognitive variables. The individual's affective state or mood (e.g., level of anxiety, depression, or anger) during or preceding the time of the symptom experience—even if unrelated to the symptom—and the emotional response to the illness or the symptom itself can serve to intensify the symptom (Chen et al., 2010; Duncan, Bott, Thompson, & Gajewski, 2009; Song, Chang, Park, Kim, & Nam, 2010). Cognitive variables that may impact the symptom experience include the degree of uncertainty surrounding it, the individual's level of knowledge about the illness or the symptom, the meaning of the symptom experience to the individual, and his or her repertoire of cognitive coping skills and perceived availability of coping resources. As psychobiological research underscores the physiological basis for mood, it becomes increasingly evident that the psychological and physiological factors impacting the symptom experience may be difficult to separate.

Situational Factors

The third category of influencing factors is situational. It encompasses the individual's environment, both social and physical. For instance, the experience of symptoms can vary by culture because there is a learned component to interpreting and expressing symptoms (Spector, 2000). Other situational factors that can influence the experience of symptoms include those that are associated with the individual's experiential background and access to resources, including the availability of financial, emotional, and instrumental help in dealing with the symptom. Examples are socioeconomic status, marital and family status, occupation, demands of work or family, access to social support, access to health care, and adequacy of health care and support provided. Alternatively, social support can be considered a psychological influencing factor, if it is conceptualized (and measured) to reflect the individual's perception about the potential availability of support, rather than as a situational factor reflecting the level of support that is actually available and/or received. The characteristics of the setting in which the individual is receiving care—whether it be an institution (e.g., policies and procedures, staffing levels) or home (e.g., equipment available, caregiver knowledge and skill)—may also be important situational considerations. The physical environment can also influence symptoms; it includes altitude, temperature, humidity, noise level, light, and presence of pollutants or irritants in the air or water. The situational factors are contextual, that is, external to the individual.

Performance Outcomes

The outcome concept in the TOUS is performance. It represents the consequences of the symptom experience. Simply stated, the theory asserts that the experience of symptoms can have an impact on the individual's ability to function or perform physically, cognitively, and in socially defined roles. In a study of elderly cancer patients receiving chemotherapy or radiotherapy, Cheng and Lee (2011) found that the symptom cluster of pain, fatigue, insomnia, and mood disturbance had a persistent effect on functional status and quality of life (QOL), even with the influence of age, gender, comorbidity, stage of illness, and treatment modality controlled. Similarly, Laird et al. (2011) found that the three-symptom cluster of pain, depression, and fatigue had a strong relationship to physical functioning of patients with advanced cancer. Similarly, Motl and McAuley (2009) found the same cluster to have a strong, negative relationship to physical activity in patients with multiple sclerosis. They found that physical limitations (a physiological influencing factor) accounted for this relationship. Role performance addresses the ability to carry out personal care and social roles, including activities of daily living and employment-related roles. Cognitive performance includes memory, comprehension, learning, concentration, and problem solving. Inclusion of performance as the key outcome of the model reflects a pragmatic orientation and a desire for relatively straightforward measurability. It is also consistent with generation of the theory from practice-based observations in maternal–infant and adult health nursing domains.

A given symptom or set of symptoms may generate a number of different performance outcomes that may occur simultaneously but also can be time ordered. Performance outcomes that are proximal in time to the symptom experience can influence more distal outcomes, particularly if the symptom is sustained for a period of time. An example would be a person with COPD who suffers from extreme dyspnea. The symptom interferes with the ability to walk uphill, climb steps, and carry groceries. As a result of these more proximal functional limitations in performance, the more distal performance outcomes might be the inability to carry out the demands of a job or being required to move to an assisted living arrangement. Another example would be that denying nicotine to smokers who are admitted to intensive care settings can result in a number of unpleasant symptoms of nicotine withdrawal that can affect cognitive functioning (e.g., delirium) and, in turn, result in increased length of hospital stay (Ely et al., 2001, 2004).

The TOUS does not explicitly include QOL as an outcome, in part because of the high degree of overlap with functional status in many QOL measures. Evidence that symptoms influence not only the physical but also the affective aspects of QOL (Dabbs et al., 2003; Fox & Lyon, 2007; Jurgens et al., 2009; Motl, Sue, & Weikert, 2010; Motl, Weikert, Suh, & Dlugonski, 2010) and that mood may both impact and be impacted by symptoms (Clayton, Mishel, & Belyea, 2006; Kugler et al., 2009) suggests the need to consider adding affective outcomes and/or QOL to the TOUS. The latter, albeit defined in many different ways, is frequently investigated as an outcome in symptom research and is included in several existing and proposed models of symptom management (Brant et al., 2009). In addition, some of the critiques of the TOUS have noted that failure to include QOL as an explicit outcome is a weakness (Brant et al., 2009). Currently, the influence of symptoms on affective variables is addressed in the TOUS by the feedback loop from the symptom experience to psychological factors, rather than an explicit outcome.

RELATIONSHIPS AMONG CONCEPTS: THE MODEL

The relationships among the major concepts of the TOUS are depicted as lines in Figure 8.1. In the original version of the theory, simplifying assumptions were made, and the relationships between the influencing factors and the symptom experience and between the symptom experience and performance were depicted as unidirectional. The revised version of the TOUS (Figure 8.1) acknowledges the complexity of the symptom experience by depicting the relationships among the three major components as reciprocal. That is, the influencing factors are assumed to impact the nature of the symptom experience, which, in turn, impacts performance. However, experiencing symptoms can also change the patient's psychological, physiological, and/or situational status. For example, experiencing the symptoms of severe pain and fatigue can negatively impact one's mood state (a psychological influencing factor) (Francoeur, 2005). Clayton et al. (2006) found that symptom bother (similar to the dimension of symptom distress) was related to mood state both directly and indirectly, with the relationship mediated by uncertainty. Likewise, performance can have a reciprocal relationship to the experience of unpleasant symptoms. For example, the experience of the multiple unpleasant symptoms stemming from use of some immunosuppressive drugs was associated with increased nonadherence to the medication regimen, which, in turn, worsened other symptoms and ultimately increased the probability of organ rejection following solid organ transplantation (Kugler et al., 2009). In a study of breast cancer patients receiving chemotherapy postoperatively, Yang, Tsai, Huang, and Lin (2011) found that an experimental group of patients who participated in a moderate-intensity, home-based walking program (physical performance) reported lower symptom severity and mood disturbance than those in the control group throughout the 12-week follow-up period.

The symptom experience can serve as a mediating or moderating variable between influencing factors and performance. A mediating relationship might be exemplified by the finding (Clayton et al., 2006) that symptoms among breast cancer survivors are a mediating variable in the relationship of age to well-being, measured by mood state and troublesome thoughts about recurrence. A mediating relationship was found by Woods, Kozachik, and Hall (2010) among women experiencing intimate partner violence; stress symptoms mediated the relationships between childhood maltreatment and sleep quality and disruptive nighttime behaviors. On the other hand, Redeker, Lev, and Ruggiero (2000) did not find fatigue and insomnia to be important mediators between psychological factors and QOL. Lee, Chung, Park, and Chun (2004) found that among Korean women with breast cancer, social support was a moderator of the relationship of mood disturbance to symptoms, such that mood disturbances were related more strongly to symptoms when social support was low than when it was high.

The most recent version of the TOUS also asserts that performance can have a feedback effect on the physiologic, psychological, and situational factors. A breast cancer patient's severe pain (symptom) can impair the desire to interact with others, hence decrease or increase the frequency of social interaction (performance). Decreased interaction with others in the social network can result not only in decreased network size as others withdraw from the network, but also in a reduction in the social support available and received from the network (situational influencing factors). Another example was provided by Kugler et al.'s (2009) compilation of findings related to the severity and distress of the symptom experience in persons undergoing solid organ transplantation.

The three categories of influencing factors are hypothesized to influence one another and to interact in their relation to the symptom experience. That is, physiological complications of surgery can interact with a patient's anxiety or depression to create more severe pain than would be experienced had the psychological factors not been operating as strongly. A common finding is that in persons with chronic illnesses, psychological factors, such as depression, anxiety, and uncertainty, mediate the relationships of physiological or situational factors to symptoms (Clayton et al., 2009). There is a positive impact of social support in mitigating the negative impact of physical illness or stress on the severity of symptoms, as found in the study by Yang et al. (2011), exemplifying the interaction of situational factors with physiological and psychological factors in their relationships to the symptoms.

The three influential factor categories are quite broad, encompassing many potential variables that can be measured in many different ways. Any given study can tap only a few of those variables and measures. Therefore, it is unlikely that all of the variables within an influential factor category will relate in the same way or with equal strength to the symptoms. It is also possible that the variables within a category relate to others in the same category in ways that mediate or moderate their effects. An example is that among postpartum women; the effects of childcare stress on postpartum fatigue were mediated by postpartum depression (Song et al., 2010).

The TOUS hypothesizes that when patients experience more than one symptom, the symptom experiences are related to one another. This hypothesis has been supported by multiple studies (Jurgens et al., 2009; Tyler & Pugh, 2009; Motl, Weikert, Suh, & Diugonski, 2010). The relationships among symptoms experienced simultaneously can be interactive, including multiplicative. That is, the experience of a given unpleasant symptom, such as pain, is exacerbated or fundamentally changed in other ways when it occurs simultaneously with another symptom, such as nausea. It is likely that the cumulative effect of multiple symptoms on function is greater than the sum of the individual symptoms; however, this conjecture has not been subjected to thorough and systematic empirical testing and is not necessarily a straightforward conclusion. For example, Fox and Lyon (2006) found in a small sample of lung cancer survivors that fatigue and dyspnea were highly correlated; the cluster of the two symptoms explained 29% of the variance in QOL; however, when the impact of each symptom in the cluster was compared, dyspnea wielded the much greater explanatory power than fatigue. Motl, McAuley, Wynn, et al. (2010) predicted that the more numerous the symptoms in a cluster, the stronger the relationship of the cluster to the outcome of physical performance among persons with multiple sclerosis. However, they found that a three-symptom cluster (fatigue, pain, and depression) had a stronger relationship to physical activity than a five-symptom cluster that also included poor sleep quality and perceived cognitive dysfunction.

USE OF THE THEORY IN RESEARCH

An increasing number of investigators are using the TOUS as the conceptual framework on which to base their studies. Other authors have cited it as a middle range theory that effectively highlights important aspects of a phenomenon for examination (Barsevick, Whitmore, Nail, Beck, & Dudley, 2006) or is consistent with the conceptualization used in or findings of a symptom-related study (Kugler et al., 2009; Franck et al., 2004). The TOUS has also been used as the basis for instrument development (Kim, Oh, & Lee, 2006; Kim, Oh, Lee, Kim, & Han, 2006; Lester, Bernhard, & Ryan-Wenger, 2012), for analyzing a concept (Farrell & Savage, 2010), or developing a more elaborate or more specific theory about one or more symptoms (Dabbs et al., 2004; Dodd et al., 2001; Henley et al., 2003; Song et al., 2010). Clinical populations in which it has been applied in research include cancer survivors and cancer patients undergoing treatment, persons who have experienced a myocardial infarction or heart failure, patients with mitral valve prolapse syndrome, patients with liver cirrhosis, those with renal failure who are on hemodialysis, stroke patients, persons with COPD, victims of intimate partner violence, and pregnant, postpartum, and breastfeeding women and their partners. The most frequent use has been in studies of persons with cancer and cancer survivors. A number of the studies based on the TOUS have been carried out in locations outside of the United States in Korea, Hong Kong, Mainland China, and Taiwan. It should be noted that the theory is also being used as the theoretical framework guiding research in other fields, such as kinesiology (Motl, McAuley, Wynn, et al. 2010). The TOUS authors continue to receive multiple inquiries from master's and doctoral students and faculty who have found the theory to be extremely relevant to the phenomena they are studying, and either plan to use or are already using it as the theoretical framework for their research.

A review of the published research based on the TOUS has provided evidence to substantiate many of the conceptualizations and hypothesized relationships in the theory. Some examples of assertions in the TOUS that have been supported empirically are described below.

1. One of the most frequently validated assertions is that the symptom experience is individualized and highly variable (Higgins, 1998). The TOUS delineation of variable dimensions of symptoms has been very useful and has been validated empirically (Jurgens et al., 2009; Liu, 2006; Kapella, Larson, Patel, Covey, & Berry, 2006; Kim et al., 2006). Most commonly measured dimensions are intensity, distress, frequency, and duration. All of these dimensions have been measured successfully and their importance as predictors of outcomes substantiated. They have been found to vary independently; for example, a symptom that occurs infrequently can be very intense and distressing (Kim et al., 2006). Quality has been studied less often than the others, but when studied qualitatively, has yielded descriptors of the symptom experience that may be helpful in differentiating different types or stages of illness and/or have proven useful for incorporation in quantitative measures (Lang et al, 2006; Parshall et al., 2001; Liu, 2006). As noted earlier, the meaning of the symptom(s) has been included in some models as an additional dimension of the symptom experience to examine (Armstrong, 2001). The TOUS incorporates meaning in the distress dimension. In an interesting departure from the TOUS model, Chen et al. (2010) identified a concept they termed symptomatic distress and conceptualized it to be categorized as a physiologic factor, rather than as a measure of the distress dimension of the symptom experience. The instrument they developed to measure the concept asked subjects to indicate the level of distress associated with each of the symptoms (from a checklist) they had experienced in the previous week. The investigators found symptomatic distress to be the strongest predictor of fatigue, which is the target symptom for their research. Regarding the dimension of time, Henley et al. (2003) have provided evidence of the complex nature of time in the symptom experience and included time as the key component of their theory, which they identify as an extension of the TOUS. The relatedness of time with the other dimensions of the symptom experience has been demonstrated, for example, by Duncan et al. (2009) and by Tzeng, Teng, Chou, and Tu (2009).

2. The revised version of the TOUS (Lenz et al., 1997) embodies the assertion that multiple symptoms can occur concurrently. As noted earlier, the current literature is replete with studies validating the existence of symptom clusters, which are defined in various ways in different disciplines, but all of which share the idea that the symptoms co-occur (Kim et al., 2005). The current literature documents that in many illness- or stress-related situations, multiple symptoms are experienced simultaneously (Barsevick, Dudley, & Beck, 2006; Jurgens et al., 2009). For example, cancer patients with solid tumors experience an average of 11 to 13 symptoms concurrently (Armstrong et al., 2004), and patients who had undergone lung or heart–lung transplantations experienced as many as 29 symptoms (Dabbs et al., 2003). Gift, Jablonski, Stommel, and Given (2004) found that fatigue, nausea, weakness, appetite and weight loss, altered taste, and vomiting formed a persistent cluster in elderly lung cancer patients. Lang et al. (2006) found that 62% of a sample of people living with chronic hepatitis C infection reported symptom clustering. The TOUS does not depict symptoms as grape-like clusters, but rather as occurring simultaneously, so in that sense, it is consistent with but differs somewhat from some definitions and depictions of symptom clusters. For example, Kim et al. (2005) stated that symptom clusters are "… composed of stable groups of symptoms, are relatively independent of other clusters, and may reveal specific underlying dimensions of symptoms" (p. 270).

   The assertion that symptoms tend to occur in clusters is viewed as a critical consideration in conceptualizing the symptom experience (Dodd et al., 2001; Kim et al., 2005). However, when a number of symptoms are experienced simultaneously, they may not all impact outcomes to the same degree. Instead, one symptom may emerge as the most important predictor, explaining a much higher proportion of the variance in outcomes than any of the others in the cluster (e.g., Reishtein, 2004). There can also be a pattern wherein symptoms occur in a sequence in which one symptom can impact other symptoms (Carpenter et al., 2004; Hutchinson & Wilson, 1998).

3. The three categories of influencing factors (physiological, psychological, and situational) varied in their importance as predictors or correlates of the symptom experience from one study to another. In some studies, a given category of factors was not related to the symptom experience; for example, situational factors, such as nursing home facility characteristics and staffing,

were not related to symptoms in the study by Duncan et al. (2009). However, such patterns are not consistent, and there is considerable evidence that all three categories are meaningful in explaining the symptom experience.

The inconsistency can be attributed, at least in part, to the specific variables chosen as indicators of the category and other methodological considerations, such as sample size and instrumentation. For example, a given concept (e.g., insomnia or poor sleep quality) in some studies is set forth as a symptom and in others as a situational factor (Barsevick, 2007; Kapella et al., 2006; Pugh, Milligan, and Lenz, 2000). Liu (2006) categorized age and gender, and Carpenter et al. (2004) categorized night-time hot flashes as situational variables; however, in the TOUS, these are included in the physiological factors category. Oh, Kim, Lee, and Kim (2004) categorized dyspnea as a physiological factor impacting the symptom of fatigue, whereas in most studies, it is considered to be a symptom. Corwin, Brownstead, Barton, Heckar, and Morin (2005) pointed out the desirability of differentiating stable from variable predictors. Stable predictors (such as psychological traits and many social environmental variables) are difficult to change and hence are less amenable to intervention than dynamic predictors.

4. The category of influencing factors that was most often documented to be associated with the symptom experience was psychological factors. Common findings, for example, were the strong association of depression with symptoms such as fatigue and dyspnea (Corwin et al., 2005; Chen et al., 2010; Motl, McAuley, Wynn, et al., 2010; Song et al., 2010), and the emergence of psychological factors as more important predictors than physiological factors in some studies (Kapella et al., 2006; Lee et al., 2010). Some issues remain to be clarified regarding the conceptualization and measurement of some of the frequently studied psychological factors, particularly depression. For example, fatigue is often included as an item on measures of depression; therefore, it is hardly surprising that the two variables have been found to be related quite strongly. Hutchinson and Wilson (1998) found that the boundaries of the three influencing factor categories in the TOUS and symptom consequences/performance outcomes to be blurred and sometimes overlapping. For example, the psychological factor component of the model (anxiety, memory loss, and depression) was difficult to differentiate from some of the symptoms themselves. They concluded that the components of

the TOUS are not necessarily mutually exclusive when applied to patients with Alzheimer's disease but are better conceptualized as fluid and possibly interchangeable depending on the context in which they occur. Redeker et al. (2000) also noted that the redundancy among measures of psychological factors, symptoms, and QOL can obscure the nature of the relationships among the TOUS components.

5. In the revised version of the TOUS, relationships among the components of the model were hypothesized to be reciprocal and potentially involve complex interactions. This assertion that the interplay among symptoms is often very complex has been substantiated (Corwin et al., 2005; Dabbs et al., 2003).

6. The outcome of interest in the TOUS is performance, conceptualized to include physical, cognitive, and social functioning. This conceptualization has been criticized as too limited (Brant et al., 2009; Dodd et al., 2001; Henely et al., 2003). The most commonly studied outcome to date has been functional performance or functional status, measured by either disease specific or general instruments. Other outcomes have included performance in occupational and caregiving roles (Scordo, 2005; Tyler & Pugh, 2009), care-seeking patterns (Jurgens, 2006; Liu, 2006), use of health resources (Scordo, 2005), health concerns (Scordo, 2005), and death/survival (Franck et al., 2004; Lee et al., 2009). Virtually all the studies that included performance outcomes revealed relationships with symptoms. An exception is the finding by Michael, Allen, and Macko (2006) that fatigue in a sample of community-dwelling subjects with chronic hemiparetic stroke was not related to ambulatory activity.

USE OF THE THEORY IN NURSING PRACTICE

To date there remains limited published evidence of the application of the TOUS in clinical practice; however, there have been several studies that have tested clinical interventions. For example, Pugh and Milligan (1995, 1998) conducted several experimental studies to test a positioning intervention, based on the TOUS, to minimize fatigue in nursing mothers because fatigue was found to be a major barrier to breastfeeding success (Milligan, Flenniken, & Pugh, 1996). The multifaceted intervention included discussions of diet and exercise, the need for sleep and rest, ways to build the mothers' self-esteem, use of social support, comfort measures such as warm compresses, and use of side-lying position while breastfeeding to conserve energy. Therefore, the intervention addressed all three TOUS categories of influential factors. It was found to be effective, in that the experimental group of mothers had lower fatigue at 14 days postpartum and sustained breastfeeding for an average of 6 weeks longer than the control group mothers. In several additional studies, similar results were found (Pugh, Milligan, & Brown, 2001; Pugh, Milligan, Frick, Spatz, & Bronner, 2002; Pugh et al., 2010).

A majority of investigators who have based their research on the TOUS have addressed the practice implications. Virtually all the studies emphasize the importance of assessing the occurrence of multiple symptoms simultaneously, because the pattern of symptom concurrence has been found across symptoms and clinical populations. They also stress the importance of routinely assessing multiple dimensions of the symptom experience. For example, the findings by Parshall et al. (2001) suggest the basis for a multifaceted assessment of dyspnea in heart failure patients, both in ambulatory care settings where these patients are managed on an ongoing basis and in emergency department settings when they seek care for dyspnea that has become particularly distressing. Such assessment can be used to identify ambulatory patients who are at risk for hospital admission, and ultimately to guide the design of interventions to decrease dyspnea and decrease hospitalization rates.

As expressed in the strategic plan of the NINR, symptom management is one of the most important problems addressed in today's clinical practice. It represents a domain that is squarely within—and perhaps even central to—nursing's practice domain. More specific models at lower levels of abstraction, such as the middle range Theory of Acute Pain Management (Good, 1998), the related middle range Theory of Pain: A Balance Between Analgesia and Side Effects (Good, 2013), or the middle range Theory of Chronotherapeutic Intervention for Postsurgical Pain Management (Auvil-Novak, 1997), can and should be applied in managing individual symptoms such as pain. Likewise more illness-specific theories and models that address multiple symptoms, such as the Model of the Symptom Experience of Acute Rejection After Lung Transplantation by Dabbs et al. (2004), and more inclusive middlerange theories make contributions to practice and may provide the advantage of a slightly different perspective than those that are highly specific. The revised Symptom Management Model (Dodd et al., 2001) is more explicit than the TOUS in addressing symptom management strategies. Brant et al. (2009) have made a plea for more explicit and expanded consideration of interventions in the symptom theories.

Although the TOUS does not explicitly include an intervention component, it does help highlight certain aspects of the symptom experience and potential strategies for symptom management that are not addressed by more symptom-specific models (Lenz, Gift, Pugh, & Milligan, 2013). For example, the TOUS stresses the importance of a multivariate assessment of the symptom experience and of possible influencing factors, and provides a rationale and framework for applying a biopsychosocial approach. It suggests that multiple management strategies may need to be applied simultaneously, given the multivariate nature of the factors influencing symptoms. It also underscores the importance of addressing the possibility of several symptom experiences occurring concurrently, because co-occurrence can affect the individual's perception of any one of the symptoms (Jurgens et al., 2009). The TOUS conceptualization also emphasizes the importance of considering the effect of co-occurrence on the patient's functioning. On the other hand, the TOUS does not address explicitly the many intervention-related concepts that Brant et al. (2009) recommend be included in theories that will help advance symptom management science; for example, self-care, self-efficacy, decision-making processes, change theory-related considerations.

According to Cooley (2000), the TOUS is valuable, because it "proposes a way to integrate information about the complexity and interactive nature of the symptom experience" (p. 146). Hutchinson and Wilson (1998) and Jurgens et al. (2009) also stressed the theory's encouragement of nurses to design interventions in a way that takes into account the multiple dimensions of symptoms and the interactive nature of symptoms, influencing factors, and consequences, thereby making them client specific. In its most recent version, the TOUS, with its emphasis on the interplay among the model's components, encourages creative thinking about new and different approaches to symptom management. Several clinicians have described it as having intuitive appeal because it is relatively straightforward, easy to understand and apply, and is focused on relevant concerns.

CONCLUSION

The TOUS, which was grounded in clinical research and practice, is a middle range theory that holds considerable promise as a basis for additional research and as a guide to nursing practice. Although it is one of the few recent middle range theories that has undergone revision based on empirical findings, the TOUS remains a work in progress. The updated version addresses several of the weaknesses of the original; however, we recognize that some aspects of the theory remain underdeveloped. Subsequent development has been piecemeal, undertaken in response to specific published critiques or applications of the theory. The authors are committed to continued development and publication of updates.

The changes that were made to the theory in the 1997 revision added to the complexity of the model but also made it more consistent with the reality that constitutes the symptom experience. The modifications have been validated in several ill (heart failure, cancer, COPD, end-stage renal failure, and solid organ transplant recipients) and well (breast-feeding mothers, pregnant women, and postpartum women) samples. Thus far the symptoms that have been described in these studies have included pain, dyspnea, nausea, vomiting, insomnia and other sleep problems, hot flashes, weakness, and fatigue. More research is needed in additional clinical populations and with additional symptoms.

The current research suggests that the symptom dimensions identified in the TOUS are both relevant and measurable; however, additional elaboration is warranted with regard to conceptualization and measurement, particularly the dimensions of quality and time. For example, it may be prudent to add abruptness of symptom onset. The theory needs to address explicitly the dynamics of the symptom experience, including the notions of possible recurrence (Brant et al., 2009; Henley et al., 2003).

The inclusion of multiple symptoms in the model introduces a number of areas of complexity that have not yet been addressed in detail; the sequence in which symptoms appear and the extent to which a given symptom tends to influence the appearance and characteristics of others is an example. The notion of primary and secondary symptoms should be included explicitly. For example, on the basis of their study of persons with multiple sclerosis, Motl, Suh, & Weikert (2010) noted that findings about the relative importance of individual symptoms within clusters in predicting outcomes have important practice implications. They suggested that targeting one symptom rather than several co-occurring symptoms may the most effective and efficient approach to improving outcomes. They recommend extending the TOUS "by examining pathways among multiple, co-occurring symptoms with performance outcomes" (p. 409).

Additional conceptual/theoretical work is needed to address several of the issues that have been pointed out by investigators who have used the theory. For example, a question exists as to whether the theory is relevant for both signs and symptoms. Likewise, its potential applicability to subjects or patients who have perceptual deficits or are unable to describe the symptom experience (e.g., infants, unconscious patients, or even the elderly) has been assumed by some investigators, but has not yet been explored fully. Another criticism of the theory is that some of the key components—specifically the antecedent influencing factors and the outcomes—need to be better defined and specific variables within the categories specified (Brant et al., 2009). The complex relationships among the three categories of influencing factors and the symptom experience need fuller elaboration and clarification.

Although the potential relevance of all three types of factors has been quite well supported, there are some inconsistencies that need to be examined. The most robust influential factors need to be identified and the nature of their complex relationships to the symptom experience explicated. Psychological influential factors have been found repeatedly to play a key role in exacerbating or mitigating symptoms; however, there is potential for conceptual and empirical overlap between psychological states (anxiety and depression in particular) and the affective or distress component of the symptom experience. There is also inconsistency as to whether mood states (anxiety, depression) are treated as symptoms themselves or as psychological influencing factors. The interplay between these two model components needs to be examined.

The performance component of the model needs additional development. Several of the investigations have revealed it to be more complex than originally thought. The notions of primary and secondary outcomes and temporally proximal and distal outcomes need to be incorporated in the model. Although the functional, pragmatic focus of the performance outcome was chosen purposefully, it does de-emphasize other, more inclusive outcomes that may be important consequences of the symptom experience. QOL, particularly the affective aspects thereof, is a prime example. Functioning is generally included as a component of QOL, but the latter is more inclusive. The possible place of QOL within the TOUS is a topic that needs to be explored conceptually and empirically.

Finally, more attention needs to be paid to symptom assessment and management. As noted earlier, the TOUS has many practice implications and recent findings suggest potentially useful interventions; however, these remain to be detailed and possible patterns discerned. The place of interventions as an explicit component of the model should be determined. Brant et al. (2009) set forth a considerable challenge in their recommendation that "future models and theories should depict the global concepts that define not only the symptom intervention but the healthcare interactions and the patient's physiological, psychological and sociocultural responses to the intervention" (p. 238). As was pointed out in the description of the process that was used to develop the TOUS, it has been and continues to be the product of exciting group interaction. Multiple practice-grounded observations, a growing body of literature documenting its application, and lively discussions with colleagues and students, have led to its continued development. Its richness can only increase as the developers continue to address the input of others who have used the theory in research and practice.

REFERENCES

Abbott, A. A., Baranson, S., & Zimmerman, L. (2010). Symptom burden clusters and their impact on psychosocial functioning following coronary artery bypass surgery. *Journal of Cardiovascular Nursing, 4,* 301–310.

Armstrong, T. S. (2001). Symptoms experience: A concept analysis. *Oncology Nursing Forum, 30,* 601–606.

Armstrong, T. S., Cohen, M. Z., Eriksen, L. R., & Hickey, J. V. (2004). Symptom clusters in oncology patients and implications for symptom research in people with primary brain tumors. *Journal of Nursing Scholarship, 36*(3), 197–206.

Auvil-Novak, S. E. (1997). A middle-range theory of chronotherapeutic intervention for postsurgical pain. *Nursing Research, 46,* 66–71.

Barsevick, A. M. (2007). The elusive concept of the symptom cluster. *Oncology Nursing Forum, 34,* 971–980.

Barsevick, A. M., Dudley, W. N., & Beck, S. L. (2006). Cancer-related fatigue, depressive symptoms, and functional status: A mediation model. *Nursing Research, 55*(5), 366–372.

Barsevick, A. M., Whitmore, K., Nail, L. M., Beck, S. L., & Dudley, W. N. (2006). Symptom cluster research: Conceptual, design, measurement and analysis issues. *Journal of Pain and Symptom Management, 31*(1), 85–95.

Brant, J. M., Beck, S., & Miaskowski, C. (2009). Building dynamic models and theories to advance the science of symptom management research. *Journal of Advanced Nursing, 66*(1), 228–240.

Carpenter, J. S., Elam, J. L., Ridner, S. H., Carney, P. H., Cherry, G. J., & Cucullu, H. L. (2004). Sleep, fatigue, and depressive symptoms in breast cancer survivors and matched health women experiencing hot flashes. *Oncology Nursing Forum, 31*(3), 591–598.

Chen, E., Nguyen, J., Cramarossa, G., Kahn, L. O., Leung, A., Lutz, S., & Chow, E. (2011). Symptom clusters in persons with lung cancer: A literature review. *Expert Review of Pharmacoeconomics & Outcomes Research, 11,* 433–439.

Chen, L.-H., Li, C.-Y., Shieh, S.-M., Yin, W.-H., & Chiou, A.-F. (2010). Predictors of fatigue in patients with heart failure. *Journal of Clinical Nursing, 19,* 1588–1596.

Cheng, K. K. F., & Lee, D. T. F. (2011). Effects of pain, fatigue, insomnia, and mood disturbance on functional status and quality of life of elderly patients with cancer. *Critical Reviews in Oncology Hematology, 78,* 127–137.

Chow, E., & Merrick, J. (2010). A critical discussion of symptom clusters in metastatic cancer. In E. Chow & J. Merrick (Eds.), *Advanced cancer: Pain and quality of life* (pp. 129–143). New York, NY: Nova Science.

Clayton, M. F., Mishel, M. M., & Belyea, M. (2006). Testing a model of symptoms, communication, uncertainty and well-being in older breast cancer survivors. *Research in Nursing & Health, 29,* 18–39.

Cooley, M. (2000). Symptoms in adults with lung cancer: A systematic research review. *Journal of Pain and Symptom Management, 19,* 137–153.

Corwin, E. J., Brownstead, J., Barton, N., Heckar, S., & Morin, K. (2005). The impact of fatigue on the development of postpartum depression. *Journal of Obstetric, Gynecologic, & Neonatal Nursing, 34*(5), 577–586.

Dabbs, A. D., Dew, M. A., Stilley, C. S., Manzetti, J., Zullo, T., McCurry, K. R., … Iacono, A. (2003). Psychosocial vulnerability, physical symptoms and physical impairment after lung and heart-lung transplantation. *The Journal of Heart and Lung Transplantation, 22*(11), 1268–1275.

Dabbs, A. D., Hoffman, L. A., Swigart, V., Happ, M. B., Iacono, A. T., & Dauber, J. H. (2004). Using conceptual triangulation to develop an integrated model of the symptom experience of acute rejection after lung transplantation. *Advances in Nursing Science, 27,* 136–149.

Dodd, M., Jansen, S., Facione, N., Faucett, J., Froelicher, E. S., Humphreys, J., & Taylor, D. (2001). Advancing the science of symptom management. *Journal of Advanced Nursing, 33,* 668–676.

Dodd, M. J., Miaskowski, C., & Lee, K. A. (2004). Occurrence of symptom clusters. *Journal of the National Cancer Institute, 32,* 76–78.

Duncan, J. G., Bott, M. J., Thompson, S. A., & Gajewski, B. J. (2009). Symptom occurrence and associated clinical factors in nursing home residents with cancer. *Research in Nursing and Health, 32,* 453–464.

Ely, E. W., Gautam, S., Margolin, R., Francis, J., May, L., Speroff, T., … Inouye, S. K. (2001). The impact of delirium in the intensive care unit on hospital length of stay. *Intensive Care Medicine, 27*(12), 1892–1900.

Ely, E. W., Shintani, A., Truman, B., Speroff, T., Gordon, S. M., Harrell, F. E., … Dittus, R. S. (2004). Delirium as a predictor of mortality in mechanically ventilated patients in the intensive care unit. *JAMA, 291*(14), 1753–1762.

Farrell, D., & Savage, E. (2010). Symptom burden in inflammatory bowel disease: Rethinking conceptual and theoretical underpinnings. *International Journal of Nursing Practice, 16,* 437–442.

Fox, S. W., & Lyon, D. E. (2006). Symptom clusters and quality of life in survivors of lung cancer. *Oncology Nursing Forum, 33*(5), 931–936.

Franck, L. S., Kools, S., Kennedy, C., Kong, S. K. F., Chen, J.-L., & Wong, T. K. S. (2004). The symptom experience of hospitalized Chinese children and adolescents and relationship to pre-hospital factors and behavior problems. *International Journal of Nursing Studies, 41,* 661–669.

Francoeur, R. B. (2005). The relationship of cancer symptom clusters to depressive affect in the initial phase of palliative radiation. *Journal of Pain and Symptom Management, 29*(2), 130–155.

Gift, A. G. (1990). Dyspnea. *Nursing Clinics of North America, 25,* 955–965.

Gift, A. G., & Cahill, C. (1990). Psychophysiologic aspects of dyspnea in chronic obstructive pulmonary disease: A pilot study. *Heart & Lung, 19,* 252–257.

Gift, A. G., Jablonski, A., Stommel, M., & Given, C. W. (2004). Symptom clusters in elderly patients with lung cancer. *Oncology Nursing Forum, 31*(2), 203–210.

Gift, A. G., & Pugh, L. C. (1993). Dyspnea and fatigue. *Nursing Clinics of North America, 28,* 373–384.

Good, M. (1998). A middle-range theory of acute pain management: Use in research. *Nursing Outlook, 436,* 120–124.

Good, M. (2013). Pain: A balance between analgesia and side effects. In S. J. Peterson & T. S. Bredow. *Middle range theories: Application to nursing research* (3rd ed., pp. 51–67). Philadelphia, PA: Wolters Kluwer/Lippincott, Williams & Wilkins.

Henley, S. M., Kallas, K. D., Klatt, C. M., & Swenson, K. K. (2003). The notion of time in symptom experiences. *Nursing Research, 52*(6), 410–417.

Higgins, P. (1998). Patient perceptions of fatigue while undergoing long-term mechanical ventilation: Incidence and associated factors. *Heart & Lung, 27*(3), 177–183.

Humphreys, J., Lee, K. A., Carrieri-Kohlman, V., Puntillo, K., Faucett, J., Janson, S., … UCSF School of Nursing Symptom Management Faculty Group. (2008). Theory of symptom management. In M. J. Smith & P. R. Liehr (Eds.), *Middle range theory for nursing* (2nd ed., pp. 145–157). New York, NY: Springer Publishing.

Hutchinson, S. A., & Wilson, H. S. (1998). The theory of unpleasant symptoms and Alzheimer's disease. *Scholarly Inquiry for Nursing Practice, 22,* 143–158.

Jurgens, C. Y. (2006). Somatic awareness, uncertainty and delay in care-seeking in acute heart failure. *Research in Nursing and Health, 29,* 74–76.

Jurgens, C. Y., Moser, D. K., Armola, R., Carlson, B., Sethares, K., Riegel, B., & the Heart Failure Quality of Life Trialist Collaborators. (2009). Symptom clusters of heart failure. *Research in Nursing & Health, 32,* 551–560.

Kapella, M. C., Larson, J. L., Patel, M. K., Covey, M. K., & Berry, J. K. (2006). Subjective fatigue, influencing variables and consequences in chronic obstructive pulmonary disease. *Nursing Research, 55*(1), 10–17.

Kim, H.-J., McGuire, D. B., Tulman, L., & Barsevick, A. M. (2005). Symptom clusters: Concept analysis and clinical implications for cancer nursing. *Cancer Nursing, 28*(4), 270–282.

Kim, S.-H., Oh, E.-G., & Lee, W.-H. (2006). Symptom experience, psychological distress, and quality of life in Korean patients with liver cirrhosis: A cross-sectional survey. *International Journal of Nursing Studies, 43,* 1047–1056.

Kim, S.-H., Oh, E.-G., Lee, W.-H., Kim, O.-S., & Han, K.-H. (2006). Symptom experience in Korean patients with liver cirrhosis. *Journal of Pain and Symptom Management, 31*(4), 325–334.

Kiser, D. W., Greer, T. B., Wilmoth, M. C., Dmochowski, J., & Naumann, R. W. (2010). Peripheral neuropathy in patients with gynecologic cancer receiving chemotherapy: Patient reports and provider assessments. *Oncology Nursing Forum, 37,* 758–764.

Kugler, C., Geyer, S., Gottlieb, J., Simon, A., Haverich, A., & Dracup, K. (2009). Symptom experience after solid organ transplantation. *Journal of Psychosomatic Research, 66,* 101–110.

Laird, B. J. A., Scott, A. C., Colvin, L. A., McKeon, A., Murray, G. D., Fearon, K. C., & Fallon, M. T. (2011). Pain, depression, and fatigue as a symptom cluster in advanced cancer. *Journal of Pain and Symptom Management, 42,* 1–11.

Lang, C. A., Conrad, S., Garrett, L., Battistutta, D., Cooksley, W. G. E., Dunne, M., & Macdonald, G. A. (2006). Symptom prevalence and clustering of symptoms in people living with chronic hepatitis C infection. *Journal of Pain and Symptom Management, 31*(4), 335–344.

Lee, E.-H., Chung, B. Y., Park, H. B., & Chun, K. H. (2004). Relationships of mood disturbance and social support to symptom experience in Korean women with breast cancer. *Journal of Pain and Symptom Management, 27*(5), 425–433.

Lee, K., Song, E. K., Lennie, T. A., Frazier, S. K., Chung, M. L., Heo, S., ... Moser, D. K. (2010). Symptom clusters in men and women with heart failure and their impact on cardiac event-free survival. *Journal of Cardiovascular Nursing, 25,* 263–272.

Lenz, E. R., Gift, A. G., Pugh, L. C., & Milligan, R. A. (2013). Unpleasant symptoms. In S. J. Peterson & T. S. Bredow (Eds.), *Middle range theories: Application to nursing research* (3rd ed., pp. 68–81). Philadelphia, PA: Wolters Kluwer/ Lippincott Williams and Wilkins.

Lenz, E. R., Pugh, L. C., Milligan, R., Gift, A., & Suppe, F. (1997). The middle-range theory of unpleasant symptoms: An update. *Advances in Nursing Science, 19*(3), 14–27.

Lenz, E. R., Suppe, F., Gift, A. G., Pugh, L. C., & Milligan, R. A. (1995). Collaborative development of middle-range nursing theories: Toward a theory of unpleasant symptoms. *Advances in Nursing Science, 17*(3), 1–13.

Lester, J., & Bernhard, L. (2009). Urogenital atrophy in breast cancer survivors. *Oncology Nursing Forum, 36,* 993–698.

Lester, B., Bernhard, L., & Ryan-Wenger, N. (2012). A self-report instrument that describes urogenital atrophy symptoms in breast cancer survivors. *Western Journal of Nursing Research, 34,* 72–96.

Liu, H. E. (2006). Fatigue and associated factors in hemodialysis patients in Taiwan. *Research in Nursing and Health, 29,* 40–50.

Miaskowski, C., Dodd, M., & Lee, K. (2004). Symptom clusters: The new frontier in symptom management research. *Journal of the National Cancer Institute Monographs, 2004*(32), 17–21.

Michael, K. M., Allen, J. K., & Macko, R. F. (2006). Fatigue after stroke: Relationship to mobility, fitness, ambulatory activity, social support and falls efficacy. *Rehabilitation Nursing, 31*(5), 210–217.

Milligan, R. A. (1989). Maternal fatigue during the first three months of the postpartum period. *Dissertation Abstracts International, 50,* 07B.

Milligan, R. A., Flenniken, P., & Pugh, L. C. (1996). Positioning intervention to minimize fatigue in breastfeeding women. *Applied Nursing Research, 9,* 67–70.

Milligan, R. A., Lenz, E. R., Parks, P. L., Pugh, L. C., & Kitzman, H. (1996). Postpartum fatigue: Clarifying a concept. *Scholarly Inquiry for Nursing Practice, 10*(3), 279–291.

Motl, R. W., & McAuley, E. (2009). Symptom cluster as a predictor of physical activity in multiple sclerosis: Preliminary evidence. *Journal of Pain and Symptom Management, 38,* 270–280.

Motl, R. W., McAuley, E., Wynn, D., Suh, S., Weikert, M., & Dlugonsky, D. (2010). Symptoms and physical activity among adults with relapsing-remitting multiple sclerosis. *Journal of Nervous and Mental Disease, 198,* 213–219.

Motl, R. W., Suh, Y., & Weikert, M. (2010). Symptom cluster and quality of life in multiple sclerosis. *Journal of Pain and Symptom Management, 39,* 1025–1032.

Motl, R. W., Weikert, M., Suh, Y., & Diugonski, D. (2010). Symptom cluster and physical activity in relapsing-remitting multiple sclerosis. *Research in Nursing and Health, 33,* 398–412.

National Institute of Nursing Research. (2011). *Bringing science to life: NINR strategic plan.* Retrieved from http://www.ninr.nih.gov/NR/rdonlyres/8BE21801-0C52-44C2-9EEA-142483657FB1/0/NINR_StratPlan_F2_508.pdf

Oh, E.-G., Kim, C.-J., Lee, W.-H., & Kim, S. S. (2004). Correlates of fatigue in Koreans with chronic lung disease. *Heart & Lung, 33*(1), 13–20.

Parse, R. R. (2005). Community of Scholars. *Nursing Science Quarterly, 18,* 119.

Parshall, M. B., Welsh, J. D., Brockopp, D. Y., Heiser, R. M., Schooler, M. P., & Cassidy, K. B. (2001). Dyspnea duration, distress and intensity in emergency department visits for heart failure. *Heart & Lung, 30*(1), 47–56.

Pugh, L. C. (1990). Psychophysiologic correlates of fatigue during childbearing. *Dissertation Abstracts International, 51,* 01B.

Pugh, L. C., & Milligan, R. A. (1993). A framework for the study of childbearing fatigue. *Advances in Nursing Science, 15*(4), 60–70.

Pugh, L. C., & Milligan, R. A. (1995). Patterns of fatigue during pregnancy. *Applied Nursing Research, 8,* 140–143.

Pugh, L. C., & Milligan, R. A. (1998). Nursing intervention to increase the duration of breastfeeding. *Applied Nursing Research, 11,* 190–194.

Pugh, L. C., Milligan, R. A., & Brown, L. P. (2001). The breastfeeding support team for low-income predominantly minority women: A pilot intervention study. *Health Care for Women International, 22,* 501–515.

Pugh, L. C., Milligan, R. A., Frick, K. D., Spatz, I. D., & Bronner, Y. (2002). Breastfeeding duration and cost effectiveness of a support program for low-income breastfeeding women. *Birth, 29*(2), 95–100.

Pugh, L. C., Milligan, R. A., & Lenz, E. R. (2000). Response to "insomnia, fatigue, anxiety, depression, and quality of life of cancer patients undergoing chemotherapy." *Scholarly Inquiry for Nursing Practice, 14,* 291–294.

Pugh, L. C., Serwint, J. R., Frick, K. D., Nanda, J. P., Sharps, P. W., Spatz, D. L., & Milligan, R. A. (2010). A randomized controlled community-based trail to improve breastfeeding rates among urban low-income mothers. *Academic Pediatrics, 10*, 14–20.

Redeker, N. S., Lev, E. L., & Ruggiero, J. (2000). Insomnia, fatigue, anxiety, depression and quality of life of cancer patients undergoing chemotherapy. *Scholarly Inquiry for Nursing Practice: An International Journal, 14*, 275–290.

Reishtein, J. L. (2004). Relationship between symptoms and functional performance in COPD. *Research in Nursing and Health, 28*, 39–47.

Rhodes, V., & Watson, P. (1987). Symptom distress-the concept past and present. *Seminars in Oncology Nursing, 3*(4), 242–247.

Roy, C. (2005). A community of scholars. *Nursing Science Quarterly, 18*, 121–122.

Scordo, K. A. (2005). Mitral valve prolapsed syndrome health concerns, symptoms and treatments. *Western Journal of Nursing Research, 27*, 390, 405.

Song, J.-E., Chang, S.-B., Park, S.-M., Kim, S., & Nam, C.-M. (2010). Empirical test of an explanatory theory of postpartum fatigue in Korea. *Journal of Advanced Nursing, 66*, 2627–2639.

Spector, R. E. (2000). *Cultural diversity in health and illness* (5th ed.). Upper Saddle River, NJ: Prentice Hall Health.

Tyler, R., & Pugh, L. C. (2009). Application of the theory of unpleasant symptoms in bariatric surgery. *Bariatric Nursing and Surgical Care, 4*, 271–276.

Tzeng, Y., Teng, Y., Chou, F., & Tu, H. (2009). Identifying trajectories of birth-related fatigue of expectant fathers. *Journal of Clinical Nursing, 18*, 1674–1683.

Waltz, C. F., Strickland, O. L., & Lenz, E. R. (2010). *Measurement in nursing and health research* (4th ed). New York, NY: Springer.

Wilmoth, M. C., Coleman, E. A., Smith, S. C., & Davis, C. (2004). Fatigue, weight gain, and altered sexuality in patients with breast cancer: Exploration of a symptom cluster. *Oncology Nursing Forum, 31*(6), 1069–1075.

Wilmoth, M. C., Hatmaker-Flanigan, E., LaLoggia, V., & Nixon, T. (2011). Ovarian cancer survivors: Qualitative analysis of the symptom of sexuality. *Oncology Nursing Forum, 38*, 699–708.

Woods, S. J., Kozachik, S. L., & Hall, R. J. (2010). Subjective sleep quality in women experiencing intimate partner violence: Contributions of situational, psychological, and physiological factors. *Journal of Traumatic Stress, 23*, 141–150.

Yang, C.-Y., Tsai, J.-C., Huang, Y.-C., & Lin, C.-C. (2011). Effects of a home-based walking program on perceived symptom and mood status in postoperative breast cancer women receiving adjuvant chemotherapy. *Journal of Advanced Nursing, 67*, 158–168.

9

Theory of Self-Efficacy

Barbara Resnick

Self-efficacy is defined as an individual's judgment of his or her capabilities to organize and execute courses of action. The core of self-efficacy theory means that people can exercise influence over what they do. Through reflective thought, generative use of knowledge and skills to perform a specific behavior, and other tools of self-influence, a person will decide how to behave (Bandura, 1997). To determine self-efficacy, an individual must have the opportunity for self-evaluation or the ability to compare individual output to some sort of evaluative criterion. This comparative evaluation process enables an individual to judge performance capability and establish self-efficacy expectation.

PURPOSE OF THE THEORY AND HOW IT WAS DEVELOPED

The Theory of Self-Efficacy is based on the social cognitive theory and conceptualizes person–behavior–environment interaction as triadic reciprocality, the foundation for reciprocal determinism (Bandura, 1977, 1986). Triadic reciprocality is the interrelationship among person, behavior, and environment; reciprocal determinism is the belief that behavior, cognitive, and other personal factors as well as environmental influences operate interactively as determinants of each other. Reciprocality does not mean that the influence of behavioral and personal factors as well as environment is equal. Depending on the situation, the influence of one factor may be stronger than the other, and these influences may vary over time.

Cognitive thought—which is a critical dimension of the person–behavior–environment interaction—does not arise in a vacuum. Bandura (1977, 1986) suggested that individuals' thoughts about themselves are developed and verified through four different processes: (1) direct experience of the effects produced by their actions, (2) vicarious experience, (3) judgments voiced by others, and (4) derivation of further knowledge of what they already know by using rules of inference. Human functioning is viewed as a dynamic interplay of personal, behavioral, and environmental influences.

Initial Theory Development and Research

In 1963, Bandura and Walters wrote *Social Learning and Personality Development*, which expanded on the social learning theory to incorporate observational learning and vicarious reinforcement. In the 1970s, Bandura incorporated what he considered to be the missing component to that theory, self-efficacy beliefs, and published *Self-Efficacy: Toward a Unifying Theory of Behavior Change* (Bandura, 1977). The work supporting self-efficacy belief was based on research testing the assumption that exposure to treatment conditions could result in behavioral change by altering an individual's level and strength of self-efficacy. In the initial study (Bandura, Adams, & Beyer, 1977; Bandura, Reese, & Adams, 1982), 33 subjects with snake phobias were randomly assigned to three different treatment conditions: (1) enactive attainment, which included actually touching the snakes; (2) role modeling or seeing others touch the snakes; and (3) the control group. The results suggested that self-efficacy was predictive of subsequent behavior, and enactive attainment resulted in stronger and more generalized (to other snakes) self-efficacy expectations.

Expansion of the early research included three additional studies (Bandura et al., 1982): (1) 10 subjects with snake phobias, (2) 14 subjects with spider phobias, and (3) 12 subjects with spider phobias. Similar to the initial self-efficacy study, enactive attainment and role modeling were effective interventions for strengthening self-efficacy expectations and impacting behavior. The study of 12 subjects with spider phobias also considered the physiological arousal component of self-efficacy. Pulse and blood pressure were measured as indicators of fear arousal when interacting with spiders. After interventions to strengthen self-efficacy expectations (enactive attainment and role modeling), heart rate decreased and blood pressure stabilized.

This early self-efficacy research used an ideal controlled setting in that the individuals with snake phobias were unlikely to seek opportunities to interact with snakes when away from the laboratory setting. Therefore, there was controlled input of efficacy information.

Although this ideal situation is not possible in the clinical setting, the theory of self-efficacy has been used to study and predict health behavior change and management in a variety of settings.

Literatures explore factors that influenced the willingness of older adults to participate in functional activities and exercises. There was a recurring theme that suggested self-efficacy and outcome expectations mattered to an individual's willingness. Therefore, the theory helps to understand behavior and guide the development of interventions to change behavior.

CONCEPTS OF THE THEORY

Bandura, a social scientist, differentiated two components of self-efficacy theory: self-efficacy expectations and outcome expectations. These two components are the major ideas of the theory. Self-efficacy expectations are judgments about personal ability to accomplish a given task, whereas outcome expectations are judgments about what will happen if a given task is successfully accomplished. Both were differentiated because individuals can believe that a certain behavior will result in a specific outcome; however, they may not believe that they are capable of performing the behavior required for the outcome to occur. For example, Mrs. White may believe that rehabilitation will enable her to go home independently; however, she may not believe that she is capable of ambulating across the room. Therefore, Mrs. White may not participate in the rehabilitation program or be willing to practice ambulation.

Bandura (1977, 1986, 1995, 1997) suggests that outcome expectations are based largely on the individual's self-efficacy expectations. People anticipate that the types of outcomes generally depend on their judgments of how well they will be able to perform the behavior. Those individuals who consider themselves highly efficacious in accomplishing a given behavior will expect favorable outcomes for that behavior. Expected outcomes are dependent on self-efficacy judgments. Therefore, Bandura postulated that expected outcomes may not add much on the prediction of behavior.

Bandura (1986) postulates that there are instances when outcome expectations can be dissociated from self-efficacy expectations. This occurs either when no action will result in a specific outcome or when the outcome is loosely linked to the level or quality of the performance. For example, if Mrs. White knows that *even if she* regains functional independence by participating in rehabilitation, she will still be discharged to a skilled nursing facility rather than back home, her behavior is likely to be influenced by her outcome expectations (discharge to the skilled nursing facility). In this situation, no matter what Mrs. White's performance, the outcome is the same; thus, outcome expectancy may influence her behavior independent of her self-efficacy beliefs.

Expected outcomes are also partially separable from self-efficacy judgments when extrinsic outcomes are fixed. For example, when a nurse provides care to 6 patients during an 8-hour shift or to 10 patients in the same shift, she receives the same salary. This could negatively impact the performance. It is also possible for an individual to believe that he or she is capable of performing a specific behavior rather than the outcome of performing that behavior is worthwhile. For example, older adults in rehabilitation may believe that they are capable of performing the exercises and activities involved in the rehabilitation process, but they may not believe that performing the exercises will result in improved functional ability. Some older adults believe that resting rather than exercising will lead to recovery. In this situation, outcome expectations may have a direct impact on performance.

Both self-efficacy and outcome expectations influence the performance of functional activities (Galik, Pretzer-Aboff, & Resnick, 2011; Harnirattisai & Johnson, 2005; Pretzer-Aboff, Galik, & Resnick, 2011; Resnick, 2011; Resnick & D'Adamo, 2011; Resnick et al., 2009), adoption and maintenance of exercise behavior (Chase, 2011; Grim, Hortz, & Petosa, 2011; Harnirattisai & Johnson, 2005; Hays, Pressler, Damush, Rawl, & Clark, 2010; Nahm et al., 2010; Qi, Resnick, Smeltzer, & Bausell, 2011), smoking cessation (Kamish & Öz, 2011), sex education for children (Akers, Holland, & Bost, 2011), and hip fracture prevention behaviors (Nahm et al., 2010). Outcome expectations are particularly relevant to older adults. These individuals may have high self-efficacy expectations for exercise, but if they do not believe in the outcomes associated with exercise (e.g., improved health, strength, or function), then it is unlikely that there will be adherence to a regular exercise program (Chase, 2011; Collins, Lee Albright, & King, 2004; Cress et al., 2005; Resnick, Luisi, & Vogel, 2008).

Generally, it is anticipated that self-efficacy will have a positive impact on behavior. However, it must be recognized that there are times when self-efficacy will have no or a negative effect on performance. Some research found that there is a negative effect of self-reported personal goals on performance such that higher personal goals can cause low performance (Vancouver & Kendell,

2006; Vancouver, Thompson, & Williams, 2001). Consistent with a multiple goal process conceptualization, self-efficacy was also found to relate positively to directing resources toward a goal but negatively to the magnitude of resources allocated for accepted goals (Vancouver, More, & Yoder, 2008). High self-efficacy expectations can actually be counterproductive. High self-efficacy may lead people to have a false sense of confidence and not put in as much effort as needed to perform optimally (Jones, Harris, Waller, & Coggins, 2005). This may be particularly true of behaviors such as exercise in which adequate resources to perform are needed (i.e., adequate physical strength), and the individual may have limited experience on which to draw and appropriately evaluate his or her self-efficacy expectations.

Sources of Self-Efficacy Judgment

Bandura (1986) suggested that judgment about one's self-efficacy is based on four informational sources: (1) enactive attainment, which is the actual performance of a behavior; (2) vicarious experience or visualizing other similar people perform a behavior; (3) verbal persuasion or exhortation; and (4) physiological state or physiological feedback during a behavior, such as pain or fatigue. The cognitive appraisal of these factors results in a perception of a level of confidence in the individual's ability to perform certain behavior. The positive performance of this behavior reinforces self-efficacy expectations (Bandura, 1995).

Enactive Attainment

Enactive attainment has been described as the most influential source of self-efficacy information (Bandura, 1977, 1986), and it is the most common intervention that is used to strengthen efficacy expectations in older adults (Estabrooks, Fox, Doerksen, Bradshaw, & King, 2005). There has been repeated empirical verification that actually performing an activity strengthens self-efficacy beliefs. Specifically, the impact of enactive attainment has been demonstrated with regard to snake phobias, smoking cessation, exercise behaviors, performance of functional activities, and weight loss. Enactive attainment generally results in greater strengthening of self-efficacy expectations compared to informational sources. However, performance alone does not establish self-efficacy beliefs. Other factors such as preconceptions of ability, the perceived difficulty of the task, the amount of effort expended, the external aid received, the situational circumstance, and past successes and failures impact the individual's cognitive appraisal of self-efficacy (Bandura, 1995). An older adult who strongly believes that he or she is able to bathe and dress independently because he or she has been doing so for 90 years will not likely alter self-efficacy expectations if he or she wakes up with severe arthritic changes one morning and is consequently unable to put on a shirt. However, repeated failures to perform the activity will impact self-efficacy expectations. The relative stability of strong self-efficacy expectations is important; otherwise an occasional failure or setback could severely impact both self-efficacy expectations and behavior.

Vicarious Experience

Self-efficacy expectations are also influenced by vicarious experiences or seeing other similar people successfully performing the same activity (Bandura, 1977; Chase, 2011; Martin et al., 2011). However, there are some conditions that impact the influence of vicarious experience. If the individual has not been exposed to the behavior of interest or has had little experience with it, vicarious experience is likely to have a greater impact. Additionally, when clear guidelines for performance are not explicated, self-efficacy will be more likely to be impacted by the performance of others. Among older adults with cognitive impairment vicarious experiences are particularly effective in increasing activity (Galik, 2007; Galik et al., 2008; Resnick, Galik, Nahm, Shaughness, & Michael, 2009).

Verbal Persuasion

Verbal persuasion involves telling an individual that he or she has the capabilities to master the given behavior. Empirical support for the influence of verbal persuasion has been documented since Bandura's early research of phobias (Bandura et al., 1977). Verbal persuasion has proven effective in supporting recovery from chronic illness and in health promotion research. Persuasive health influences lead people with a high sense of self-efficacy to intensify efforts at self-directed change of risky health behavior. Verbal encouragement from a trusted, credible source in the form of counseling and education has been used alone and with performance behavior to strengthen efficacy expectations (Bennett et al., 2011; Chase, 2011; Gau, Chang, Tian, & Lin, 2011; Irvine et al., 2011; Kamish & Öz, 2011; Martin et al., 2011; Oberg, Bradley, Allen, & McCrory, 2011; Pretzer-Aboff, Galik, & Resnick, 2009; Resnick,

Gruber-Baldini, Zimmerman, et al., 2009; Rosal et al., 2011; Skinner et al., 2011; Utz et al., 2008; van Stralen, de Vress, Mudde, Bolman, & Lechner, 2011; Williams, 2011). For example, verbal encouragement through telephone calls was successful in increasing physical activity among older adults (King et al., 2007; Skinner et al., 2011) and encouragement through the computer was effective in strengthening self-efficacy associated with behaviors to prevent unintended pregnancy and infections (Swartz et al., 2011) and in improving coping self-efficacy associated with HIV (Brown, Vanable, Carey, & Elin, 2011).

Physiological Feedback

Individuals rely in part on information from their physiological state to judge their abilities. Physiological indicators are especially important in relation to coping with stressors, physical accomplishments, and health functioning. Individuals evaluate their physiological state or arousal, and if aversive, they may avoid performing the behavior. For example, if the older adult has a fear of falling or getting hurt when walking, a high arousal state associated with the fear can limit the performance and decrease the individual's confidence in ability to perform the activity. Similarly, if the rehabilitation activities result in fatigue, pain, or shortness of breath, these symptoms may be interpreted as physical inefficacy and the older adult may not feel capable of performing the activity.

Interventions can be used to alter the interpretation of physiological feedback and help individuals to cope with physical sensations, enhancing self-efficacy and resulting in improved performance. Interventions include (a) visualized mastery, which eliminates the emotional reactions to a given situation (Bandura et al., 1977); (b) enhancement of physical status (Bandura, 1995); and (c) altering the interpretation of bodily states (Li, Fisher, Harmer, & McAuley, 2005; McAuley et al., 2006; Resnick, Galik, Gruber-Baldini, & Zimmerman, 2011; Resnick, Gruber-Baldini, Galik, et al., 2009; Resnick, Gruber-Baldini, Zimmerman, et al., 2009; Resnick, Luisi, et al., 2008; Schnoll et al., 2011). Interventions that decrease the pain associated with the use of pain medication or ice treatments and interventions focused on decreasing fear of falling have been shown to increase participation in rehabilitation and exercise among older adults (Rejeski, Katula, Rejeski, Rowley, & Sipe, 2005; Rejeski et al., 2005; Resnick et al., 2011; Resnick, Gruber-Baldini, Galik, et al., 2009; Resnick, Gruber-Baldini, Zimmerman, et al., 2009; Resnick, Luisi, et al., 2008; Schnoll et al., 2011).

RELATIONSHIPS AMONG THE CONCEPTS: THE MODEL

The theory of self-efficacy was derived from the social cognitive theory and must be considered within the context of reciprocal determinism. The four sources of experience (direct experience, vicarious experience, judgments by others, and derivation of knowledge by inference) that can potentially influence self-efficacy and outcome expectations interact with characteristics of the individual and the environment. Ideally, self-efficacy and outcome expectations are strengthened by these experiences and subsequently moderate behavior. Since self-efficacy and outcome expectations are influenced by performance of a behavior, it is likely that there is a reciprocal relationship between performance and efficacy expectations (see Figure 9.1).

Measurement of Self-Efficacy and Outcome Expectations

Operationalization of self-efficacy constructs is based on Bandura's (1977) early work with snake phobias. Self-efficacy measures were developed as paper and pencil measures that list activities—from least to most difficult—in a specific behavioral domain. In Bandura's (1977, 1986) early work, participants were asked to indicate whether they could perform the activity (magnitude of self-efficacy expectations) and then evaluated the level of confidence they had in performing the given activity (strength of self-efficacy).

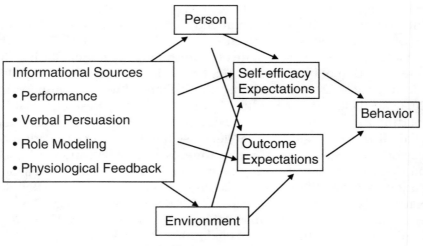

FIGURE 9.1   Self-Efficacy

Traditionally in the development of self-efficacy measures, items are derived based on the combined quantitative and qualitative research exploring factors that influenced adherence to a specific behavior, such as exercise (Bandura, 1986; Resnick & Jenkins, 2000). For example, the self-efficacy for exercise scale includes nine items, with each item reflecting a commonly recognized challenge associated with exercise for older individuals (Resnick & Jenkins, 2000). Participants then responded by indicating that they have no confidence (0) or are very confident (10).

Development of outcome expectation measures has been less well-defined, although the process of establishing appropriate items is the same as it is for self-efficacy expectations. However, there is increasing evidence of measurement of outcome expectations across a few behaviors, such as physical activity, specifically exercise (Harnirattisai & Johnson, 2002; Merrill, Shields, Wood, & Beck, 2004; Millen & Bray, 2009; Resnick, 2005; Resnick, Galik, Petzer-Aboff, Rogers, & Gruber-Baldini, 2008; Resnick, Wehren, & Orwig, 2003; Resnick, Zimmerman, Orwig, Furstenberg, & Magaziner, 2000; Resnick, Zimmerman, Orwig, Furstenberg, & Magaziner, 2001a, 2001b; Shaughnessy, Resnick, & Macko, 2004; Wilcox, Castro, & King, 2006), function (Harnirattisai & Johnson, 2002), medication adherence (Qi et al., 2011; Resnick et al., 2003), and breast cancer treatment (Rogers et al., 2005).

USE OF THE THEORY IN NURSING RESEARCH

The theory of self-efficacy has been used in nursing research focusing on clinical aspects of care, education, nursing competency, and professionalism. The number of studies exploring the relationship between self-efficacy and exercise or testing the impact of exercise interventions on exercise behavior over the past 5 years was approximately 650. Of these, 150 were published in nursing journals. As noted, fewer studies have addressed outcome expectations associated with behaviors.

Self-efficacy expectations are used in cross-sectional work to describe the sample and consider the relationship between demographic factors and self-efficacy, psychosocial factors, performance of behaviors and/ or outcome expectations. Alternatively, self-efficacy expectations are used to predict behavior in longitudinal research and to guide interventions and change behavior in intervention studies. These studies cover behaviors associated with exercise, physical activity, function, parenting, nursing skills, health promotion behaviors, and management of chronic illness among others. The majority of these studies have been done within the United States, although there is an increasing literature supporting the use of this theory among Asians as well as other cultural groups. The most important with regard to the use of the theory of self-efficacy in nursing research is that the researcher maintains the behavioral specificity by developing a specific fit between the behavior that is being considered and efficacy and outcome expectations. If the behavior of interest is walking for 20 minutes every day, the self-efficacy measure should focus on the challenges related to this specific behavior (time, fatigue, pain, or fear of falling).

Self-Efficacy Studies Related to Managing Chronic Illness

Self-efficacy is commonly used to explain and improve the management of chronic illnesses (Horowitz, Eckhardt, Talavera, Goytia, & Lorig, 2011). Gortner and colleagues were some of the first nurses to initiate self-efficacy intervention research in chronic illness management with the focus of the work being on cardiovascular disease (Gortner & Jenkins, 1990; Gortner, Rankin, & Wolfe, 1988). Jenkins's work built off that of Gortner et al., and she tested a self-efficacy intervention on recovery of 156 patients following cardiac surgery (Gortner & Jenkins, 1990). The use of self-efficacy theory to help individuals manage chronic illness continues to be prevalent in patients with congestive heart failure (Granger, Moser, Germino, Harrell, & Ekman, 2006; Han, Lee, Park, Park, & Cheol, 2005; Johansson, Dahlström, & Bromström, 2006), hypertension (Martin et al., 2011; Resnick et al., 2009), those with diabetes (Lorig et al., 2010; Oberg et al., 2011; Rosal et al., 2011), rheumatoid arthritis (Niedermann et al., 2011), stroke (Shaughnessy & Resnick, 2009), cancer (McCorkle et al., 2011), renal disease (Curtin, Mapes, Schatell, & Burrows-Hudson, 2005), and mental illness (Druss et al., 2010) among others. In addition, the self-efficacy work in chronic illness has focused on self-management of the symptoms associated with chronic problems such as pain (Bennett et al., 2011; Gustavsson, Denison, & von Koch, 2011).

Consistently, self-efficacy expectations have been associated with outcome behavior (e.g., management of pain, medication use) (Harnirattisai & Johnson, 2002; Qi et al., 2011; Resnick, Galik, et al., 2008; Resnick & Jenkins, 2000; Resnick et al., 2003; Shaughnessy et al., 2004) and more recent work focuses on interventions geared to strengthening self-efficacy and associated outcome behavior relevant for the chronic medical problem. For example, following a 12-week individualized and group dietary education program delivered in a naturopathic primary care clinic to improve management of diabetes, there was a decline in HbA1c and an improvement in dietary intake, physical activity, self-efficacy and self-management of diabetes (Oberg et al., 2011). Another study addressing diabetes self-management tested a series of culturally sensitive educational sessions for Latinos with diabetes. The intervention strengthened self-efficacy expectations, improved knowledge, and increased adherence to monitoring of blood sugar among other outcomes (Rosal et al., 2011). Many innovative interventions using technology have also been established to manage chronic illness. An example of this is the pilot work testing a computerized stress management training for women with HIV (Brown et al., 2011).

Self-Efficacy for Health Promoting Activities Such as Exercise and Weight Loss

Self-efficacy approaches have been commonly used to influence exercise and diet behaviors. Self-efficacy expectations have generally been positively associated with exercise (Chase, 2011; Grim et al., 2011; Nahm et al., 2010; Resnick, 2005; van Stralen et al., 2011). Specifically, findings noted that self-efficacy was significantly associated with the adoption and maintenance of exercise behavior (Irvine et al., 2011; McAuley et al., 2006; Pretzer-Aboff et al., 2011; Qi et al., 2011; Resnick, Luisi, et al., 2008; Resnick et al., 2007). Expected outcomes in the form of perceived benefits from exercise were likewise associated with exercise behavior among older adults (Resnick, Luisi, et al., 2008; Wilcox et al., 2006).

Using the theory of self-efficacy, interventions have been developed and tested to increase exercise behavior in healthy community-dwelling adults (King et al., 2007; Resnick et al., 2009; Resnick, Luisi, et al., 2008) as well as those who have sustained a hip fracture or orthopedic event (Hays et al., 2010; Orwig et al., 2011), or among those who have cardiac disease (Duncan, Pozehl, Norman, & Hertzog, 2011; Gary, 2006; Padula, Yeaw, & Mistry, 2009; Resnick et al., 2007), in cancer survivors (Bennett, Lyons, Winters-Stone, Nail, & Scherer, 2007; Bennett et al., 2011; McCorkle et al., 2011; Rogers et al., 2004), in patients with chronic obstructive pulmonary disease (Donesky et al., 2011; Hospes, Bossenbroek, Ten Hacken, van Hengel, & de Greef, 2009), in patients with diabetics (Collins et al., 2011), and to help manage pain during childbirth (Gau et al., 2011). For example, a comprehensive self-efficacy-based intervention, the Exercise Plus Program, which incorporated all four sources of self-efficacy information (mastery, verbal persuasion, self-modeling, and physiological feedback) to increase exercise self-efficacy and behavior for hip fracture patients has been repeatedly tested (Orwig et al., 2011; Resnick et al., 2007). Consistently this 12-month intervention—provided in home settings by exercise trainers—was noted to result in increased time spent in physical activity over the first 12 months post hip fracture.

Another example of a self-efficacy–based exercise intervention was a study that focused on older adults with lower-extremity neuropathy. Specifically, exercise and balance training activities were provided and participants were evaluated to determine if the level of physical activity provided could be tolerated and increased among these individuals (Kruse, LeMaster, & Madsen, 2010). This exercise program resulted in increasing the time spent in physical activity but did not alter performance (e.g., gait speed).

Dietary interventions have also been developed and tested to improve the dietary intake and maintain or facilitate the weight loss (Huang, Yeh, & Tsai, 2011; Oberg et al., 2011; Rejeski, Mihalko, Ambrosius, Bearon, McClelland, 2011; Rosal et al., 2011). For example, a group-mediated intervention for weight loss among older, obese adults were tested to determine if it resulted in changes in self-regulatory self-efficacy for eating behavior and weight loss (Rejeski et al., 2011). A significant treatment effect was observed for self-efficacy for weight loss as well as weight among those who were exposed to both the diet intervention and physical activity. Similarly a dietary intervention that was not focused on weight loss but rather on improving dietary intake for individuals with diabetes was noted to be effective. This intervention resulted in strengthening self-efficacy around healthy eating and improved hemoglobin A1c levels among those exposed to the intervention (Oberg et al., 2011).

Self-Efficacy Interventions for Symptom Management

In addition to using self-efficacy–based interventions to increase adherence to healthy behaviors, such as exercise and healthy diets, self-efficacy interventions have been developed and tested to manage symptoms across a variety of areas. Most commonly these focus on symptoms, such as pain management (Bennett et al., 2011; Gustavsson et al., 2011), fear of falling (Yoo, Jun, & Hawkins, 2010; Zijlstra et al., 2011), and memory changes (McDougall, Becker, Acee, Vaughan, & Delville, 2011; Williams, 2011). For example, a multicomponent cognitive behavioral group intervention was tested with a sample of 540 community-dwelling adults aged 70 years or older who reported a fear of falling and avoided physical activity (Zijlstra et al., 2011). Testing showed that the multicomponent cognitive behavioral intervention improved control beliefs, self-efficacy, outcome expectations, and social interactions. Moreover, these variables mediated the association between the intervention and concerns about falling or daily activity in community-dwelling older adults.

Another example of symptom-focused interventions recently reported was focused on memory in cancer survivors 65 years of age and older who experience treatment-induced memory impairments. This study compared a memory versus health training intervention in a convenience sample of older adults (McDougall et al., 2011). The memory training was designed to increase cognitive performance, reduce anxiety, decrease negative attributions, promote health, and increase memory self-efficacy. Moderate to large effects were revealed in everyday and verbal memory performance scores, memory self-efficacy, strategy use, and memory complaints. There were also moderate effects for group-by-time interactions on the visual memory performance, memory self-efficacy, depression, trait anxiety, and complaints. The memory intervention group tended to improve more than the health training group, although this was not always consistent.

Self-Efficacy Interventions for Education of Health Care Providers

In addition to a clinical focus, self-efficacy–based research has also guided the exploration of education techniques for nurses. Studies of undergraduates have focused on self-efficacy expectations related to academic performance (Ravert, 2004), clinical skills (Darkwah, Ross, Williams, & Madill, 2011; Sherriff, Burston, & Wallis, 2011), and the impact of self-efficacy expectations for assessment skills related to cardiovascular status of patients on behaviors among nurse practitioner students (Jeffries et al., 2011). An example of one study focused on undergraduate education (Sherriff et al., 2011) and evaluated the effect of an on-line, medication calculation education and testing program. The outcome measures used with the nursing students included medication calculation proficiency and self-efficacy expectations associated with medication calculation. Participants were registered nurses and nursing students who were working as supervised nursing students. Outcome measures included number of test attempts, self-efficacy, medication calculation error rates, and satisfaction with the program. Medication calculation scores at first test attempt showed improvement following 1 year of access to the program. Two of the self-efficacy subscales improved over time and nurses reported satisfaction with the online program.

An example of the type of self-efficacy–based interventions used with advanced practice nurses includes the simulation-based cardiovascular assessment curriculum (Jeffries et al., 2011). The educational interventions included faculty-led, simulation-based case presentations using the Harvey® cardiopulmonary patient simulator (CPS), and independent learning sessions using the CPS and a multimedia, computer-based CD-ROM program. Outcome measures included a cognitive written exam, a skills checklist, learner self-efficacy, and a satisfaction survey. The 36 students who received the simulation-based training showed statistically significant pre- to post-test improvement in cognitive knowledge and cardiovascular assessment skills.

A few examples are provided on the types of self-efficacy–based interventions used in nursing as related to care of patients across the life span, in community-based health promotion activities, and in education of patients and providers. There are numerous other studies both within and outside of nursing that likewise provide effective examples of self-efficacy–based interventions that change behavior and improve clinical and knowledge-related outcomes among health care providers. Clearly, the theory is used extensively to guide nursing research and clinical practice.

Self-Efficacy Expectations, Outcome Expectations, and Behavior

Bandura postulates that self-efficacy and outcome expectations increase following self-efficacy–based interventions, particularly performance of the behavior of interest (Bandura, 1995). However, the theory is not always supported by multiple studies in which older adults have been exposed to self-efficacy–based interventions for exercise, which resulted in no change in efficacy expectations, even though there were improvements in behavior (Orwig et al., 2011; Resnick et al., 2009; Resnick, Galik, Gruber-Baldini, & Zimmerman, 2009; Resnick, Gruber-Baldini, Zimmerman, et al., 2009; Resnick, Luisi, et al., 2008). These findings may, in part, be due to measurement issues in that the individuals who volunteered for these exercise intervention studies generally had strong self-efficacy and outcome expectations at baseline and thus there was a ceiling effect. In addition, the measures used may not have been specific enough for the behavior of interest. For example, in many of these studies self-efficacy was measured in light of the challenges that can influence engaging in an exercise activity rather than simply asking about confidence in, for example, walking 10 feet, 20 feet, and so on. It is also possible that the intervention was not strong enough to result in a change in self-efficacy and outcome expectations.

Alternative explanations for a lack of significant increase in self-efficacy or outcome expectations following an intervention have been proposed by McAuley (McAuley et al., 2006). Specifically, he suggested that a decline in self-efficacy following exposure to an exercise intervention can also occur when there is a decrease in exposure to exercise classes, when exposed to a new exercise that is challenging, when there is a change in clinical condition or ability so that the exercise program is perceived to be more difficult, or when the exercise program is progressively more challenging. Therefore, it is critical to consider these aspects when implementing exercise intervention studies.

USE OF THE THEORY IN NURSING PRACTICE

Translation of research findings into practice is not often done in a timely fashion. This is particularly true of research findings that focus on behavior change. However, there is evidence to demonstrate that the theory of self-efficacy can help direct nursing care. The theory has been particularly helpful with regard to motivating individuals to participate in health-promoting activities, such as regular exercise, smoking cessation, weight loss, and going for recommended cancer screenings. For example, Resnick and her research teams [(Galik et al., 2008; Resnick et al., 2009; Resnick, Galik, et al., 2009; Resnick, Luisi, et al., 2008) (Nahm et al., 2010; Orwig et al., 2011; Resnick, Gruber-Baldini, Galik, et al., 2009; Resnick, Gruber-Baldini, Zimmerman, et al., 2009) (Qi et al., 2011; Shaughnessy & Resnick, 2009)] have used self-efficacy theory as a foundation for programs that encourage exercise and physical activity in older adults. Among these interventions, the function-focused care (FFC) approach has been tested the most extensively and will be described as an exemplar.

Function-Focused Care

FFC, also referred to as restorative care, is a philosophy of care that focuses on evaluating the older adult's underlying capability with regard to function and physical activity and helping him or her to optimize and maintain abilities and continually increase time spent in physical activity. Implementation of FFC is guided overall by a social ecological model. This model provides an overarching framework for understanding the interrelations among diverse personal and environmental factors that can influence behavior change and specifically addresses intrapersonal, interpersonal, environmental, and policy factors. At the interpersonal level, self-efficacy–based interventions are used to facilitate a FFC approach and change behavior among caregivers as well as older individuals. The ultimate goal is to optimize function and physical activity among older adults.

FFC is implemented using the following four components: (I) environment and policy/procedure assessments; (II) education; (III) developing function-focused goals; and (IV) mentoring and motivating. Component I involves completing assessments of the environment and policies/procedures relevant to function and physical activity within the settings. The findings from these assessments guide environmental and policy/procedure change, such as making pleasant walking areas on units or in facilities, establishing transportation policies that allow patients/residents to ambulate to tests or procedures, or allowing residents to walk in outside areas when living in long-term care settings.

Component II involves teaching nursing staff, other members of the interdisciplinary team (e.g., social work, physical therapy), patients, and families about the philosophy of FFC. Teaching is done both formally and informally in small groups or one-on-one and incorporates self-efficacy techniques including verbal encouragement, use of role models, and actual performance of skills and activities (e.g., use of demonstrations by caregivers for how to interact with older individuals using a FFC approach).

Component III involves establishing individualized goals for the older individuals who are geared toward increasing his or her function and time spent in the physical activity. Goals are established after evaluating that older adult's underlying function and ability (e.g., ability to follow a one- two-, or three- step command, ability to get up from a chair). Individualized goals provide important encouragement as they indicate to the older individual that the goal established is something that the health care team or family in the home setting believe he or she is capable of achieving.

Component IV is implemented using all four sources of self-efficacy–based information for both the caregivers being exposed to FFC and the patient/resident. Building off the initial education done with caregivers (this includes nurses, nursing assistants, home health care workers, and family caregivers, and other members of the interdisciplinary team including physicians, social workers, physical therapists, etc.), an identified champion in a facility or home setting will provide the ongoing verbal encouragement, support, recognition, and positive reinforcement around performing FFC with the older individual. For example, this might be a simple "it was terrific that you worked with Mrs. Jones to have her walk to the dining room today"; or "that was great this morning when you led the residents in a few minutes of dance prior to eating breakfast." The champion also can provide one-on-one mentoring and role modeling as needed. This might include intervening in a situation in which FFC is not occurring. For example, a nursing assistant or a family might be pushing Mrs. Jones to the dining room in a wheelchair because she wanted to get a ride. The champion might interrupt and role model FFC interactions by indicating to Mrs. Jones that she did a great job walking to the dining room this morning and encourage her to "show Jane [the caregiver] how well you can do it!" Other formalized activities the champion might do include: (a) observing performance of caregivers within a setting and providing one-on-one mentoring of ways in which to incorporate FFC into routine care, (b) providing caregivers with positive reinforcement for doing FFC interactions, (c) meeting in groups or informally with caregivers to address their beliefs about physical activity and feelings and experiences associated with providing FFC, (d) reinforcing the benefits associated with FFC for both caregivers and older adults as a way to strengthen outcome expectations, (e) highlighting role models (other caregivers who successfully implemented the program), and (f) identifying change-aides and positive opinion leaders to help with dissemination and implementation of FFC and eliminate the influence of negative opinion leaders.

In addition, caregivers are taught to implement self-efficacy–based approaches to motivate older adults to engage in function and physical activity. As with all types of behaviors, actual performance is the best way to strengthen self-efficacy and outcome expectations. Therefore, the caregivers are taught to engage the resident in an activity he or she is capable of performing well and without uncomfortable sensations such as fear or pain. Once performance occurs when the caregivers are taught to provide critically important positive reinforcement to older individuals for engaging in the activity. This might be a hug, a smile, or a round of applause! Goals are set with the older individual, working even with cognitively impaired individuals to learn from them what is important and what they want to be able to do functionally and physically. This might be working toward going out on a trip or going to a granddaughter's wedding. Activities and goals are individualized and should reflect what the person has done and enjoyed throughout his or her lifetime. Walking, shopping, delivering televisions, or working on a nursing unit can all be used to motivate the older individual to engage in those well-known activities yet again.

Role modeling is very useful as is self-modeling as a way to motivate older individuals. The role model may be the caregiver versus a peer and may be as simple as showing the older individual what to do. This is particularly true among those with cognitive impairment who may not remember multiple steps or commands. Likewise, reminding the older individual that he or she was able to walk to the bathroom successfully yesterday and thus can do so today is a form of self-modeling that is often effective.

For older adults, the experience of engaging in functional and physical activity must occur free of uncomfortable physiological feedback. Given the high prevalence of musculoskeletal disease, associated pain and fear of falling among older adults are two primary areas that must be acknowledged and addressed. It is extremely challenging to eliminate these sensations and yet maintain function and physical activity; thus, acknowledging the sensations, talking about them, and assuring the individual that we "won't let them fall" or "won't have them do anything that will cause them more pain" are important. Pain medications and use of ice or heat to a joint are other ways to manage the pain before ambulation or a given activity.

In addition to addressing the uncomfortable sensations associated with an activity, the positive and pleasant outcomes and sensations can be highlighted. Making function and physical activity fun is important—music, dance, and the use of humor through what may be slower and more tedious personal care activities are useful interventions. Associating exercise activities with improvements in blood pressure readings, blood sugars, and weight loss are other ways to demonstrate the benefits of activity.

CONCLUSION

The studies that nurse researchers have done using the theory of self-efficacy provide support for the importance of self-efficacy and outcome expectations with regard to behavior change. The studies also provide support for the effectiveness of specific interventions that have been tested to strengthen both self-efficacy and outcome expectations and thereby improve behavior. However, it is important to note that studies have also demonstrated that self-efficacy and outcome expectations may not be the only predictors of behavior. Other variables, such as genetic predispositions, tension/anxiety, barriers to behavior, and other psychosocial experiences impact behavior. Bandura (1986) recognized that expectations alone would not result in behavior change if there were no incentives to perform or if there were inadequate resources or external constraints. Certainly an individual may believe that he or she can participate in a rehabilitation program but may not have the resources (i.e., transportation or money) to do so. In addition, when considered over time, it is possible that self-efficacy and outcome expectations will not get stronger. Rather, the individual may recognize that it is not as easy to perform a given behavior, and self-efficacy and outcome expectations may actually weaken.

Self-efficacy theory is situation specific. Therefore, it is difficult to generalize an individual's self-efficacy from one type of behavior to the other. If an individual has high self-efficacy with regard to diet management, this may or may not generalize to persistence in an exercise program. Future nursing research needs to focus on the degree to which specific self-efficacy behaviors can be generalized. To what degree is self-efficacy a dimension of individual humanness, distinct for each person but consistent across a range of related behaviors for one person? Future consideration should also be given to the relationship between self-efficacy and resilience, particularly with regard to specific areas. Resilience refers to the capacity to spring back from a physical, emotional, financial, or social challenge. Self-efficacy is an important component of resilience. Future research should also begin to consider the genetic variability in individuals and how this may impact self-efficacy. For example, it is now believed that a common variant in a single gene (the angiotensin-1 converting enzyme gene) is associated with older individuals who are more likely to benefit from physical activity (Nicklas, 2010). These individuals will tend to have stronger self-efficacy and thus be more likely to engage in the activity on a regular basis.

Measurement of self-efficacy and outcome expectations requires the development of situation-specific scales with a series of activities listed of increasing difficulty or by a contextual arrangement in nonpsychomotor skills such as dietary modification (Bandura, 1997). It is important to carefully construct these scales and establish evidence of reliability and validity. Behavior-specific scales can be used as the foundation for assessing an individual's self-care abilities in a particular area. Interventions can then be developed that are relevant for that individual.

A persistent problem with the use of the theory of self-efficacy in nursing research has been the lack of consideration of outcome expectations. In particular, with regard to exercise in older adults, outcome expectations have been noted to be better predictors of exercise behavior than self-efficacy expectations (Resnick, Luisi, et al., 2008; Wilcox et al., 2006). The influence of self-efficacy expectations and outcome expectations as they relate to initiation versus long-term adherence to behaviors is currently not well understood and ongoing research in this area is needed. Social cognitive theory and the theory of self-efficacy have helped guide nursing research related to behavior change. Ongoing studies are needed to continue to build and utilize this work to improve the health of individuals in this country and globally.

REFERENCES

Akers, A. Y., Holland, C. L., & Bost, J. (2011). Interventions to improve parental communication about sex: A systematic review. *Pediatrics, 127*(3), 494–510.
Bandura, A. (1977). Self-efficacy: Toward a unifying theory of behavioral change. *Psychological Review, 84*, 191–215.
Bandura, A. (1986). *Social foundations of thought and action*. Upper Saddle River, NJ: Prentice Hall.
Bandura, A. (1995). *Self-efficacy in changing societies*. New York, NY: Cambridge University Press.
Bandura, A. (1997). *Self-efficacy: The exercise of control*. New York, NY: W. H. Freeman and Company.
Bandura, A., Adams, N., & Beyer, J. (1977). Cognitive processes mediating behavioral change. *Journal of Personality and Social Psychology, 35*(3), 125–149.
Bandura, A., Reese, L., & Adams, N. (1982). Microanalysis of action and fear arousal as a function of differential levels of perceived self-efficacy. *Journal of Personality and Social Psychology, 43*, 5–21.
Bennett, J., Lyons, K. S., Winters-Stone, K., Nail, L. M., & Scherer, J. (2007). Motivational interviewing to increase physical activity in long-term cancer survivors: A randomized controlled trial. *Nursing Research, 56*(1), 18–27.
Bennett, M., Bagnall, A. M., Raine, G., Closs, S. J., Blenkinsopp, A., Dickman, A., & Ellershaw, J. (2011). Educational interventions by pharmacists to patients with chronic pain: Systematic review and meta-analysis. *Clinical Journal of Pain, 27*(7), 623–630.
Brown, J., Vanable, P. A., Carey, M. P., & Elin, L. (2011). Computerized stress management training for HIV+ women: A pilot intervention study. *AIDS Care, 23*(12), 1525–1532.
Chase, J. (2011). Systematic review of physical activity intervention studies after cardiac rehabilitation. *Journal of Cardiovascular Nursing, 26*(5), 351–358.

Collins, R., Lee, R. E., Albright, C. L., & King, A. C. (2004). Ready to be physically active? The effects of a course preparing low-income multiethnic women to be more physically active. *Health Education & Behavior, 31*(1), 47–64.

Collins, T., Lunos, S., Carlson, T., Henderson, K., Lightbourne, M., Nelson, B., & Hodges, J. S. (2011). Effects of a home-based walking intervention on mobility and quality of life in people with diabetes and peripheral arterial disease: A randomized controlled trial. *Diabetes Care, 34*(10), 2174–2179.

Cress, M., Buchner, D. M., Prohaska, T., Rimmer, J., Brown, M., Macera, C., ... Chodzko-Zajko, W. (2005). Best practices for physical activity programs and behavior counseling in older adult populations. *Journal of Aging & Physical Activity, 13*(1), 61–74.

Curtin, R., Mapes, D., Schatell, D., & Burrows-Hudson, S. (2005). Self-management in patients with end stage renal disease: Exploring domains and dimensions. *Nephrology Nursing Journal, 32*(4), 389–395.

Darkwah, V., Ross, C., Williams, B., & Madill, H. (2011). Undergraduate nursing student self-efficacy in patient education in a context-based learning program. *Journal of Nursing Education, 50*(10), 579–582.

Donesky, D., Janson, S. L., Nguyen, H. Q., Neuhaus, J., Neilands, T. B., & Carrieri-Kohlman, V. (2011). Determinants of frequency, duration, and continuity of home walking in patients with COPD. *Geriatric Nursing, 32*(3), 178–187.

Druss, B., Zhao, L., von Esenwein, S. A., Bona, J. R., Fricks, L., Jenkins-Tucker, S., ... Lorig, K. (2010). The Health and Recovery Peer (HARP) program: A peer-led intervention to improve medical self-management for persons with serious mental illness. *Schizophrenia Research, 118*(1–3), 264–270.

Duncan, K., Pozehl, B., Norman, J. F., & Hertzog, M. (2011). A self-directed adherence management program for patients with heart failure completing combined aerobic and resistance exercise training. *Applied Nursing Research, 24*(4), 207–214.

Estabrooks, P., Fox, E. H., Doerksen, S. E., Bradshaw, M. H., & King, A. C. (2005). Participatory research to promote physical activity at congregate-meal sites. *Journal of Aging and Physical Activity, 13*(2), 121–144.

Galik, E. (2007). Behavior change: Innovative interventions to optimize function in the cognitively impaired. *Advance for Nurses, 9*(20), 35.

Galik, E., Pretzer-Aboff, I., & Resnick, B. (2011). Nurses perspective of function focused care in acute care. *International Journal of Older Adults, 15*(1), 48–55.

Galik, E., Resnick, B., Gruber-Baldini, A., Nahm, E., Pearson, K., & Pretzer-Aboff, I. (2008). Pilot testing of the restorative care intervention for the cognitively impaired. *Journal of the American Medical Directors Association, 9*(7), 516–522.

Gary, R. (2006). Exercise self-efficacy in older women with diastolic heart failure: Results of a walking program and education intervention. *Journal of Gerontological Nursing, 32*(7), 31–41.

Gau, M., Chang, C. Y., Tian, S. H., & Lin, K. C. (2011). Effects of birth ball exercise on pain and self-efficacy during childbirth: A randomised controlled trial in Taiwan. *Midwifery, 27*(6), e293–e300.

Gortner, S., & Jenkins, L. (1990). Self-efficacy and activity level following cardiac surgery. *Journal of Advanced Nursing, 15,* 1132–1138.

Gortner, S., Rankin, S., & Wolfe, M. (1988). Elders' recovery from cardiac surgery. *Progress in Cardiovascular Nursing, 3*(2), 54–61.

Granger, B., Moser, D., Germino, B., Harrell, J., & Ekman, I. (2006). Caring for patients with chronic heart failure: The trajectory model. *European Journal of Cardiovascular Nursing, 5*(3), 222–227.

Grim, M., Hortz, B., & Petosa, R. (2011). Impact evaluation of a pilot web-based intervention to increase physical activity. *American Journal of Health Promotion, 25*(4), 227–230.

Gustavsson, C., Denison, E., & von Koch, L. (2011). Self-management of persistent neck pain: Two-year follow-up of a randomized controlled trial of a multicomponent group intervention in primary health care. *Spine, 36*(25), 2105–2115.

Han, K., Lee, S. J., Park, E. S., Park, Y., & Cheol, K. H. (2005). Structural model for quality of life in patients with chronic cardiovascular disease in Korea. *Nursing Research, 54,* 85–96.

Harnirattisai, T., & Johnson, R. (2002). *Reliability of self-efficacy and outcome expectations scales for exercise and functional activity in Thai elder.* Paper presented at the Health Science Research Day, University of Missouri-Columbia.

Harnirattisai, T., & Johnson, R. (2005). Effectiveness of a behavioral change intervention in Thai elders after knee replacement. *Nursing Research, 54*(2), 97–107.

Hays, L., Pressler, S., Damush, T., Rawl, S., & Clark, D. (2010). Exercise adoption among older, low-income women at risk for cardiovascular disease. *Public Health Nursing, 27*(1), 79–88.

Horowitz, C., Eckhardt, S., Talavera, S., Goytia, C., & Lorig, K. (2011). Effectively translating diabetes prevention: A successful model in a historically underserved community. *Translational Behavioral Medicine, 1*(3), 443–452.

Hospes, G., Bossenbroek, L., Ten Hacken, N. H., van Hengel, P., & de Greef, M. H. (2009). Enhancement of daily physical activity increases physical fitness of outclinic COPD patients: Results of an exercise counseling program. *Patient Education & Counseling, 75*(2), 274–278.

Huang, T., Yeh, C. Y., & Tsai, Y. C. (2011). A diet and physical activity intervention for preventing weight retention among Taiwanese childbearing women: A randomised controlled trial. *Midwifery, 27*(2), 257–264.

Irvine, A., Philips, L., Seeley, J., Wyant, S., Duncan, S., & Moore, R. W. (2011). Get moving: A web site that increases physical activity of sedentary employees (includes abstract). *American Journal of Health Promotion, 25*(3), 199–206.

Jeffries, P. R., Beach, M., Decker, S. I., Dlugasch, L., Groom, J., Settles, J., & O'Donnell, J. M. (2011). Multi-center development and testing of a simulation-based cardiovascular assessment curriculum for advanced practice nurses. *Nursing Education Perspectives, 32*(5), 316–322.

Johansson, P., Dahlström, U., & Bromström, A. (2006). Consequences and predictors of depression in patients with chronic heart failure: Implications for nursing care and future research. *Progress in Cardiovascular Nursing, 21*(4), 202–211.

Jones, F., Harris, P., Waller, H., & Coggins, A. (2005). Adherence to an exercise prescription scheme: The role of expectations, self-efficacy stage of change and psychological well-being. *British Journal of Health Psychology, 10*, 359–378.

Kamish, S., & Öz, F. (2011). Evaluation of a smoking cessation psychoeducational program for nurses. *Journal of Addictions Nursing, 22*(3), 117–123.

King, A. C., Friedman, R., Marcus, B., Castro, C., Napolitano, M., Ahn, D., & Baker, L. (2007). Ongoing physical activity advice by humans versus computers: The Community Health Advice by Telephone (CHAT) trial. *Health Psychology, 26*(6), 718–727.

Kruse, R., LeMaster, J. W., & Madsen, R. W. (2010). Fall and balance outcomes after an intervention to promote leg strength, balance, and walking in people with diabetic peripheral neuropathy: "feet first" randomized controlled trial. *Physical Therapy, 90*(11), 1568–1579.

Li, F., Fisher, K. J., Harmer, P., & McAuley, E. (2005). Falls self-efficacy as a mediator of fear of falling in an exercise intervention for older adults. *Journal of Gerontology B Psychological Sciences and Social Sciences, 60*(1), 34–40.

Lorig, K., Ritter, P. L., Laurent, D. D., Plant, K., Green, M., Jernigan, V. B., & Case, S. (2010). Online diabetes self-management program: A randomized study. *Diabetes Care, 33*(6), 1275–1281.

Martin, M. Y., Kim, Y. I., Kratt, P., Litaker, M. S., Kohler, C. L., Schoenberger, Y. M., … Williams, O. D. (2011). Medication adherence among rural, low-income hypertensive adults: A randomized trial of a multimedia community-based intervention. *American Journal of Health Promotion, 25*(6), 372–378.

McAuley, E., Konopack, J. F., Motl, R. W., Morris, K. S., Doerksen, S. E., & Rosengren, K. R. (2006). Physical activity and quality of life in older adults: Influence of health status and self-efficacy. *Annals of Behavioral Medicine, 31*(1), 99–103.

McCorkle, R., Ercolano, E., Lazenby, M., Schulman-Green, D., Schilling, L. S., Lorig, K., & Wagner, E. H. (2011). Self-management: Enabling and empowering patients living with cancer as a chronic illness. *CA: A Cancer Journal for Clinicians, 61*(1), 50–62.

McDougall, G., Becker, H., Acee, T. W., Vaughan, P. W., & Delville, C. L. (2011). Symptom management of affective and cognitive disturbance with a group of cancer survivors. *Archives of Psychiatric Nursing, 25*(1), 24–35.

Merrill, R. M., Shields, E. C., Wood, A., & Beck, R. E. (2004). Outcome expectations that motivate physical activity among world senior games participants. *Perceptions and Motor Skills, 99*(3), 1277–1289.

Millen, J., & Bray, S. R. (2009). Promoting self-efficacy and outcome expectations to enable adherence to resistance training after cardiac rehabilitation. *Journal of Cardiovascular Nursing, 24*(4), 316–327.

Nahm, E., Barker, B., Resnick, B., Covington, B., Magaziner, J., & Brennan, P. (2010). Effects of a social cognitive theory-based hip fracture prevention web site for older adults. *Computers, Informatics, Nursing, 28*(6), 371–377.

Nicklas, B. (2010). Heterogeneity of physical function responses to exercise in older adults: Possible contribution of variation in the angiotensin-1 converting enzyme (ACE) gene? *Perspectives on Psychological Science, 5*, 575–584.

Niedermann, K., de Bie, R. A., Kubli, R., Ciurea, A., Steurer-Stey, C., Villiger, P. M., & Büchi, S. (2011). Effectiveness of individual resource-oriented joint protection education in people with rheumatoid arthritis. A randomized controlled trial. *Patient Education & Counseling, 82*(1), 42–48.

Oberg, E. B., Bradley, R., Allen, J., & McCrory, M. A. (2011). CAM: Naturopathic dietary interventions for patients with Type 2 diabetes. *Complementary Therapies in Clinical Practice, 17*(3), 157–161.

Orwig, D., Hochberg, M., Yu-Yahiro, J., Resnick, B., Hawkes, W. G., Shardell, M., … Magaziner, J. (2011). Delivery and outcomes of a yearlong home exercise program after hip fracture: A randomized controlled trial. *Journal of Archives of Internal Medicine, 171*(4), 323–331.

Padula, C., Yeaw, E., & Mistry, S. (2009). A home-based nurse-coached inspiratory muscle training intervention in heart failure. *Applied Nursing Research, 22*(1), 18–25.

Pretzer-Aboff, I., Galik, E., & Resnick, B. (2009). Parkinson's disease: Barriers and facilitators to optimizing function. *Rehabilitation Nursing, 34*(2), 55–63.

Pretzer-Aboff, I., Galik, E., & Resnick, B. (2011). Testing the impact of res-care Parkinson's disease. *Nursing Research, 60*(4), 276–283.

Qi, B., Resnick, B., Smeltzer, S. C., & Bausell, B. (2011). Self-efficacy enhanced education program in preventing osteoporosis among chinese immigrants: A randomized controlled trial. *Nursing Research, 60*(6), 393–404.

Ravert, P. (2004). *Use of a human patient simulator with undergraduate nursing students: A prototype evaluation of critical thinking and self-efficacy.* Doctoral Dissertation, University of Utah.

Rejeski, W. J., Fielding, R., Blair, S., Guralnik, J., Gill, T., Hadley, E., … Pahor, M. (2005). The lifestyle interventions and independence for elders (LIFE) pilot study: Design and methods. *Contemporary Clinical Trials, 26*(2), 141–154.

Rejeski, W. J., Katula, J., Rejeski, A., Rowley, J., & Sipe, M. (2005). Strength training in older adults: Does desire determine confidence? *Journal of Gerontology B Psychological Sciences and Social Science, 60*(6), P335–P337.

Rejeski, W. J., Mihalko, S. L., Ambrosius, W. T., Bearon, L. B., & McClelland, J. W. (2011). Weight loss and self-regulatory eating efficacy in older adults: The cooperative lifestyle intervention program. *Journals of Gerontology Series B: Psychological Sciences & Social Sciences, 66B*(3), 279–286.

Resnick, B. (2005). Reliability and validity of the outcome expectations for exercise scale-2. *Journal of Aging and Physical Activity, 13*(4), 382–394.

Resnick, B. (2011). *Implementing restorative care nursing in all setting.* New York, NY: Springer.

Resnick, B., & D'Adamo, C. (2011). Wellness center use and factors associated with physical activity among older adults in a retirement community. *Rehabilitation Nursing, 36*(2), 47–53.

Resnick, B., Galik, E., Gruber-Baldini, A., & Zimmerman, S. (2009). Implementing a restorative care philosophy of care in assisted living: Pilot testing of Res-Care-AL. *Journal of the American Academy of Nurse Practitioners, 21*(2), 123–133.

Resnick, B., Galik, E., Gruber-Baldini, A., & Zimmerman, S. (2011). Testing the impact of function focused care in assisted living. *Journal of the American Geriatrics Society, 59*(12), 2233–2240.

Resnick, B., Galik, E., Nahm, E., Shaughnessy, M., & Michael, K. (2009). Optimizing adherence in older adults with cognitive impairment. In J. Okene, S. Shumaker, & K. Riekert's (Eds.), *The handbook of health behavior change* (3rd ed.). New York, NY: Springer Publishing.

Resnick, B., Galik, E., Petzer-Aboff, I., Rogers, V., & Gruber-Baldini, A. (2008). Testing the reliability and validity of self-efficacy and outcome expectations of restorative care performed by nursing assistants. *Journal of Nursing Care Quality, 23*(2), 162–169.

Resnick, B., Gruber-Baldini, A., Galik, E., Pretzer-Aboff, I., Russ, K., Hebel, J., & Zimmerman, S. (2009). Changing the philosophy of care in long-term care: Testing of the restorative care intervention. *The Gerontologist, 49*(2), 175–184.

Resnick, B., Gruber-Baldini, A., Zimmerman, S., Galik, E., Pretzer-Aboff, I., Russ, K., & Hebel, J. R. (2009). Nursing home resident outcomes from the Res-Care intervention. *Journal of the American Geriatrics Society, 57*(7), 1156–1165.

Resnick, B., & Jenkins, L. (2000). Reliability and validity testing of the self-efficacy for exercise scale. *Nursing Research, 49*, 154–159.

Resnick, B., Luisi, D., & Vogel, A. (2008). Testing The Senior Exercise Self-Efficacy Pilot Project (SESEP) for use with urban dwelling minority older adults. *Public Health Nursing, 25*(3), 221–234.

Resnick, B., Orwig, D., Yu-Yahiro, J., Hawkes, W., Shardell, M., Hebel, J., ... Magaziner, J. (2007). Testing the effectiveness of the exercise plus program in older women post hip fracture. *Annals of Behavioral Medicine, 34*(1), 67–76.

Resnick, B., Shaughnessy, M., Galik, E., Scheve, A., Fitten, R., Morrison, T., ... Agness, C. (2009). Pilot testing of the PRAISEDD intervention among African American and low income older adults. *Journal of Cardiovascular Nursing, 24*(5), 352–361.

Resnick, B., Wehren, L., & Orwig, D. (2003). Reliability and validity of the self-efficacy and outcome expectations for osteoporosis medication adherence scales. *Orthopaedic Nursing, 22*(2), 139–147.

Resnick, B., Zimmerman, S., Orwig, D., Furstenberg, A., & Magaziner, J. (2000). Outcome expectations for exercise scale: Utility and psychometrics. *Journal of Gerontology Social Sciences, 55B*(6), S352–S356.

Resnick, B., Zimmerman, S., Orwig, D., Furstenberg, A. L., & Magaziner, J. (2001a). Model testing for reliability and validity of the outcome expectations for exercise scale. *Nursing Research, 50*(5), 293–299.

Resnick, B., Zimmerman, S. I., Orwig, D., Furstenberg, A. L., & Magaziner, J. (2001b). Building evidence of reliability and validity of the outcome expectations for exercise scale through model testing. *Nursing Research, 50*(5), 293–300.

Rogers, L., Matevey, C., Hopkins-Price, P., Shah, P., Dunnington, G., & Courneya, K. S. (2004). Exploring social cognitive theory constructs for promoting exercise among breast cancer patients. *Cancer Nursing, 27*(6), 462–473.

Rogers, L., Shah, P., Dunnington, G., Greive, A., Shanmugham, A., Dawson, B., & Courneya, K. S. (2005). Social cognitive theory and physical activity during breast cancer treatment. *Oncology Nursing Forum, 32*(4), 807–815.

Rosal, M. C., Ockene, I. S., Restrepo, A., White, M. J., Borg, A., Olendzki, B., ... Reed, G. (2011). Randomized trial of a literacy-sensitive, culturally tailored diabetes self-management intervention for low-income latinos: Latinos en control. *Diabetes Care, 34*(4), 838–844.

Schnoll, R., Martinez, E., Tatum, K. L., Glass, M., Bernath, A., Ferris, D., & Reynolds, P. (2011). Increased self-efficacy to quit and perceived control over withdrawal symptoms predict smoking cessation following nicotine dependence treatment. *Addictive Behaviors, 36*(1–2), 144–147.

Shaughnessy, M., & Resnick, B. (2009). Using theory to develop an exercise intervention for patients post stroke. *Topics in Stroke Rehabilitation, 16*(2), 140–146.

Shaughnessy, M., Resnick, B., & Macko, R. (2004). Testing reliability and validity of the stroke self-efficacy and outcome expectations measures for exercise. *Journal of Stroke Cerebrovascular Disease, 2004 Sep–Oct; 13*(5), 214–219.

Sherriff, K., Burston, S., & Wallis, M. (2011). Effectiveness of a computer based medication calculation education and testing programme for nurses. *Nurse Education Today, 32*(1), 46–51.

Skinner, C., Buchanan, A., Champion, V., Monahan, P., Rawl, S., Springston, J., ... Bourff, S. (2011). Process outcomes from a randomized controlled trial comparing tailored mammography interventions delivered via telephone vs. DVD. *Patient Education & Counseling, 85*(2), 308–312.

Swartz, L., Sherman, C. A., Harvey, S. M., Blanchard, J., Vawter, F., & Gau, J. (2011). Midlife women online: Evaluation of an internet-based program to prevent unintended pregnancy & STIs. *Journal of Women & Aging, 23*(4), 342–359.

Utz, S., Williams, I., Jones, R., Hinton, I., Alexander, G., Yan, G., ... Oliver, M. N. (2008). Culturally tailored intervention for rural African Americans with type 2 diabetes. *The Diabetes Educator, 34*(5), 854–865.

van Stralen, M. M., de Vress, H., Mudde, A. N., Bolman, C., & Lechner, L. (2011). The long-term efficacy of two computer-tailored physical activity interventions for older adults: Main effects and mediators. *Health Psychology, 30*(4), 442–452.

Vancouver, J. B., & Kendell, L. (2006). When self-efficacy negatively relates to motivation and performance in a learning context. *The Journal of Applied Psychology, 91*(5), 1146–1153.

Vancouver, J. B., More, K., & Yoder, R. J. (2008). Self-efficacy and resource allocation: Support for a nonmonotonic, discontinuous model. *The Journal of Applied Psychology, 93*(1), 35–47.

Vancouver, J. B., Thompson, C., & Williams, A. A. (2001). The changing signs in the relationships among self-efficacy, personal goals and performance. *Journal of Applied Psychology, 86*(4), 605–620.

Wilcox, S., Castro, C., & King, A. (2006). Outcome expectations and physical activity participation in two samples of older women. *Journal of Health Psychology, 11*(1), 65–77.

Williams, K. N. (2011). Targeting memory improvement in assisted living: A pilot study. *Rehabilitation Nursing, 36*(6), 225–232.

Yoo, E., Jun, T. W., & Hawkins, S. A. (2010). The effects of a walking exercise program on fall-related fitness, bone metabolism, and fall-related psychological factors in elderly women. *Research in Sports Medicine, 18*(4), 236–250.

Zijlstra, G., van Haastregt, J. C., van Eijk, J. T., de Witte, L. P., Ambergen, T., & Kempen, G. I. (2011). Mediating effects of psychosocial factors on concerns about falling and daily activity in a multicomponent cognitive behavioral group intervention. *Aging & Mental Health, 15*(1), 68–77.

10

Story Theory

Mary Jane Smith and Patricia R. Liehr

*O*ur belief in the healing potential of story and recognition of the importance of building theory at the intersection of practice and research have been essential to the development of Story Theory. The theory was first published in 1999 (Smith & Liehr) with the name "attentively embracing story." Since that time, after discussion with colleagues and students, most of whom questioned the complexity of the name, we simplified the name to "story theory," which has always been the essence of the theory. The central ontology and epistemology of the theory remains as Reed (1999) described it over a decade ago. The ontology affirms that "story is an inner human resource for making meaning," and the epistemology is based on the understanding that "middle range theory bonds research and practice in a method of knowledge development" (p. 205).

PURPOSE OF THE THEORY AND HOW IT WAS DEVELOPED

Stories are a fundamental dimension of the human experience. They bind humans to other humans and times to other times (Taylor, 1996). Stories express who people are, where they've been, and where they are going. The purpose of story theory is to describe and explain story as the context for a nurse–person health-promoting process. The theory was developed to provide a story-centered structure for guiding nursing practice and research. The core nursing process for practice and research is intentional dialogue occurring in a nurse–person relationship. In this relationship, the nurse gathers a story about a health challenge that matters to the person.

The authors have had a long-term relationship that started in an educational program and cultivated discussion of common values about nursing practice and research. Smith began studying rest in 1975 with her dissertation research (Smith, 1975). Later, she conceptualized rest as "easing with the flow of rhythmic change in the environment" (Smith, 1986, p. 23). Liehr's (1992) dissertation examined the blood pressure effects of talking about the usual day and listening to a story. These early works were harbingers of what was to come in collaboration.

Years passed and we both pursued our own work. A serendipitous meeting at a nursing conference led to discussion of the importance of story for promoting health and human development. In talking about our individual work, we were struck by the commonalities that surfaced when we gathered stories. It became clear that story was a context for guiding practice and research. This clarity demanded articulation of a theory as a basis for further work. It was important that the theory be at the middle range level of abstraction to ensure applicability. The theory was developed in an enthusiastic discourse that fits the description by Belenky, Clinchy, Goldberger, and Tarule (1996) "as a place where people work at the very edges of their abilities, constantly pushing each other's thinking into new territory, giving names to things that have gone unnamed, dreaming of better ways, describing common ground and finding ways to realize shared dreams" (p. 13).

We began trying to name the theory to reflect our experience with patients and research participants. We had an image of the way story-sharing mattered to people when we listened with full attention. It took time to engage in the creative process of naming the theory. After several months and many names, we had the name that we believed accurately captured what we were describing. Once the theory was named, each of us began to view practice and research situations through the lens of attentively embracing story. As we used this lens to consider practice and research and discussed the theory with colleagues and students, we reflected on the theory name. We came to recognize that all people do not attentively embrace their story even when given the opportunity for story sharing with someone who truly cares to listen. Readiness for embracing story and experiencing ease varies from individual to individual. The attentively embracing part of the theory name came from our early work with pregnant teens and persons in cardiac rehabilitation (Smith & Liehr, 2003). People who embraced their story of pregnancy or broken heart were people who moved on to purposeful living.

The original name limited expression of the complexity that is naturally inherent in the emergent human health story. We changed the name between 2003 and 2006. Although the process of attentive embracing is incorporated into the theory's meaning, the words were removed from the theory name. The current name, story theory, is more precise, parsimonious, and at the middle range level of discourse while still reflecting the basic nature and the complex process described in the theory. The name change is consistent with the original intent of theory applicability to any situation where a nurse engages a person to intentionally dialogue about what matters most to him or her about the complicating health challenge.

In our earliest writing on middle range theory (Smith & Liehr, 1999), we emphasized the importance of naming the theory in a way that describes the central core shaping the structure of the theory. What we did not address was that the theory name, like any other element or dimension of a theory, is a work in progress. When authors of a theory find that an element or dimension, such as a designated name, is not consistent with the core meaning of the theory, a change is in order. It is essential that the name be appropriate to the theory and offer a unique identity that clearly represents the theory.

We describe story as a narrative happening of connecting with self-in-relation through intentional dialogue to create ease. Ease emerges in the midst of accepting the whole story as one's own … a process of attentive embracing.

Foundation Literature and Assumptions

Story theory is at the middle range level of abstraction, holding assumptions congruent with unitary and neomodernist perspectives (Parse, 1981; Reed, 1995; Rogers, 1994). In these nonreductionistic views, human beings are transforming and transcending in mutual process with their environment. The mutual, ever-changing motion of creating meaning is essential to the unitary perspective depicting the narrative happening of story in and through time. Developmental personal history and human potential for health and healing are essential to the neomodernist perspective. In this view, the healing power of story is a manifestation all through life.

The human story is a health story in the broadest sense. It is a recounting of one's current life situation to clarify present meaning in relation to the past with an eye toward the future, all in the present moment. The idea of story is not new to nursing. Several extant nursing theories explicitly or implicitly incorporate dimensions of story (Boykin & Schoenhofer, 2001; Newman, 1999; Parse, 1981; Peplau, 1991; Watson, 1997). The nursing literature frequently addresses the importance of the nurse's story (Benner, 1984; Chinn & Kramer, 1999; Ford & Turner, 2001), and Banks-Wallace (2002) emphasizes the place of story for researchers seeking to understand African American culture, which is embedded in an oral tradition. In her discussion about story as a vehicle for research, Banks-Wallace (2002) also notes the therapeutic value of storytelling.

Sandelowski has evaluated both the research (1991) and practice (1994) merits of the human story. Burkhardt and Nagai-Jacobson (2002) call attention to the power of story: "In the process of telling and hearing stories, persons often come to new insights and deeper understandings of themselves because stories include not only events in our lives, but also the meanings and interpretations that define the significance of the events for particular lives" (p. 296). McAdams (1993) describes processes occurring when interpreted meaning supports healing: "Stories help us organize our thoughts, providing a narrative for human intentions and interpersonal events that is readily remembered and told. In some instances, stories may also mend us when we are broken, heal us when we are sick" (p. 31). Arthur Frank (1997) refers to stories as ways to repair the damage caused by illness so that one's life path is reconstructed in the context of illness; he refers to "redrawing maps and finding new destinations" (p. 53).

There is a body of literature that calls attention to "narrative" in health care (Charon, 2006; Charon & Montello, 2002). Charon and Montello (2002) address the role of narrative in medical ethics and interchangeably use the terms "narrative" and "story." However, in later work, Charon (2006) distinguishes the terms and simultaneously ties them together. "The word *narrate* itself combines roots meaning 'to count' and 'to tell' … narrative contains, almost like a repository or reliquary, aspects of human knowledge and experience that can, once stored—and *storied*—be drawn on again and again" (p. 60). Paley and Eva (2005) affirm Charon's distinction noting the emotional nature of story as a distinguishing quality and reminding the reader that "all stories are narratives but not all narratives are stories" (p. 88). Bruner (2002) reminded readers that both "telling" and "knowing in some particular way" are implicit in roots of "to narrate," and these roots are twisted together in complex connection.

For the purposes of our work, we refer to stories within the context of narrative … story is a narrative happening of connecting with self-in-relation through intentional dialogue to create ease. Story expresses the narration of events-as-remembered while infusing unique personal perspectives that give a glimpse of thoughts and feelings, shape meaning, and guide choices in-the-moment. Charon (2012) posits that stories connect person-to-person at the social membrane of patient–clinician engagement. The ongoing attention to narrative and story in disciplines outside of nursing confirms our belief about the significance of story and reminds us that this core dimension of nursing practice is now being recognized by other disciplines. The multidisciplinary perspectives have contributed to more precise understanding and inspired continued effort to articulate the meaning of story for nursing practice.

Nightingale (1946) called for a rejection of mindless chattering and a devotion to listening to the patient: "He feels what a convenience it would be, if there were any single person to whom he could speak simply and openly ... to whom he could express his wishes and directions" (p. 96). Nurses have long known the importance of listening and they have known how to listen so that they could understand what matters most. Story theory articulates the implicit wisdom of practicing nurses ... enabling guidance for practice and a framework for research. The assumptions that underlie story theory create a value-laden niche where the theory emerges.

The assumptions of the theory are that persons (1) change as they interrelate with their world in a vast array of flowing connected dimensions, (2) live an expanded present where past and future events are transformed in the here and now, and (3) experience meaning as a resonating awareness in the creative unfolding of human potential. The first assumption grounds sensitivity to the complexity of entangled health story dimensions to highlight persons moving with, through, and beyond their unfolding story. The second assumption invites a focus on the storyteller's present health experience with the listener's understanding that the storyteller's unique perspective incorporates the past and future in the here and now. The third assumption supports the human propensity to create meaning through awareness of thoughts, feelings, behavior, bodily experience, and other human expressions, all in the rhythm of the unfolding health story.

CONCEPTS OF THE THEORY

Story theory is composed of three interrelated concepts: (1) intentional dialogue, (2) connecting with self-in-relation, and (3) creating ease. According to the theory, story is a narrative happening of connecting with self-in-relation through intentional dialogue to create ease. Ease emerges in the midst of accepting the whole story as one's own.

Intentional Dialogue

Intentional dialogue is purposeful engagement with another to summon the story of a complicating health challenge. There is intention to engage in dialogue about the unique life experience of one's pain, confusion, joy, broken relationships, satisfaction, or suffering as a catalyst to seek a message and begin a process of change. Telling one's story happens in a trusting relationship with another where the nurse walks with the storyteller along a path, journeying a little further along to uncover what is happening, and paying attention to the unfolding movement of story, where both the storyteller and the nurse come to know better who they are (Campbell, 1988; Keen & Valley-Fox, 1989). Intentional dialogue energizes the experience of being alive by touching that which matters most to the storyteller. Throughout the flow of the story, the nurse holds fast to what has real meaning for the person who is recollecting what is past in the here and now, and accepting self as truly alive in the present moment of hopes, dreams, and expectations. In giving full attention to the other, the nurse "conveys to the speaker that his contribution is worth listening to, that as a person he is respected enough to receive the undivided attention of another" (Rogers, 1951, p. 34).

There are two processes of intentional dialogue: true presence and querying emergence. True presence is the nurse's nonjudgmental rhythmical focusing/refocusing of energy on the other, which is open to what was, is, and can be. It is "bringing one's humanness to the moment while simultaneously giving self over to the other who is exploring the meaning of the situation" (Liehr, 1989, p. 7). True presence is crucial to walking with the other who is sharing story. It is the substance of the nurse's activity during story sharing. Attending to the emergence of the unfolding health story assumes true presence and focuses on seeking clarification of the patterns that connect the beginning, middle, and end of a story. The nurse lives true presence by staying in while staying out. There is an all-at-once staying close to the story rhythm from the perspective of the storyteller while simultaneously distancing to discern patterns of connectedness. If the story is told over many encounters, it helps the nurse to make notes about story progress, possible patterns, and hunches about meaning.

Querying the emergence of the health story is clarification of vague story directions. Both the nurse and the storyteller attend to the story of the complicating health challenge. The nurse concentrates and tries to understand the story from the other's perspective. Nothing can be assumed about the story; only the storyteller knows the details. The story is never finished. There is always more to the story, including parts that the individual may not want to tell. The nurse in true presence stays with the longing to tell and the desire to tell only so much at a time.

Connecting With Self-in-Relation

Connecting with self-in-relation is the active process of recognizing self as related with others in a story plot. Hall and Allan (1994) identified self-in-relation as a central concept in their model for nursing practice and focused on the meaning of the concept for nurse–client interaction, noting that the "self is created in relation to others" (p. 112). Surrey (1991), who has developed a theory of self-in-relation, proposes it as the primary developmental process for women. The conceptualizations of Hall, Allan, and Surrey fit with our ideas in some places and misfit in others, but their ideas confirm a common ground of valuing self-in-relation as a dimension of human development and caring processes.

In story theory, connecting with self-in-relation is composed of personal history and reflective awareness. Personal history is the unique narrative uncovered when individuals reflect on where they have come from, where they are now, and where they are going in life. Venturing into the story is following the path of life as recollected. In the recollection, the nurse invites an awareness of self-in-relation to the context of a unique life. In following the story path, the nurse encourages reckoning with a personal history by traveling to the past to arrive at the story beginning, moving through the middle, and into the future all in the present, thus going into the depths of the story to find unique meanings that often lie hidden in the ambiguity of puzzling dilemmas. Self is affirmed in recognition and acceptance of nuances, faults, and strengths, as well as understanding of how one has lived and how one envisions future hopes and dreams.

Reflective awareness, which is the opposite of taking life for granted, is being in touch with bodily experience, thoughts, and feelings. It relates to being in touch with one's view of and place in the world and, more concretely, in the moment (Kabat-Zinn, 1994). Reflective awareness enables thoughtful observation of self so that bodily experience, thoughts, and feelings are recognized for what they are, as separate and distinct entities rather than personal defining qualities. For instance, when people in pain recognize that their pain is separate and distinct from who they are, they simultaneously recognize that they are more than their pain; that the pain is not a personal life-defining entity; and that they can be with the pain rather than being defined by it. With this mindful way of being in the moment, there is "a profound shift in one's relationship to thoughts and emotions, the result being greater clarity, perspective, objectivity and ultimately, equanimity" (Shapiro, Carlson, Astin, & Freedman, 2006, p. 379).

As the nurse guides reflective awareness on bodily experiences, thoughts, and feelings in a given moment of story, the storyteller becomes present to what is known and unknown, allowing unrecognized meaning to surface. Maslow (1967) describes the desire to know and the simultaneous fear of knowing. He states, "It is certainly demonstrable that we need the truth and we love to seek it. And yet it is just as easy to demonstrate that we are also simultaneously afraid to know the truth" (p. 167). Meaning changes when the unknown comes to light as known in an expanded present moment where there is coherence and integration. In sharing the story, the person is telling the story to the nurse who is attentively present and at the same time telling the story to self. Reflective awareness on the personal history of story enlivens one's connection with self-in-relation to others and the world. It establishes an environment for creating ease.

Creating Ease

Creating ease is an energizing release experienced as the story comes together in movement toward resolving. It happens in the context of a person's search for ease and the nurse's intention to enable ease. The two dimensions of creating ease are remembering disjointed story moments and flow in the midst of anchoring. Remembering disjointed story moments is connecting events in time through the realization, acceptance, and understanding that come as health story fragments sort and converge as a meaningful whole. Polanyi (1958) discusses understanding as "a grasping of disjointed parts into a comprehensive whole" (p. 28). In the nurse–person dialogue, there is a remembering of disconnected moments as the nurse moves with the person through the story. Patterns surface as individuals shed a momentary light on the meaning of important experiences. Often, the nurse does not divert attention to the highlighted experiences when they are first introduced but tucks them into the background while staying with the foreground story. With focused presence over time, the nurse enables the other to illuminate issues, values, ideas, and context, uncovering coherent patterns of meaning in the tapestry of life experience. Disjointed moments are woven together as the storyteller remembers the health story in the presence of a caring nurse.

Flow is an experience of dynamic harmony, and anchoring is an experience of comprehending meaning. As patterns are discerned, named, and made explicit, anchoring and flowing occur all at the same time. Meaning surfaces while anchoring in a moment of pattern clarity, allowing a sense of flow and calmness. "Flow is the way people describe their state of mind when consciousness is harmoniously ordered and they want to pursue whatever they are doing for its own sake" (Csikszentmihalyi, 1990, p. 6). Csikszentmihalyi describes the harmony that ensues when one anchors to meanings, which capture purposeful unity and focus on life direction. He provides descriptions of individuals who used changing health situations to achieve clarity of purpose, noting that "a person who knows how to find flow from life is able to enjoy even situations that seem only to allow despair" (Csikszentmihalyi, 1990, p. 193). The defining feature of flow is "intense experiential involvement in moment-to-moment activity" (Csikszentmihalyi, 2005, p. 600).

As disjointed story moments come together, a whole story surfaces, encompassing moments of gladness and melancholy, restriction and freedom, fear and security, and discrepancy and coherence, to name only a few of the juxtaposed realities that characterize any and every whole story. No story is one sided. The person experiencing loss is also experiencing gain and the one who is lonely often has uplifting interactions with others. When story sharing becomes a vehicle for healing, "embracing story" happens. Embracing story energizes release from the confines of a disjointed story where story moments are scattered making it difficult to discern a plot. Ease is resonating energy, enabling vision even for only a moment—a powerful moment creating possibilities for human development.

RELATIONSHIPS AMONG THE CONCEPTS: THE MODEL

The theory comes to life in practice and research through traditional dimensions of story. Franklin (1994) asserts that stories are composed of complicating, developmental, and resolving processes. When gathering health story data, the complicating process focuses on a health challenge that arises when there is a change in the person's life; the developmental process is composed of the story plot that links to the health challenge and suffuses it with meaning; and the resolving process is a shift in view that enables progressing with new understanding. The relationships among the concepts of the theory are depicted in Figure 10.1. This model is different from the first model of the theory (Smith & Liehr, 1999), which attempted to show the dynamic nature of the theory but failed to capture the all-at-once nature of intentional dialogue, connecting with self-in-relation and creating ease. In a recent chapter (Liehr & Smith, 2011), we addressed the evolution of the model and the challenge of depicting complexity within the limited dimensionality of the printed page.

The current model attempts to depict a common flow of energy between nurse and person where story emerges. In this shared flux of energy, all the concepts of story come together. The model incorporates story processes (complicating health challenge, developing story plot, movement toward resolving) that provide a base for gathering story in research and practice. Story plot is the organizing theme that brings events of the story together in a meaningful whole (Polkinghorne, 1988). It is proposed that developing story plot about a complicating health challenge facilitates movement toward resolving.

Story is a narrative happening of connecting with self-in-relation through intentional dialogue to create ease. Ease emerges in the midst of accepting the whole story as one's own. Implicit in the description is the suggestion that story process begins with intentional dialogue to support connecting with oneself in relationship with others and with one's world with the possibility of experiencing ease. There is no doubt that the relationship among the concepts appears on the printed page as linear. However, the intent is that these concepts are in a dynamic interrelationship, a quality that is difficult to depict in a model. For example, moments of ease surface when the nurse first

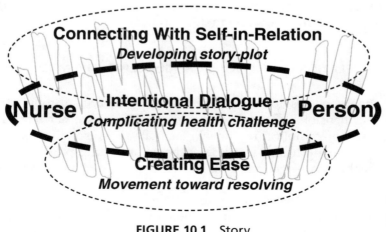

FIGURE 10.1 Story

engages the person in a caring way to identify what really matters. Even a brief encounter with a caring nurse enables a connection before story parts come together as a whole. Needless to say, the complexity of human interaction defies linearity. As nurse scientists we are called to fit language to the relationships among the concepts as best we can, recognizing that the simplicity necessary for models conflicts with the complexity recognized in most nursing phenomena.

Theory-Guided Story Gathering

The theory proposes common processes for gathering a story, whether the nurse is doing research or practice. To gather a story is to engage in intentional dialogue and to invite telling the story of a complicating health challenge through the developing plot and movement to resolve the health challenge. The common processes of story are complicating health challenge, developing story plot, and movement toward resolving.

Complicating Health Challenge

A complicating health challenge is any circumstance where life change or pattern disruption generates uneasiness in everyday living. The health challenge may be an obvious illness-related phenomenon, such as the diagnosis of a serious illness, or it may be a naturally occurring developmental event like sending a youngest child off to college. It may be discomfort brought on by bullying or by the demand for lifestyle change. Whatever the health challenge, story gathering begins when the nurse asks about "what matters most" to the storyteller. Attentive presence to "what matters" is a way of "being with," which places the storyteller at the center of attention. It carries the storyteller into the moment so that the present moment can be explored as mystery. Movement into the moment calls for connecting with the clear and centered intention to listen and hear the story with the storyteller leading the direction.

Developing Story Plot

The nurse invites a reflection on the past, focusing on issues that have importance for the complicating health challenge in the present moment. These issues are the beginnings of the developing story plot and are critical to understanding self-in-relation. For instance, issues of changing life circumstances, cited by the storyteller when talking about a complicating health challenge, will generally be recognized as story-plot turning points. At the empirical level, story plot may be documented as high points, low points, and turning points synthesized in the description of the complicating health challenge. High points include times when things are going well, low points are times when things are not going so well, and turning points can be important decisions or twists in the story all in the expanded present of the unfolding health story. Csikszentmihalyi (1997) believes that "the only path to finding out what life is about is a patient, slow attempt to make sense of the realities of the past and the possibilities of the future as they can be understood in the present" (p. 4). This path is a synthesis of high points, low points, and turning points that characterize critical moments of the story plot.

Sometimes, the high points, low points, and turning points that create the story plot can be uncovered by taking pen to paper and drawing relationship structures. For instance, a family tree can be used to note important relationships and serve as a base for understanding connecting with self-in-relation. The authors have described the use of a story path (Liehr & Smith, 2000) as a relationship structure that links present, past, and future of an unfolding story plot. When using this approach, the nurse generally begins with a line on a blank piece of paper and labels the line "the story of ...." to orient the person sharing the story to the dialogue. The story will always be about a health challenge. Most often, the story begins with the present ... asking the storyteller to identify where he or she is right now, today, on the life/health journey. Then, attention turns to the past and finally to the future. When using the story path for research, we have found that the time-oriented dimension of this approach is more important than the actual line on a piece of paper. Sometimes participants engage with the researcher to "populate" the line, marking meaningful life events, and sometimes the line is seemingly dismissed by the participant as the present–past–future story unfolds. When this approach for gathering stories was first described (Liehr & Smith, 2000), its utility for collecting practice evidence was emphasized. As a research approach, story path enables collection of stories about a particular health challenge with the consistent structure of present–past–future focus. To this point, researchers who have used the story path approach have collected focused stories in 20–40 minutes, and they have collected larger numbers of stories than might be traditional for qualitative studies. Therefore, researchers have usually sampled a broad range of participants before being assured of redundancy in the stories of health challenge. This pattern has led to a greater number of shorter stories for analysis. Researchers have used the story path approach to gather data in studies of: lifestyle change for hemodialysis patients (Hain, 2008); the experience of nurses caring for SARS patients (Liu & Liehr, 2009); the experience of caregiving when a loved one has cancer (Whisenant, 2011; Williams, 2007); and the experience of living with migraine headache (Ramsey, 2012).

Another promising approach to story gathering is photovoice, where people are encouraged to document a particular experience through photographs, which are then used as a foundation for story sharing about the experience. Carlson, Engebretson, and Chamberlain (2006) described the use of photovoice to collect stories about things that generated pride and things that needed to be changed in a lower-income African American urban community. Possible vehicles for story gathering are limited only by the imagination of the nurse scholar. The underlying principles to keep in mind when identifying a story-gathering structure is the meaning of the structure for the person from whom the story is being gathered, and the potential of the structure to stay true to the intent of story gathering. For instance, use of a linear story path may be confusing for people from cultures who view time as overlapping/extending in the moment. Also, people at the end-of-life may have difficulty talking about a future. The nurse will adjust the story-gathering approach to allow for cultural and situational qualities that reflect appreciation of each unique storyteller.

Movement Toward Resolving

Resolving happens in keeping the storyteller immersed in the "now" health experience. Finding a center of stillness and letting go of busyness and distractions energizes mindful attention to the story and propels movement toward resolving. Kunz (1985) contends that "centering quiets both the mind and emotions and thereby helps develop the power of focusing and intent" (p. 299). The experience of flow happens when the person is fully engaged in overcoming a challenge "that is just about manageable" (Csikszentmihalyi, 1997, p. 30). In a centered-present focus, one is free to take on the complicating health challenge and to view it in a manageable way. Oftentimes, this shift to a manageable view energizes a sense of ease as a person attentively embraces the fullness of life emerging in the moment. It is an opportunity to change thinking and feeling and to move on differently.

Over the years, we have learned that movement toward resolving emerges along a spectrum including subtle recognition as well as all-out embracing the now moment. Resolution does not close when the storytelling ends; it occurs in its own time. On some occasions, subtle recognition is a huge step along the path of human development, opening doors and pointing directions, and enabling next steps.

USE OF THE THEORY IN NURSING RESEARCH

Since story theory was first published over a decade ago, we have explored ways to measure what is learned from practice stories and we have debated the best qualitative approach as well as the value of a quantitative approach for analyzing story data when guided by the theory. We have learned that there is neither a simple destination for the exploration nor an answer to the debate. To some extent, we ourselves, our students, our colleagues, and anyone who uses story theory to guide research is pushing the edge of understanding about how nursing practice stories collected through research can best be gathered and analyzed to access their inherent wisdom. Several examples of published research will be presented, highlighting the place that story theory has had in the research process. In these examples, the reader will find that the theory has been used to guide a story-centered care intervention, and used to guide story analysis with both quantitative and qualitative methods. Regardless of the place of story theory in a study design, health story gathered for the purpose of scholarly inquiry requires an analysis strategy based on a research question. It is the wording of the question that guides the method of analysis. Therefore, for each example, the research question will be made explicit.

Research on a Story-Centered Care Intervention

In an effort to assess the power of story gathering guided by story theory, Liehr et al. (2006) tested story-centered care for people with stage one hypertension. In this instance, story-centered care was an intervention randomly assigned to people who were receiving structured exercise and nutritional counseling after being diagnosed with stage one hypertension. The research question was: what is the difference in 24-hour ambulatory blood pressure (BP) when story-centered care is added to structured exercise and nutrition counseling for people with stage one hypertension? None of the participants was medicated for hypertension; rather, before entering the study, they had been instructed by their health care providers to adjust their diet and increase exercise. The major outcome variable, 24-hour ambulatory BP, was measured twice before and twice after the intervention over a 6-month period. Participants who received story-centered care in addition to the structured exercise and nutrition counseling had statistically significant lower systolic BP while awake than those who received only the exercise and nutrition intervention ($p < 0.05$). During story-centered care, advanced practice nurses engaged participants in four 1-hour dialogue sessions about the health challenge of integrating lifestyle change into their everyday patterns. This study was conducted with a small number of participants ($N = 24$), but the significant findings suggest that story-centered care guided by story theory shows promise for enhancing the effect of structured exercise and nutrition counseling for people with stage one hypertension.

Analyzing Story Data: Quantitative

The association of quantitative indicators for story words may raise questions about the fit between the analysis strategy and the paradigmatic and theoretical underpinnings. A quantitative analysis that captures story progression offers congruence, as does relationship analysis where word use is analyzed in association with health outcome indicators to expand understanding of a health challenge. Pennebaker and Stone (2003) refer to word-use analysis as a tool for accessing a window into personality. If one accepts this vision of word use, a relationship analysis has potential to tie together personality–health qualities in an informative way. When word use in a story about a health challenge is quantified, quantification is not intended to represent a measure of the story but rather a numeric chronicle of story word qualities (e.g., negative emotion words; positive emotion words; cognitive process words; linguistic elements) over time or an opportunity for understanding story–health outcome connections.

Hain (2008) studied 63 people undergoing hemodialysis and she analyzed story data using a quantitative approach. One research question was: "What is the relationship between word use in stories of lifestyle change and cognitive function for older adults undergoing hemodialysis?" She considered word count, big words, words per sentence, and cognitive process words in her analysis. Story path was used to collect the stories about living with the challenge of lifestyle change.

Cognitive function was measured with the modified minimental state (3MS) exam, which measures global cognitive function including orientation, attention, recall, and language. Word use was analyzed with Linguistic Inquiry and Word Count (LIWC), a software program developed by Pennebaker, Francis, and Booth (2001). The LIWC program is word-based computerized text analysis software that discerns linguistic elements (word count and sentence punctuation); affective, cognitive, sensory, and social words; and words that reflect relativity and personal concerns. Seventy-two dimensions of language use comprise the LIWC structure for narrative evaluation. The structure has had psychometric testing, and reliability and validity estimates are reported by Pennebaker and King (1999).

Preparation of the nurse–participant transcripts for analysis included deletion of the nurse's words, correction of spelling errors, and removal of utterances that did not constitute recognizable words. After cleaning the data in this way, each transcript was saved as a text file. The LIWC program computes the percentage of words used for each word category and linguistic element. Hain's research questions the relationship between LIWC outcome indicators and cognitive function. The story data were considered in relation to the cognitive data, with the intent that word use in stories of lifestyle change would enhance understanding of cognitive function. Hain found statistically significant relationships between global cognitive function and the linguistic elements of words per sentence ($r = 0.41$; $p < 0.01$) and use of big words ($r = 0.37$, $p < 0.01$). In her discussion of the findings, she suggests that these linguistic elements could be indicators readily detected by nurses who work with hemodialysis patients, allowing referral for cognitive assessments, which could contribute to better quality of care and improved adherence to lifestyle prescriptions (Hain, 2008).

Analyzing Story Data: Qualitative

Stories are the substance of qualitative research, and traditional approaches can be used when analyzing stories gathered with the guidance of story theory. For instance, phenomenological analysis is an example of an established way to analyze story data when the research question addresses the human experience (Giorgi, 1985; Smith & Liehr, 1999; Van Manen, 1990). Narrative inquiry may be another way to analyze story data. Clandinin and Connelly (2000) propose narrative inquiry for analysis when the researcher wishes to understand experience emerging in a social context over time. Their simple definition of narrative inquiry is "stories lived and told" (p. 20).

Ramsey (2012) addressed the question, what is the structure of meaning for women living with migraine headache? The study was guided by story theory (Liehr & Smith, 2008) and phenomenology (van Manen, 1990). The two perspectives describe the surfacing of meaning in the conscious reflection of telling a story of a significant lived experience. Data were gathered using story path and analyzed using a phenomenological approach. The seven interrelated themes in the structure of meaning were that living with migraine headache is (a) recalling the significant experience that reshaped life; (b) experiencing self as vulnerable, with unmet expectations, unfulfilled relationships, and regrets; (c) being overcome by unrelenting torturous pain magnified by intrusion from the outside world; (d) pushing through to hold self together to do what needs to be done, in spite of torturous pain; (e) surrendering to the compelling call to focus on self in order to relieve the torturous pain; (f) making the most of pain-free time to get on with life and navigate the aftermath of the headache experience; and (g) being on guard against an unpredictable attack and yet hopeful that it is possible to outsmart the next attack.

We recently refined the story inquiry research method (Liehr & Smith, 2011) based on experience analyzing story data guided by the method. Since story inquiry was first introduced five years ago (Liehr & Smith, 2007), three studies have reported findings guided by the method (Hains, Wands, & Liehr, 2011; Kelley & Lowe, 2012; Liehr, Nishimura, Ito, Wands, & Takahashi, 2011). Each study will be briefly described culminating with the lessons learned about using the story inquiry method.

When using the story inquiry method, the researcher will pose a research question related to a complicating health challenge, story plot (high points, low points, turning points), and/or movement toward resolving the health challenge (Liehr & Smith, 2011). The five inquiry method processes are as follows: (1) gather stories about a complicating health challenge using a meaningful consistent structure to encourage story sharing; (2) begin deciphering the dimensions of the complicating health challenge; (3) describe the developing story plot (high points, low points, turning points); (4) identify movement toward resolving; and (5) synthesize findings to address the research question. In any single study, a researcher may address all of the story analysis processes (health challenge; story plot; approaches for resolving challenges) or only select one through articulation of the research questions.

Hain et al. (2011) posed the questions: (1) What are the health challenges of making lifestyle change for older adults undergoing hemodialysis and (2) how do they resolve the challenges? Data were analyzed to address the first research question using a traditional inductive approach, beginning with the words of the 64 participants, isolating the excerpts related to health challenges, grouping like statements together, eliminating redundancy, and naming each of the groups. The health challenge themes described by participants were living a restriction-driven existence; balancing independence/dependence; and struggling with those providing care. A similar inductive approach was used to analyze data addressing the second research question. Approaches used by participants to resolve the health challenges were unhappy passive acceptance; taking lifestyle change in stride; active attitudinal effort to accept reality; and assertive behavior to get what you want.

Lessons learned from the use of story inquiry method in this study primarily focused on analysis of the health challenge. The three themes that arose from health challenge analysis were dimensions of the health challenge of making lifestyle change for older adults undergoing hemodialysis. When the researcher identifies a focus for study, such as making lifestyle change, being obese, or being admitted to a nursing home, the health challenge is named. To arrive at the nuances and complexities of the health challenge, inductive analysis occurs. Therefore, the research question will more appropriately address the dimensions of any given health challenge to get at the nature of the health challenge as experienced by participants. This lesson is reflected in the latest description of the story inquiry method (Liehr & Smith, 2011).

In a study of survivors from Pearl Harbor and Hiroshima, Liehr et al. (2011) posed the research questions: (1) What turning points marked movement over time in stories of health for survivors? and (2) what turning point–associated thoughts, feelings, sensations, and interpretations created meaning for them? Data were analyzed using standard inductive processes as described earlier. Turning points for Hiroshima survivors were (1) facing the disorienting aftermath with fall of the A-bomb; (2) becoming Hibakusha (A-bomb survivor); and (3) reaching out to create meaning/purpose consistent with peace. For the Pearl Harbor survivors, the turning points were (1) coming to grips with the reality of a Japanese attack; (2) honoring the memory of their war experience and moving on; and (3) embracing connection as a source of comfort. Each of these turning points was imbued with themes that enriched the meaning and contributed to understanding (Liehr et al., 2011).

The major lesson learned about story inquiry method while conducting the study with Pearl Harbor (n = 23) and Hiroshima

($n = 28$) survivors was related to the importance of defining "turning points" for use by all analysts. This is especially important when more than one researcher is engaged in analyzing but it is even important when one researcher is conducting the analysis over time. Liehr et al. (2011) defined turning points as "twists in the stories, where there was a shift in living through and with wartime trauma" (p. 219). Staying true to the definition at the start of each analysis session is critical to the integrity of the data analysis.

One final study that used story inquiry method was reported by Kelley and Lowe (2012), who analyzed stories of stress for 50 Cherokee-Keetoowah adolescents ranging in age from 14 to 18 years. The research questions posed were as follows: (1) What is the health challenge of stress experienced by Cherokee-Keetoowah adolescents? and (2) how do these adolescents resolve stress? As previously discussed, dimensions of the health challenge of stress became the focus for the first research question. Data were analyzed using an inductive approach. Cherokee-Keetoowah adolescents identified the burden of expectations, relationship disruption, and imposing feelings and actions of others as dimensions of the health challenge of stress. They described connecting with valued others, engaging in meaningful activities, and choosing a positive attitude about change as the approaches they used to manage stress.

One implicit lesson in this work with Cherokee adolescents relates to the potential of story methods to ensure cultural sensitivity. Issues of cultural sensitivity in research are addressed if people are approached with humility and intention to understand. Story-gathering guided by the theory is a vehicle for humble understanding. Bessarab and Ng'andu (2010) describe the use of yarning, an indigenous cultural conversation approach, when conducting research with indigenous people. Banks (2011) advocates the use of story to advance health equity research, emphasizing the beauty of a level playing field of researcher–participant when stories are shared and honored.

A second lesson from the Kelley and Lowe (2012) study relates to the method for story exchange. Stories were written rather than collected in a face-to-face format in this study. Adolescents were given instructions to write for 15 minutes about their stress and how they managed it without regard for punctuation, spelling, or sentence structure. Their stories were anonymous, perhaps contributing to the authenticity of what was shared, particularly for adolescents. The potential for story-centered writing sessions that cultivate personal reflection warrants further exploration in future research using the story inquiry method.

USE OF THE THEORY IN NURSING PRACTICE

The question leading the story when the foremost intention is caring–healing is "what matters" to the client about the complicating health challenge. In eliciting the story, the nurse leads the client along, clarifying meaningful connections about what is happening in everyday living in the context of the client's complicating health challenge. Sharing the health challenge story brings developing story plot and movement toward resolving to the surface. The resulting story about "what matters" to the client provides distinct information about how one person lived the presenting health challenge.

Stories are so integral to nursing practice that they are often gathered by nurses and used to guide health care decision making without a second thought about their potential for knowledge development. In 2005, Smith and Liehr introduced an approach for analyzing practice stories guided by story theory. Seven phases of inquiry were proposed to direct practicing nurses wishing to use stories as practice evidence contributing to knowledge development. The phases of inquiry are (1) gather a story about a complicating health challenge, (2) compose a reconstructed story, (3) connect existing literature to the health challenge, (4) refine the name of the complicating health challenge, (5) describe the developing story plot, (6) identify movement toward resolving, and (7) collect additional stories about the complicating health challenge (Smith & Liehr, 2005).

Health stories collected through application of story theory during nursing practice include those about patients with dementia who expressed disagreement through behavioral messages (Ito, Takahashi, & Liehr, 2007) and coming to know the voice of vulnerable adolescents in an urban practice setting (Jolly, Weiss, & Liehr, 2007). Summers (2002) used the theory as a foundation for mutual timing, a concept she believes is critical for effective health care encounters.

More recently, Rateau (2010) described her personal story of a catastrophic loss from a house fire and explosion. Through recounting her story, she experienced an increased understanding of the event leading to a transformation of meaning and a deepened level of well-being. She offers implications for using story theory guided practice for persons experiencing traumatic catastrophic loss to reflect on self and relationships with others in finding meaning to move beyond the loss.

Two scholars used story theory to provide culturally sensitive care. Attending to the person's story in true presence created a caring relationship in which cultural perspectives were honored and infused in the practice encounter. Millender (2011) described the application of story theory for a hospitalized Guatemalin Mayan patient to develop a culturally relevant plan of care. She found that the medical history did not offer evidence of the patient's cultural beliefs and values, and concluded that engaging in intentional dialogue guided by story theory provided the nurse with useful cultural information. In reference to the Appalachian culture, Gobble (2009) described application of story theory to uncover religious and cultural perspectives that guided culturally sensitive advanced practice nursing for a woman living in a rural community. An understanding of rural culture and religious beliefs was the context in which the story of the complicating health challenge unfolded. Through listening attentively to what mattered most to the person, a caring/healing health promoting process was fostered.

Performance Excellence and Accountability in Kidney Care (PEAK) is a voluntary movement to reduce mortality among first-year dialysis patients at a national level. On their website at www.kidneycarequality. com/CampLearnCenter.htm, under Best Practice 2, practitioners are referred to the story theory as a means to achieve this best practice. The best practice is stated as follows: Enhance and maintain quality of life by incorporating an individual holistic educational approach about the physical and psychosocial impact of dialysis on patient lives. Theory-based website guidance for health professionals engaging with dialysis patients includes the following dialogue-leading questions and statements:

1. Tell me about the challenges you are facing as you begin dialysis.
2. What is most important to you right now?
3. Can you think of a past challenge or "difficult time" that you "got through." Tell me about that time and what helped you get through it.
4. Tell me about your future hopes and dreams.

According to Hain (2011), story theory-guided practice acknowledges the power of stories for nursing practice. She goes on to say "By coming to know a 'person through story' the nurse can identify what is most important and develop goals that the person is likely to embrace, which may result in better health outcomes" (p. 252).

Use of the Theory in Nursing Education

Carpenter (2010) described applying story theory to structure an undergraduate clinical course for a student in the honor's program. The result was an innovative teaching strategy that increased the quality for all students in the practicum experience. This was accomplished by guiding students to develop skill in intentional dialogue and the use of story path. It was concluded that taking the course beyond the bio-medical/technical aspects of care to show the importance of nursing presence through gathering the patient's story enriched the practice experience.

These beliefs about the importance of story for health and human caring have recently been confirmed by the Carnegie Foundation report (Benner, Sutphen, Leonard, & Day, 2010), calling for a radical transformation in nursing education. In their guidelines for improving nursing education, the authors say:

> Because injuries and illness occur in the context of a person's life, the nurse must formulate a narrative of the patient's immediate clinical history, his concerns, and even an account of his life and lifeworld. Reasoning across time involves the ability to construct a sensible story of immediate events, their sequence, and their consequences in terms of illness trajectory and life concerns. (p. 225)

As nursing moves toward educating greater and greater numbers of nurses with practice doctorates, it is important to honor the wisdom found in practice stories; to consider the potential of practice stories for advancing nursing practice scholarship; and to identify systematic approaches for using practice stories for nursing knowledge development. Story theory provides one systematic approach for viewing practice stories, where the stories create the foundation for knowledge development.

CONCLUSION

Collaborative work on story theory began in 1996, and the theory was first published in 1999. In the years since we first began thinking through the meaning of story for health, we have accomplished a great deal and have moved a short distance from where we began. Development and publication of the theory led to further consideration and description of use in practice (Liehr & Smith, 2000; Smith & Liehr, 2005). We believe that story is central to nursing practice and to nursing practice scholarship, and we are committed to providing a structure enabling ready access to the wisdom of practice stories. Story theory provides a substantive guide for story gathering in research and practice. Story processes focused on the complicating health challenge, developing story plot, and movement toward resolving have an inherent potential for growing nursing knowledge and guiding nursing practice.

Both quantitative and qualitative analyses have been applied to story data. We believe that several methods are appropriate for the qualitative analysis of story data, and we have recently refined the story inquiry method (Liehr & Smith, 2011), which is relevant when the researcher is pursuing understanding of a complicating health challenge. Linguistic analysis, using software programs such as LIWC, shows promise for quantitative analysis. Each time we share another dimension of our thinking on story theory with the nursing community, we learn more about the theory and formulate next directions. Middle range theory development is scholarship in progress with practice and research. As these thoughts are shared, new questions are realized, and so the story goes.

REFERENCES

Banks, J. (2011). Storytelling to access social context and advance health equity research. *Preventative Medicine, 55*(5), 394–397. doi:1016/j.ypmed.2011.10.015

Banks-Wallace, J. (2002). Talk the talk: Storytelling and analysis rooted in African-American oral tradition. *Qualitative Health Research, 12*(3), 410–426.

Belenky, M. F., Clinchy, B. M., Goldberger, N., & Tarule, J. M. (1996). *Women's ways of knowing: The development of self, voice, and mind.* New York, NY: Basic Books.

Benner, P. (1984). *From novice to expert.* Menlo Park, CA: Addison-Wesley.

Benner, P., Sutphen, M., Leonard, V., & Day, L. (2010). *Educating nurses: A call for radical transformation.* San Francisco CA: Jossey-Bass.

Bessarab, D., & Ng'andu, B. (2010). Yarning about yarning as a legitimate method in indigenous research. *International Journal of Critical Indigenous Studies, 3*(1), 37–50.

Boykin, A., & Schoenhofer, S. (2001). The role of nursing leadership in creating caring environments in health care delivery systems. *Nursing Administration Quarterly, 25*(3), 1–7.

Bruner, J. (2002). *Making stories: Law, literature, life.* New York, NY: Farrar, Straus & Giroux.

Burkhardt, M. A., & Nagai-Jacobson, M. G. (2002). *Spirituality: Living our connectedness.* Albany, NY: Delmar.

Campbell, J. (1988). *The power of myth.* New York, NY: Doubleday.

Carlson, E. D., Engebretson, J., & Chamberlain, R. M. (2006). Photovoice as a social process of critical consciousness. *Qualitative Health Research, 16*(6), 836–852.

Carpenter, R. (2010). Using Story Theory to create an innovative honors level nursing course. *Nursing Education Perspectives, 31*(1), 28–32.

Charon, R. (2006). *Narrative medicine: Honoring the stories of illness.* New York, NY: Oxford University Press.

Charon, R. (2012). At the membranes of care: Stories in narrative medicine. *Academic Medicine, 87*(3), 342–347.Charon, R., & Montello, M. (Eds.). (2002). *Stories matter: The role of narrative in medical ethics.* New York, NY: Routledge.

Chinn, P. L., & Kramer, M. K. (1999). *Theory and nursing integrated knowledge development.* New York, NY: Mosby.

Clandinin, D. J., & Connelly, F. M. (2000). *Narrative inquiry: Experience and story in qualitative research.* San Francisco, CA: Jossey-Bass.

Csikszentmihalyi, M. (1990). *Flow: The psychology of optimal experience.* New York, NY: Harper & Row.

Csikszentmihalyi, M. (1997). *Finding flow.* New York, NY: Basic Books.

Csikszentmihalyi, M. (2005). Flow. In A. J. Elliot & C. S. Dweck (Eds.), *Handbook of competence and motivation* (pp. 598–608). New York, NY: Guilford.

Ford, K., & Turner, D. (2001). Stories seldom told: Pediatric nurses' experiences of caring for hospitalized children with special needs and their families. *Journal of Advanced Nursing, 33,* 288–295.

Frank, A. W. (1997). *The wounded storyteller: Body, illness, and ethics.* Chicago, IL: University of Chicago Press.

Franklin, J. (1994). *Writing for story.* Middlesex, UK: Penguin.

Giorgi, A. (1985). *Phenomenology and psychological research.* Pittsburgh, PA: Duquesne University Press.

Gobble, C. D. (2009). The value of story theory in providing culturally sensitive advanced practice nursing in rural Appalachia. *Online Journal of Rural Nursing and Health Care, 9*(1), 94–105.

Hain, D. (2008). Cognitive function and adherence of older adults undergoing hemodialysis. *Nephrology Nursing Journal, 35*(1), 23–30.

Hain, D. (2011). Response to "Modeling the complexity of story theory for nursing practice." In A. W. Davidson, M. A. Ray, & M. C. Turkel (Eds.), *Nursing, caring, and complexity science* (pp. 249–252). New York, NY: Springer.

Hain, D. J., Wands, L. M., & Liehr, P. (2011). Approaches to resolve health challenges in a population of older adults undergoing hemodialysis. *Research in Gerontological Nursing, 4*(1), 53–62.

Hall, B. A., & Allan, J. D. (1994). Self in relation: A prolegomenon for holistic nursing. *Nursing Outlook, 15,* 110–116.

Ito, M., Takahashi, R., & Liehr, P. (2007). Heeding the behavioral message of elders with dementia in day care. *Holistic Nursing Practice, 21*(1), 12–18.

Jolly, K., Weiss, J. A., & Liehr, P. (2007). Understanding adolescent voice as a guide for nursing practice and research. *Issues in Comprehensive Pediatric Practice, 30*(3), 3–13.

Kabat-Zinn, J. (1994). *Wherever you go, there you are.* New York, NY: Hyperion.

Keen, S., & Valley-Fox, A. (1989). *Your mythic journey.* Los Angeles, CA: Jeremy P. Tarcher.

Kelley, M., & Lowe, J. (2012). The health challenge of stress experienced by Native American adolescents. *Archives in Psychiatric Nursing, 26*(1), 71–73.

Kunz, D. (1985). Compassion, rootedness and detachment: Their role in healing. In D. Kunz (Ed.), *Spiritual aspects of the healing arts* (pp. 289–305). Wheaton, IL: The Theosophical Publishing House.

Liehr, P. (1989). A loving center: The core of true presence. *Nursing Science Quarterly, 2*, 7–8.

Liehr, P. (1992). Uncovering a hidden language: The effects of listening and talking on blood pressure and heart rate. *Archives of Psychiatric Nursing, 6*, 306–311.

Liehr, P., Meininger, J. C., Vogler, R., Chan, W., Frazier, L., Smalling, S., & Fuentes, F. (2006). Adding story-centered care to standard lifestyle intervention for people with Stage 1 hypertension. *Applied Nursing Research, 19*, 16–21.

Liehr, P., Nishimura, C., Ito, M., Wands, L. M., & Takahashi, R. (2011). A lifelong journey of moving beyond wartime trauma for survivors from Hiroshima and Pearl Harbor. *Advances in Nursing Science, 34*(3), 215–228.

Liehr, P., & Smith, M. J. (2000). Using story theory to guide nursing practice. *International Journal of Human Caring, 4*, 13–18.

Liehr, P., & Smith, M. J. (2007). Story inquiry: A method for research. *Archives of Psychiatric Nursing, 21*(2), 120–121.

Liehr, P., & Smith, M. J. (2008). Story theory. In M. J. Smith & P. L. Liehr (Eds.), *Middle range theory for nursing* (2nd ed., pp. 205–224). New York, NY: Springer Publishing.

Liehr, P., & Smith, M. J. (2011). Modeling the complexity of story theory for nursing practice. In A. W. Davidson, M. A. Ray, & M. C. Turkel (Eds.), *Nursing, caring, and complexity science* (pp. 241–248). New York, NY: Springer Publishing.

Liehr, P., & Smith, M. J. (2011). Refining story inquiry as a method for research. *Archives of Psychiatric Nursing, 25*(1), 74–75.

Liu, H., & Liehr, P. (2009). Instructive messages from Chinese nurses' stories of caring for SARS patients. *Journal of Clinical Nursing, 18*, 2880–2887.

Maslow, A. H. (1967). Neurosis as a failure of personal growth. *Humanitas, 8*, 153–169.

McAdams, D. P. (1993). *The stories we live by.* New York, NY: Guilford.

Millender, E. (2011). Using stories to bridge cultural disparities, one culture at a time. *Journal of Continuing Education in Nursing, 42*(1), 37–42.

Newman, M. A. (1999). The rhythm of relating in a paradigm of wholeness. *Image: Journal of Nursing Scholarship, 31*, 227–230.

Nightingale, F. (1946). *Notes on nursing: What it is and what it is not.* Philadelphia, PA: J.B. Lippincott.

Paley, J., & Eva, G. (2005). Narrative vigilance: The analysis of stories in health care. *Nursing Philosophy, 6*, 83–97.

Parse, R. R. (1981). *Man-living-health: A theory of nursing.* New York, NY: Wiley.

PEAK: Performance Excellence and Accountability in Kidney Care. Patient "Tools of Engagement." Best practice 2. Retrieved from http://www.kidneycarequality.com/CampLearnCenter.htm

Pennebaker, J. W., Francis, M. E., & Booth, R. J. (2001). *Linguistic inquiry and word count: LWIC2001.* Mahwah, NJ: Erlbaum.

Pennebaker, J. W., & King, L. A. (1999). Linguistic styles: Language use as an individual difference. *Journal of Personality and Social Psychology, 77,* 1296–1312.

Pennebaker, J. W., & Stone, L. (2003). Words of wisdom: Language use over the life span. *Journal of Personality and Social Psychology, 85*(2), 291–301.

Peplau, H. (1991). *Interpersonal relations in nursing.* New York, NY: Springer Publishing.

Polanyi, M. (1958). *The study of man.* Chicago, IL: University of Chicago Press.

Polkinghorne, D. E. (1988). *Narrative knowing and the human sciences.* Albany, NY: State University of New York Press.

Ramsey, A. R. (2012). Living with migraine headache: A phenomenological study of women's experiences. *Holistic Nursing Practice, 26*(6), 297–307.

Rateau, M. R. (2010). A story of transformation following catastrophic loss. *Archives in Psychiatric Nursing, 24*(4), 260–265.

Reed, P. A. (1995). Treatise on nursing knowledge development for the 21st century: Beyond postmodernism. *Advances in Nursing Science, 17,* 70–84.

Reed, P. A. (1999). Response to "Attentively embracing story: A middle-range theory with practice and research implications." *Scholarly Inquiry for Nursing Practice: An International Journal, 13,* 205–209.

Rogers, C. R. (1951). *Client-centered therapy.* Boston, MA: Houghton Mifflin.

Rogers, M. E. (1994). The science of unitary human beings: Current perspectives. *Nursing Science Quarterly, 7,* 33–35.

Sandelowski, M. (1991). Telling stories: Narrative approaches in qualitative research. *Image: Journal of Nursing Scholarship, 23,* 161–166.

Sandelowski, M. (1994). We are the stories we tell. *Journal of Holistic Nursing, 12,* 23–33.

Shapiro, S. L., Carlson, L. E., Astin, J. A., & Freedman, B. (2006). Mechanisms of mindfulness. *Journal of Clinical Psychology, 62*(3), 373–386.

Smith, M. J. (1975). Changes in judgment of duration with different patterns of auditory information for individuals confined to bed. *Nursing Research, 24,* 93–98.

Smith, M. J. (1986). Human-environment process: A test of Rogers' principle of integrality. *Advances in Nursing Sciences, 9,* 21–28.

Smith, M. J., & Liehr, P. (1999). Attentively embracing story: A middle-range theory with practice and research implications. *Scholarly Inquiry for Nursing Practice: An International Journal, 13,* 187–204.

Smith, M. J., & Liehr, P. (2003). The theory of attentively embracing story. In M. J. Smith & P. R. Liehr (Eds.), *Middle range theory for nursing* (pp. 167–187). New York, NY: Springer Publishing.

Smith, M. J., & Liehr, P. (2005). Story theory: Advancing nursing practice scholarship. *Holistic Nursing Practice, 19*(6), 272–276.

Summers, L. (2002). Mutual timing: An essential component of provider/patient communication. *Journal of the Academy of Nurse Practitioners, 14,* 19–25.

Surrey, J. L. (1991). The self-in-relation: A theory of women's development. In J. Jordan, A. G. Kaplan, B. Miller, I. P. Stiver, & J. L. Surrey (Eds.), *Women's growth in connection: Writings from the Stone Center* (pp. 51–66). New York, NY: Guilford.

Taylor, D. (1996). *The healing power of stories.* New York, NY: Doubleday.

van Manen, M. (1990). *Researching lived experience.* Albany, NY: State University of New York Press.

Watson, J. (1997). The theory of human caring: Retrospective and prospective. *Nursing Science Quarterly, 10,* 49–52.

Whisenant, M. (2011). Informal caregiving in patients with brain tumors. *Oncology Nursing Forum, 38*(5), E373–E381.

Williams, L. (2007). Whatever it takes: Informal caregiving dynamics in blood and marrow transplantation. *Oncology Nursing Forum, 34*(2), 379–387.

11

Theory of Transitions

Eun-Ok Im

Nursing phenomena occur around various life transitions such as during pregnancy and at midlife. There are transitions from a critical care unit to a long-term care facility, from hospital to community, from one country to a different country, and within a hospital due to changes in administrators. People sometimes go through transitions smoothly and successfully, but frequently have issues, concerns, and/or problems in transitions due to the disequilibrium caused by changes (Meleis, 2010). Nurses have played a central role in providing care for people in transitions, especially for individuals, families, and communities experiencing changes that trigger new roles, losses of networks, and support systems (Meleis, 2010, p. xv). Nurses could facilitate successful transitions by providing information, support, and/or direct care, which subsequently help prevent diseases, reduce health risks, enhance health/well-being, and facilitate rehabilitation of those in transitions. Meleis (2010) asserted that transitions are central to the mission of nursing.

Transitions Theory started from the point of view that nursing phenomena could be explained as a health/illness experience during life changes. The theory has frequently been used to explain nursing phenomena across diverse circumstances related to change in health/illness, life situations, developmental stages, and organizations (Im, 2009; Meleis, 2010). Furthermore, transitions theory has provided a structure for nursing curriculum, a framework for research questions/hypotheses, and directions for nursing care (Im, 2009). In this chapter, the purpose and development process of transitions theory are described. Then, the major concepts of transitions theory and the relationships among the concepts are described. Finally, the current use of transitions theory in nursing research and practice is presented.

PURPOSE OF THE THEORY AND HOW IT WAS DEVELOPED

Purpose of the Theory

The purpose of this middle range theory is to describe, explain, and predict human beings' experiences in various types of transitions including health/illness transitions, situational transitions, developmental transitions, and organizational transitions. Because nursing phenomena frequently involve transition, transitions theory has been used in nursing research and practice (Im, 2011). Furthermore, due to its comprehensiveness, transitions theory has been widely accepted in nursing research and practice (Im, 2011). An entire issue of *Advances in Nursing Science* (2012) was recently dedicated to transitions, and in her editorial, Chinn recognizes Meleis's contribution, noting the central importance of transitions for the discipline: "I believe that the concept of transitions, along with the central concept of caring, forms a core around which the practice of nursing is constructed" (p. 191). Transitions theory was formulated with the goal of integrating what is known about transition experience across different types of life change to provide direction for nursing therapeutics. This theory also provides a framework guiding direction about integrating the results of previous research related to transitions and manipulating transition-related concepts for further study.

How It Was Developed

The development of transitions theory can be characterized by the following descriptors (Im, 2011): a borrowed view; research program and collaborative works; and mentoring.

From a Borrowed View

The theory has been developed over the past 50 years. Meleis (2007) initiated her conceptualization of transitions theory in her master's and PhD dissertation research. Then, through her early theoretical works on role supplementation theory and her research on immigrant health, she began to inquire about the nature of transitions and the human experience of transitions. Thus, we can say that development of transitions theory started with the role insufficiency theory (Meleis, 1975, 2007; Meleis & Swendsen, 1978; Meleis, Swendsen, & Jones, 1980), which has its theoretical roots in symbolic interactionism and role theories in sociology. In her first theoretical work, Meleis claimed role insufficiency was a result of unhealthy transitions. Role insufficiency was defined as any difficulty in the cognizance and/or performance of a role or in the attainment of its goals, as well as difficulty in the sentiments associated with the role behavior, as perceived by the self or by significant others (Meleis, 1975; Meleis & Swendsen, 1978; Meleis et al., 1980). In the early work, the goal of healthy transitions was the mastery of behaviors, sentiments, cues, and symbols associated with new roles and identities and nonproblematic processes (Meleis, 1975). Meleis (2007) later mentioned her difficulties in conceptualizing the nature of transitions and the nature of responses to different transitions, but also thought that the goal of nursing knowledge development should be on developing nursing therapeutics (Jones, Zhang, & Meleis, 1978; Meleis, 1975; Meleis & Swendsen, 1978). Her work in the 1970s shows her efforts to develop the idea of role supplementation with a focus on defining the components, processes, and strategies that may be related to role supplementation.

From a Research Program and Collaborative Works

Meleis's well-known research interests were on immigrant populations and their health (Jones et al., 1978; Im & Meleis, 2000; Im, Meleis, & Lee, 1999; Lipson & Meleis, 1983, 1985; Lipson, Reizian, & Meleis, 1987; Meleis, 1981; Meleis, Lipson, & Dallafar, 1998; Meleis & Rogers, 1987; Meleis & Sorrell, 1981). Most of her publications in the 1980s and 1990s focused on the health/illness experience of Arab immigrants in the United States. Through her research, immigration was conceptualized as a situational transition (Budman, Lipson, & Meleis, 1992; Im et al., 1999; Laffrey, Meleis, Lipson, Solomon, & Omidian, 1989; Lipson & Meleis, 1983, 1985; Lipson et al., 1987; Meleis, 1981; Meleis et al., 1998; Meleis & La Fever, 1984; Meleis & Rogers, 1987; Meleis & Sorrell, 1981).

This is also the period when Chick and Meleis (1986) conceptualized transition as a concept central to nursing. While working as a faculty member at the University of California, San Francisco (UCSF), Meleis met Chick—who was a visiting scholar at UCSF at that time—and they worked together to develop transitions as a concept (Chick & Meleis, 1986). This was the first theoretical work on transitions theory. In addition, Meleis's collaborative works with international colleagues helped conceptualize transitions as central to nursing (Lane & Meleis, 1991; May & Meleis, 1987; Meleis, Arruda, Lane, & Bernal, 1994;

Meleis, Douglas, Eribes, Shih, & Messias, 1996; Meleis, Kulig, Arruda, Beckman, 1990; Meleis, Mahidal, Lin, Minami, & Neves, 1987; Shih et al., 1998; Stevens, Hall, & Meleis, 1992).

From Mentoring

The development of transitions theory also results from the mentoring process. Meleis's first major paper on transitions theory in 1997 (Schumacher & Meleis, 1994) resulted from working with and mentoring a student. Based on the work of Chick and Meleis, Schumacher, who was a doctoral student at UCSF at that time, worked with Meleis to conduct an extensive literature review on transitions in nursing and developed the transition framework based on 310 articles (Schumacher & Meleis, 1994). This integrated literature review led to a definition of transitions and creation of a conceptual framework in nursing. This framework was well received by nursing researchers, and a few researchers began to use it in their studies.

Transitions theory was later developed based on the research studies by Meleis's former students who investigated diverse populations in various types of transitions. Former students of Meleis conducted an analysis of their research findings related to transition experiences and responses, and integrated similarities and differences to further develop transitions as a middle range theory. As a group, the researchers compared, contrasted, and integrated the findings, and developed transitions theory through extensive reading, reviewing, and dialoguing with constant analysis and comparison of the findings related to the major concepts of the theory.

With the emergence of situation-specific theories as a new type of nursing theory (Meleis, 1997), several situation-specific theories were developed based on transitions theory by Meleis's former students (Im, 2006; Im & Meleis, 1999a, 1999b; Schumacher, Jones, & Meleis, 1999). These situation-specific theories include the situation-specific theory of low-income Korean immigrant women's menopausal transition (Im & Meleis, 1999a), the situation-specific theory of elderly transition (Schumacher, Dodd, & Paul, 1993; Schumacher, Jones, & Meleis, 1999), and the situation-specific theory of Caucasian cancer patients' pain experience (STOP) (Im, 2006). As a whole, Meleis (2010) published all the theoretical works related to transitions theory and Im (2011) recently published a literature review on transitions theory to provide direction for future theoretical development.

CONCEPTS OF THE THEORY

The major concepts of transitions theory suggested by Meleis, Sawyer, Im, Schumacher, and Messias (2000) include the following: types and patterns of transitions, properties of transition experiences, transition conditions (facilitators and inhibitors), patterns of response/process and outcome indicators, and nursing therapeutics. The definitions of each of these concepts were described in two manuscripts (Meleis et al., 2000; Schumacher & Meleis, 1994) more than a decade ago. The definitions are summarized here.

Types and Patterns of Transitions

Types of Transitions

The concept of types of transitions includes four different types: developmental transitions, health and illness transitions, situational transitions, and organizational transitions. Developmental transitions are those due to developmental events including birth, adolescence, menopause, aging (or senescence), and death. Health and illness transitions are events such as a recovery process, hospital discharge, and diagnosis of chronic illness (Meleis & Trangenstein, 1994). Situational transitions are those due to changes in life circumstances such as entering an educational program, immigrating from one country to another, and moving from home to a nursing home (Chick & Meleis, 1986). Organizational transitions are those related to changing environmental conditions that affect the lives of clients and workers (Schumacher & Meleis, 1994).

Patterns of Transitions

In the transitions theory (Meleis et al., 2000), patterns of transitions include multiplicity and complexity. Multiple transitions frequently occur simultaneously; people experience several different types of transitions at the same time rather than experiencing a single transition. Meleis et al. (2000) suggested that multiple transitions could happen sequentially or simultaneously, and the degree of overlap among multiple transitions and the associations between separate events that initiate different transitions should be considered because of the complexities involved.

Properties of Transition Experience

In the transitions theory (Meleis et al., 2000), the properties of transition experiences include awareness, engagement, change and difference, time span, and critical points and events. These properties of transition experience are interrelated as a complex process.

Awareness

Awareness is perception, knowledge, and recognition of a transition experience (Meleis et al., 2000, p. 18). The level of awareness could be reflected in the degree of congruency between what is known about processes and responses and what constitutes an expected set of responses and perceptions of individuals undergoing similar transitions (Meleis et al., 2000, p. 18). According to Chick and Meleis (1986), a person's awareness of change may not necessarily mean that the person has begun his or her transition. Meleis et al. (2000) proposed later that a lack of the awareness also does not always mean that the transition has not begun.

Engagement

Properties of transitions also include engagement (Meleis et al., 2000). Engagement is the degree to which a person demonstrates involvement in the process of transition (Meleis et al., 2000, p. 19). According to Meleis et al. (2000), the level of awareness influences the level of engagement, and there will be no engagement without awareness.

Changes and Differences

The properties of transition also include changes and differences (Meleis et al., 2000). Changes in a person's identities, roles, relationships, abilities, and behaviors result in a sense of movement or direction in internal and external processes (Schumacher & Meleis, 1994). All transitions are considered to be associated with change although not all change indicates a transition. In the theory, Meleis et al. (2000) proposed that disclosing and explaining the meaning, influence, and scope of change (e.g., nature, temporality, perceived importance or severity, personal, familial, and societal norms and expectations) are essential in understanding transition. Differences are conceptualized as a property of transitions. Unsatisfied or atypical expectations, feeling dissimilar, being realized as dissimilar, or viewing the world and others in dissimilar ways could mean challenging differences. Transitions theory suggests that nurses need to consider a client's level of comfort and mastery in dealing with changes and differences to provide adequate and appropriate care for people in transitions.

Time Span

Another property of transitions is time span (Meleis et al., 2000). Transitions theory indicates that all transitions could be characterized as flowing and moving over time (Meleis et al., 2000). Actually, transition refers to a span of time with an identifiable starting point, extending from the first signs of anticipation, perception, or demonstration of change; moving through a period of instability, confusion, and distress; and to an eventual ending with a new beginning or period of stability (Meleis et al., 2000). However, Meleis et al. (2000) also warned that framing the time span of some transition experiences can be problematic or even impossible.

Critical Points and Events

Critical points and events are markers such as birth, death, the cessation of menstruation, or the diagnosis of an illness (Meleis et al., 2000). In transitions theory, it was acknowledged that some transitions may not have specific marker events although most transitions have critical marker points and times. The critical points and times are frequently associated with an awareness of changes or challenging engagement in transition processes. Final critical points are identified by a sense of comfort in new schedules, competence, lifestyles, and self-care behaviors.

Transition Conditions

Transition conditions are those circumstances that influence the way a person moves through a transition that facilitate or hinder progress toward achieving a healthy transition (Schumacher & Meleis, 1994). Transition conditions are the personal, community, or societal factors that may facilitate or inhibit the transition processes and outcomes.

Personal Conditions

Personal conditions refer to meanings, cultural beliefs and attitudes, socioeconomic status, preparation, and knowledge (Meleis et al., 2000). The meaning attached to a transition and the transition process facilitates or inhibits successful transitions. Personal conditions also include cultural beliefs and attitudes (e.g., stigma associated with cancer), socioeconomic status, anticipatory preparation, or lack of preparation.

Community and Societal Conditions

Community conditions and societal conditions could facilitate or inhibit successful transitions. An example of community conditions is community resources and an example of societal conditions is marginalized immigrants' status in the host country (Meleis et al., 2000).

Patterns of Response–Process and Outcome Indicators

In the framework by Schumacher and Meleis (1994), indicators of healthy transitions were included as a major concept. In transitions theory, indicators of healthy transitions were replaced with patterns of response that include process indicators and outcome indicators (Meleis et al., 2000). Process indicators lead clients toward health or vulnerability and risk. Thus, process indicators help nurses assess and intervene to facilitate healthy transitions. Outcome indicators can be used to assess if a transition is healthy or not. However, outcome indicators can sometimes be linked to events in people's lives if they are assessed early in a transition process. The process indicators include feeling connected, interacting, being situated, and developing confidence and coping. The need to feel and stay connected is included as a process indicator of a healthy transition because immigrants are usually in a healthy transition when they add new contacts to their old contacts with their family members and friends. The meaning of the transition and the resulting behaviors can be discovered, analyzed, and understood, and this interactive process may result in a healthy transition. In most transitions, place, time, space, and relationships indicate whether the person is in the process of a healthy transition. The extent of increased confidence that people in transition have indicates whether the person is in the process of a healthy transition. As an outcome indicator, mastery and fluid integrative identities are included in the theory. A healthy transition can be indicated by the extent of mastery of skills and behaviors that people in transition use to manage changes in their situations. Integrative identities through which identities are reformulated can also indicate a healthy transition.

Nursing Therapeutics

In the framework by Schumacher and Meleis (1994), nursing therapeutics are described as three measures that are widely applicable to therapeutic intervention during transitions. The three measures include assessment of readiness, preparation of transition, and role supplementation (Schumacher & Meleis, 1994). Assessment of readiness requires multidisciplinary efforts and should be based on a comprehensive understanding of the client. This requires the evaluation of each transition condition to produce a comprehensive sketch of people's readiness during transitions and helps determine various patterns of different transition experiences. The preparation for transition refers to education to produce the best condition/situation through which people in transition could be ready for a transition. Role supplementation as the last nursing therapeutic was originally suggested by Meleis (1975) and used by several researchers (Brackley, 1992; Dracup, Meleis, Clark, Clyburn, Shields, & Stanley, 1985; Gaffney, 1992; Meleis & Swendsen, 1978).

RELATIONSHIPS AMONG THE CONCEPTS: THE MODEL

The relationships among the major concepts can be illustrated as in Figure 11.1 (Meleis et al., 2000). This relationship is based on the transition framework by Schumacher and Meleis (1994) and the middle range theory of transitions by Meleis et al. (2000). The following statements regarding the relationships have been explicated by Im (2011, p. 423):

- Transitions are complex and multidimensional. Transitions have patterns of multiplicity and complexity.
- All transitions are characterized by flow and movement over time.
- Transitions cause changes in identities, roles, relationships, abilities, and patterns of behavior.
- Transitions involve a process of movement and change in fundamental life patterns, which are manifested in all individuals.

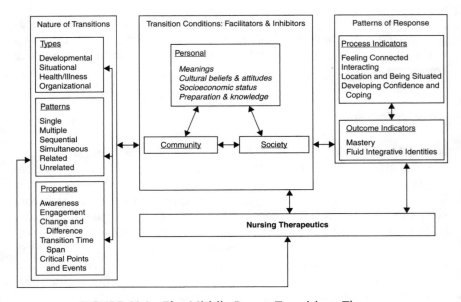

FIGURE 11.1   The Middle Range Transitions Theory
Source: Reprinted with permission from Meleis, A. I., Sawyer, L. M.,
Im, E. O., Messias, D. K. H., & Schumacher, K. (2000). Experiencing
transitions: An emerging middle range theory. *Advances in Nursing Science*,
23(1), 12–28.

- Change and difference are neither interchangeable nor synonymous with transition. Transitions result in change and are the result of change.
- The daily lives of clients, environments, and interactions are shaped by the nature, conditions, meanings, and processes of transition experiences.
- Vulnerability is related to transition experiences, interactions, and environmental conditions that expose individuals to potential damage, problematic or extended recovery, or delayed or unhealthy coping.
- Nurses are the primary caregivers of clients and their families who are undergoing transitions.

Transitions theory also has the following theoretical assertions (Schumacher & Meleis, 1994; Meleis et al., 2000; Im, 2011, p. 424):

- Developmental, situational, health and illness, and organizational transitions are central to nursing practice.

- Patterns of transition include whether the client is experiencing a single transition or multiple transitions; whether multiple transitions are sequential or simultaneous; the extent of overlap among transitions; and the nature of the relationship between the different events that are triggering transitions for a client.
- Properties of transition experience are interrelated parts of a complex process.
- The level of awareness influences the level of engagement, in which engagement may not happen without awareness.
- Humans' perceptions of and meanings attached to health and illness situations are influenced by and in turn influence the conditions under which a transition occurs.
- Healthy transition is characterized by both process and outcome indicators.
- Negotiating successful transitions depends on the development of an effective relationship between the nurse and the client (nursing therapeutic). This relationship is a highly reciprocal process that affects both the client and the nurse.

Derivatives of Transitions Theory

In this section, three situation-specific theories that were derived from transitions theory are presented: Situation-specific theory of Caucasian cancer patients' pain experience (STOP), situation-specific theory of pain experience for Asian American cancer patients (SPEAC), and situation-specific theory of Asian immigrant women's menopausal symptom experience in the United States (AIMS).

The Situation-Specific Theory of Caucasian Cancer Patients' Pain Experience

The STOP (Im, 2006) is a derivative of transitions theory. The reason for developing the STOP was to provide a better theoretical basis for the explanation of ethnic-specific cancer pain experience by narrowing the scope of the theory specifically to the pain experience of Caucasian cancer patients. STOP was developed to be a comprehensive theory that could be easily applied to nursing research and practice for management of Caucasian cancer patients' pain. To derive and develop STOP, an integrative approach was used. First, several assumptions were made, which include the following: The theory development process considered the diversity and complexity of the phenomenon from a nursing perspective; it was based on philosophical, theoretical, and methodological plurality; Caucasian cancer patients' pain experience occurred in a specific sociopolitical context; and it was based on a feminist nursing perspective. Multiple theorizing sources were used, which included a systematic literature review and research findings from a multiethnic study on cancer pain experience and transitions theory.

Deduction From Transitions Theory

Transitions theory provided the theoretical basis for development of STOP. Caucasian cancer patients' pain experience can be easily linked to the health/illness transition. The major concepts of transitions theory are related to the pain experience of Caucasian cancer patients. For instance, the concept of transition conditions includes personal, community, and societal conditions (Meleis et al., 2000): Socioeconomic status can influence selection of pain management strategies; community resources can influence support for pain management; and societal conditions can make women's pain experience different from that of men.

Induction Through a Literature Review and a Research Study

To develop STOP, a systematic integrated literature review was conducted and used as a source for theorizing. PubMed was searched for the years of 1995 to 2000 using keywords of Caucasian, White, cancer, pain, and/or experience. A total of 114 articles were included in the literature review (78 retrieved articles and 36 from the reference lists of the retrieved articles). All the articles were sorted by the major concepts of STOP. The literature review findings were analyzed and incorporated into the theorizing process.

In addition to the literature review, findings of a study on cancer pain that developed a decision support computer program for cancer pain management (DSCP study) (Im, Guevara, & Chee, 2007; Im et al., 2007, 2009; Im, Liu, Kim, & Chee, 2008; Im, Lim, Clark, & Chee, 2008) were used as a source for theorizing. The overall purpose of the study was to explore gender and ethnic differences in cancer pain experience among 480 cancer patients from four major ethnic groups in the United States. The study included a quantitative Internet survey and four qualitative ethnic-specific online forums. Multiple measurement scales, including questions on sociodemographic characteristics and health/illness status, three unidimensional cancer pain scales, two multidimensional cancer pain scales, the Memorial Symptom

Assessment Scale, and the Functional Assessment of Cancer Therapy Scale-General, were used for the quantitative Internet survey. Nine online forum topics were used for the qualitative online forums. The quantitative data were analyzed using descriptive and inferential statistics including analysis of variance (ANOVA) and hierarchical multiple regression analyses, and the qualitative data were analyzed using a thematic analysis.

The relationships among the five major concepts of STOP (Im, 2006) are the nature of transition, transition conditions, patterns of response, Caucasian cancer patients' pain experience, and nursing therapeutics. These five concepts are basically those of the transitions theory except the concept of Caucasian cancer patients' pain experience, the focus of STOP. Through the literature review and the findings of the DSCP study, all major concepts are confirmed to impact Caucasian cancer patients' pain experience. For instance, the nature (terminal or chronic) of transitions influences Caucasian cancer patients' pain experience. Cancer patients' religion can influence the patients' attitudes toward pain, which subsequently influences their pain experience.

Uniqueness of STOP

Compared with the middle range transitions theory, STOP has unique subconcepts (under the major concepts), which are frequently ethnic specific. For example, although cancer experience could be a health/illness transition that all ethnic groups go through in a common way, most Caucasian cancer patients tend to perceive the health/illness transition as a highly individualistic transition. In other words, depending on individual situations, they perceive health/illness transitions differently. Some experience horrible pain during the transition, while others rarely notice pain. Similarly, under the concept of patterns of response, the STOP has several ethnic-specific subconcepts such as control and transcendence. In the DSCP study, many patients thought they did not have control of their pain and/or disease and needed to bear the experience. On the contrary, others tried to control their pain and/or disease by selecting a specific health care provider whom they wanted to work with. In the DSCP study, the participants tried to transcend their cancer and cancer pain experience by "living life to the fullest" or by "not sweating the small things" (Im, 2006, p. 242). Because of these ethnic-specific subconcepts, STOP can be directly applied in nursing research and practice for Caucasian cancer patients' pain experience.

The Situation-Specific Theory of Pain Experience for Asian American Cancer Patients

The SPEAC (Im, 2008) was also derived from transitions theory. An integrative approach was used to develop the SPEAC. The theoretical development started from the following multiple assumptions: There are diversity and complexity in cancer pain experience; theory development is cyclic and evolutionary; the pain experience of Asian American cancer patients occurs in specific sociopolitical contexts; and a feminist nursing perspective is different from other perspectives. The SPEAC was developed using the following multiple sources: transitions theory, an integrative literature review, and research findings from a research study on cancer pain.

Deduction From Transitions Theory

Transitions theory was used for the development of the SPEAC primarily because Asian American cancer patients' pain experience can be easily linked to the health/illness transition. Also, the major concepts of transitions theory are appropriate to a theory about the pain experience of Asian American cancer patients. For example, Asian American cancer patients' pain experience could be linked to their health/illness transition. Transitions theory has a major concept of properties of transitions that includes awareness, engagement, change and difference, time span, and critical points and events (Meleis et al., 2000). All these properties can be easily linked to Asian American cancer patients' pain experience (Im, 2008). For example, Asian American cancer patients have an awareness of their health/illness transition, are engaged in the diagnosis and treatment process during the transition, experience changes in their physical, psychological, and social selves due to the health/illness transition, and have specific critical points in their transition process (e.g., diagnosis as a start point of the transition, death or ultimate survival as an ending point of the transition) (Im, 2008).

Induction Through a Literature Review and a Research Study

A systematic integrated literature review was conducted to provide the basis for theorizing. First, the literature was searched through PubMed from 1998 to 2008 with the key words of Asian American, cancer pain, and experience; Asian American, cancer, and pain; and Asian American and cancer. There were 24 retrieved articles and 15 additional articles from the reference lists of the retrieved articles. All the articles were sorted by the major concepts that were the focus of the SPEAC, and major findings were analyzed and incorporated into the theory development process.

The findings of the DSCP study were also used as the basis for the theorizing process of the SPEAC. As mentioned above, the overall goal of the DSCP study was to explore differences in cancer pain experience by gender and ethnicity. The study was conducted among 480 cancer patients from four major ethnic groups in the United States using multiple measurement scales and nine online forum topics. Then data were analyzed using descriptive and inferential statistics and a thematic analysis. Only the findings among Asian American cancer patients were the focus of the SPEAC.

The SPEAC includes five major concepts (Im, 2008): (1) the nature of transition, (2) transition conditions, (3) patterns of response, (4) Asian American cancer patients' pain experience, and (5) nursing therapeutics. These major concepts are identical to those of the transitions theory except for the concept of Asian American cancer patients' pain experience. All major concepts were found to influence Asian American cancer patients' pain experience in the literature review or in the DSCP study findings. The nature of transitions (terminal or chronic) can influence Asian American cancer patients' pain experience. Transition conditions such as background characteristics can also influence Asian American cancer patients' pain experience; for example, cancer patients' gender can influence the patients' cultural attitudes toward pain, which subsequently influence pain experience in their unique culture.

Uniqueness of the SPEAC

The unique aspects of the SPEAC compared to the transitions theory are the subconcepts (under the major concepts) that are ethnic specific. For example, although cancer experience is a universal health/illness transition, most Asian American cancer patients tend to experience the health/illness transition with a situational transition (immigration transition), which is a unique aspect of the SPEAC. Similarly, under the major concept of transition conditions, the SPEAC includes several ethnic-specific subconcepts such as being Asian American, country of birth, and subethnicity. Finally, the major concept of pattern of response includes ethnic-specific subconcepts such as tolerance, natural, normal, and mind control. In the DSCP study, Asian American cancer patients tended to tolerate pain instead of treating it aggressively.

They also tended to consider their pain experience natural, and they tried to normalize or minimize their conditions to overcome cultural stigma attached to cancer. Many of them also tried to manage their pain through mind control by having a strong will, hope, and positive thinking. These ethnic-specific subconcepts give the SPEAC the power to uniquely explain Asian American cancer patients' pain experience, and the SPEAC can be directly applied to nursing research or practice related to Asian Americans' cancer pain experience.

The Situation-Specific Theory of Asian Immigrant Women's Menopausal Symptom Experience in the United States

The AIMS (Im, 2010; Im, Lee, & Chee, 2010; Im, Lee, & Chee 2011) was also derived from transitions theory. The AIMS was developed using an integrative approach like STOP and SPEAC. The theorizing process began with multiple assumptions of theorizing (Im, 2010, p. 145):

- There are diversities and complexities in Asian immigrant women's menopausal symptom experience.
- The theory development process is cyclical and evolutionary and occurs in specific sociopolitical contexts.
- The inadequate management of menopausal symptoms reported by Asian immigrant women stems from biology and women's continuous interactions with their environments.
- The menopausal symptom experience is influenced by ethnicity and thus significantly interacts with gender, race, and class to structure relationships among individuals.

Deduction From the Transitions Theory

The reason for developing the AIMS beginning with transitions theory was that Asian immigrant women's menopausal symptom experience could be linked to the health/illness and developmental transitions that they experience in their menopausal transition and to the situation transition due to their immigration from one country to another. The major concepts of transitions theory are relevant to a theory about Asian immigrant women's menopausal symptom experience. For example, transitions theory has a subconcept of critical points and events under a major concept of properties of transitions (Meleis et al., 2000). This subconcept can be easily linked to the nature of menopausal symptom experience that Asian immigrant women go through.

Women's menopausal symptom experience has a specific beginning point with physical and psychological changes and a specific ending point that can be vague to some women (Im, 2010).

Induction Through a Literature Review and a Research Study

A systematic integrated literature review was also conducted to provide the basis for theorizing. A literature search through PubMed, PsycINFO, and CINAHL for the past 5 years was conducted using various key words including midlife, women, menopause, symptom, Asian, immigrant, Chinese, Korean, Japanese, predictors, and/or factors. The literature review included a total of 75 articles written in English and published in nursing and clinical journals. The articles were sorted by the major foci of AIMS to explain the menopausal symptom experience of Asian immigrant women in the United States. Finally, the major findings of the retrieved articles were analyzed and incorporated into the AIMS theory.

A study on menopausal symptom experience of four major ethnic groups of midlife women in the United States (MOMS) provided another element of foundation for the AIMS (Im, Lee, & Chee, 2011; Im, Lee, Chee, Brown, & Dormire, 2010; Im, Lee, Chee, Dormire, & Brown, 2010). The overall goal of the study was to explore ethnic differences in menopausal symptom experience among four major ethnic groups of midlife women in the United States (White, African American, Asian, and Hispanic). The study included a quantitative Internet survey and four qualitative ethnic-specific online forums. For the Internet survey, the questions on background, self-reported ethnic identity, and health and menopausal status and the Midlife Women's Symptom Index were used. For the online forums, seven online forum topics related to the menopausal symptom experience were used. The data analysis process included descriptive and inferential statistics including ANOVA and hierarchical multiple regression analyses for the Internet survey data and thematic analysis for the qualitative online forum data.

The AIMS includes three major concepts illustrated in Figure 11.2 (Im, 2010): (1) transition conditions, (2) patterns of response, and (3) nursing therapeutics. These major concepts came from transitions theory; however, the subconcepts under the major concepts are different. Transition conditions include five subconcepts: (1) demographic factors, (2) genetic factors, (3) ethnic-related factors, (4) health and menopausal status, and (5) lifestyle factors. These subconcepts are different from the subconcepts of transition conditions in transition

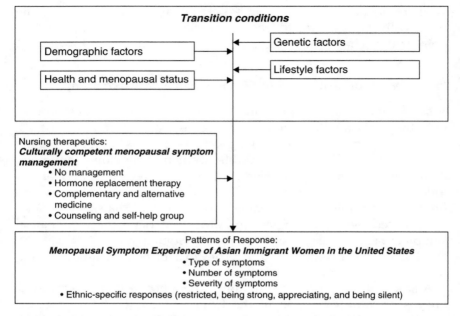

FIGURE 11.2   The Situation-Specific Theory of Asian Immigrant
Women's Menopausal Symptom Experience in the United States
Source: Reprinted with permission from Im, E. O. (2010). A situation specific
theory of Asian immigrant women's menopausal symptom experience in the
U.S. *Advances in Nursing Science, 33*(2), 143–157.

theory (personal and community transition conditions). The subconcepts under the pattern of response for AIMS include the type,
number, and severity of symptoms, and ethnic-specific response to
menopausal transition. Process and outcome indicators are not sepa-
rated because they tend to be mingled in the symptom experience.
For instance, the types of the symptoms (e.g., hot flash) experienced
during the menopausal transition could indicate both the process of
menopausal transition and the outcome of the menopausal transition. The subconcept of ethnic-specific response includes four major
themes from the MOMS study: restricted, being strong, appreciating,
and being silent. In the MOMS study, women perceived certain restrictions in their menopausal symptom experience; for example, women
perceived some restrictions given that their cultural heritage limits
behaviors, emotions, and actions related to menopausal symptom
experience. Women thought that the difficulties in their menopausal
transition were nothing compared with what they had gone through

with their immigration transition and that they became strong and faced their menopausal transition without problems. Women also considered menopause a relief and benefit because they would not need to worry about potential pregnancies or purchase feminine products for their menstrual periods. Finally, women considered silence the best strategy to cope with their menopausal symptoms. The concept of nursing therapeutics includes the following subconcepts: no management, hormone replacement therapy, complementary and alternative therapies, and counseling and self-help groups (Im, 2010). Finally, transition conditions influence menopausal symptom experience and nursing therapeutics to intervene and influence (enhance/worsen) the menopausal symptom experience of Asian immigrant women in the United States.

Uniqueness of the AIMS

The AIMS is unique from transitions theory because the specific subconcepts can be applied only to Asian immigrant women in menopausal transition. For example, menopausal transition could be a universal health/illness transition, but Asian immigrant women's menopausal transition is different from other ethnic groups because of their unique cultural attitudes and values related to women's health and menopausal symptoms. Thus, AIMS includes several ethnic-specific subconcepts such as responses like restricted, being strong, appreciating, and being silent. As in the SPEAC, these ethnic-specific subconcepts give AIMS the power to explain the menopausal symptom experience of Asian immigrant women in the United States. Also, the ethnic specificity makes the AIMS directly applicable to nursing research and practice with Asian immigrant women in the United States.

USE OF THE THEORY IN NURSING RESEARCH

Transitions theory has been nationally and internationally used in research studies across a broad spectrum of life transitions (Davies, 2005; Weiss et al., 2007). In addition, the theory was often used as the parent theory for situation-specific theories (Im & Meleis, 1999a; Im, 2006; Schumacher et al., 1999). The theory has been translated for use in Sweden, Taiwan, and many other countries (Im, 2009). After testing transitions theory in her investigation of transition experience of relatives related to older people's move to nursing homes, Davies (2005) concluded that the nature of transitions, transition conditions, and patterns of response could be helpful in explaining diverse factors that influence each person's transition and her or his unique experience. Weiss et al. (2007) concluded that their study findings supported transitions theory as a useful theoretical basis for conceptualizing and investigating predictors and outcomes of adult medical-surgical patients' perceptions of their readiness for hospital discharge. In addition, Weiss and Lokken (2009) concluded that transitions theory was a useful basis to determine predictors and outcomes of postpartum mothers' perceived readiness for hospital discharge.

USE OF THE THEORY IN NURSING PRACTICE

Transitions theory has been widely used in nursing practice for people across unique health-related transitions, including illness, recovery, birth, death, loss, and immigration (Meleis & Trangenstein, 1994). It has been used with geriatric populations, psychiatric populations, maternal populations, family caregivers, menopausal women, Alzheimer's patients, immigrant women, and people with chronic illness (Aroian & Prater, 1988; Brackley, 1992; Im, 1997; Kaas & Rousseau, 1983; Schumacher, Dodd, & Paul, 1993; Shaul, 1997). The theory has provided a comprehensive perspective on the nature and type of transitions, transition conditions, and process and outcome indicators of patterns of response to transitions. In addition, the theory can be used to develop nursing therapeutics that are congruent with the unique experience of clients and their families, to facilitate healthy successful transitions.

Other than clinical practice, transitions theory has been nationally and internationally used in nursing education (Meleis, personal communication, December 29, 2011). It has been incorporated into university nursing curricula (Meleis, personal communication, January 2008), including the University of Connecticut and Clayton State University in Morrow, Georgia. At UCSF, Meleis taught an independent graduate elective course on transitions and health to address student learning needs and requests of graduate students. In 2007, a center called Transitions and Health was established at the University of Pennsylvania (Mary Naylor, Director), which is the first center of its kind based on transitions theory. In addition, transitions theory has been used in a number of doctoral dissertations.

CONCLUSION

The middle range transitions theory has evolved from a borrowed perspective—through research studies and international and national collaborative works—and from the mentoring process. The theory has been developed based on multiple sources including research studies among diverse groups of people in various types of transitions. Several situation-specific theories were derived from transitions theory. Also, transitions theory can guide nursing education and practice in current health care systems that are characterized by diversities and complexities. However, as Meleis et al. (2000, p. 27) mentioned, transitions theory is an emerging framework that needs to be further developed, tested, and refined. Transitions theory could be further developed through research studies, nursing practice, and nursing education. The theory also needs to be further refined and tested to explain the major concepts and relationships among the major concepts with diverse populations in both common human transitions and unique health transitions. This testing will increase the theory's explanatory and predictive power. Most of all, future studies need to specifically aim to develop and test interventions based on the theory, through which it will gain prescriptive power to direct nursing practice.

REFERENCES

Aroian, K., & Prater, M. (1988). Transitions entry groups: Easing new patients' adjustment to psychiatric hospitalization. *Hospital and Community Psychiatry, 39*, 312–313.

Brackley, M. H. (1992). A role supplementation group pilot study: A nursing therapy for potential parental caregivers. *Clinical Nurse Specialist, 6*(1), 14–19.

Budman, C. L., Lipson, J. G., & Meleis, A. I. (1992). The cultural consultant in mental health care: The case of an Arab adolescent. *The American Journal of Orthopsychiatry, 62*(3), 359–370.

Chick, N., & Meleis, A. I. (1986). Transitions: A nursing concern. In P. L. Chin (Ed.), *Nursing research methodology: Issues and implantation.* Gainsburg, MD: Aspen Publishers.

Chinn, P. (2012). Transitions: A core nursing concept. *Advances in Nursing Science, 35*(3), 191.

Davies, S. (2005). Meleis's theory of nursing transitions and relatives' experiences of nursing home entry. *Journal of Advanced Nursing, 52*(6), 658–671.

Dracup, K., Meleis, A. I., Clark, S., Clyburn, A., Shields, L., & Staley, M. (1985). Group counseling in cardiac rehabilitation: Effect on patient compliance. *Patient Education and Counseling, 6*(4), 169–177.

Gaffney, K. F. (1992). Nurse practice-model for maternal role sufficiency. *Advances in Nursing Sciences, 15*(2), 76–84.

Im, E. O. (1997). *Negligence and ignorance of menopause within gender multiple transition context: Low income Korean immigrant women* (Unpublished doctoral dissertation). University of California, San Francisco, CA.

Im, E. O. (2006). A situation-specific theory of Caucasian cancer patients' pain experience. *Advances in Nursing Science, 29*(3), 232–244.

Im, E. O. (2008). The situation specific theory of pain experience for Asian-American cancer patients. *Advances in Nursing Science, 31*(4), 319–331.

Im, E. O. (2009). Meleis transition theory. In M. R. Alligood & A. M. Tomey (Eds.), *Nursing theorists and their work* (7th ed., pp. 416–433). Mosby: St. Louis, MO.

Im, E. O. (2010). A situation specific theory of Asian immigrant women's menopausal symptom experience in the U.S. *Advances in Nursing Science, 33*(2), 143–157.

Im, E. O. (2011). Transitions theory: A trajectory of theoretical development in nursing. *Nursing Outlook, 59*(5), 278–285.

Im, E. O., Chee, W., Guevara, E., Liu, Y., Lim, H. J., Tsai, H., ... Shin, H. (2007). Gender and ethnic differences in cancer pain experience: A multiethnic survey in the U.S. *Nursing Research, 56*(5), 296–306.

Im, E. O., Guevara, E., & Chee, W. (2007). The pain experience of Hispanic patients with cancer in the United States. *Oncology Nursing Forum, 34*(4), 861–868.

Im, E. O., Lee, S. H., & Chee, W. (2010). Sub-ethnic variations in the menopausal symptom experience: Asian American midlife women. *Journal of Transcultural Nursing, 21*(2), 123–33.

Im, E. O., Lee, S. H., & Chee, W. (2011). Be conditioned, but empowered: Asian American midlife women in menopausal transition. *Journal of Transcultural Nursing, 22*(3), 290–299.

Im, E. O., Lee, B. I., Chee, W., Brown, A., & Dormire, S. (2010). Menopausal symptoms among four major ethnic groups in the United States. *Western Journal of Nursing Research, 32*(4), 540–565.

Im, E. O., Lee, B. I., Chee, W., Dormire, S., & Brown, A. (2010). A national multiethnic online forum study on menopausal symptom experience. *Nursing Research, 59*(1), 26–33.

Im, E. O., Lee, S. H., Liu, Y., Lim, H. J., Guevara, H., & Chee, W. (2009). A national online forum on ethnic differences in cancer pain experience. *Nursing Research, 58*(2), 86–94.

Im, E. O., Lim, H. J., Clark, M., & Chee, W. (2008). African-American cancer patients' pain experience. *Cancer Nursing, 31*(1), 38–46.

Im, E. O., Liu, Y., Kim, Y. H., & Chee, W. (2008). Asian–American cancer patients' pain experience. *Cancer Nursing, 31*(3), E17–E23.

Im, E. O., & Meleis, A. I. (1999a). Situation-specific theories: Philosophical roots, properties, and approach. *Advances in Nursing Science, 22*(2), 11–24.

Im, E. O., & Meleis, A. I. (1999b). A situation-specific theory of Korean immigrant women's menopausal transition. *Journal of Nursing Scholarship, 31*(4), 333–338.

Im, E. O., & Meleis, A. I. (2000). Meanings of menopause: Low-income Korean immigrant women. *Western Journal of Nursing Research, 22*(1), 84–102.

Im, E. O., Meleis, A. I., & Lee, K. (1999). Symptom experience of low-income Korean immigrant women during menopausal transition. *Women and Health, 29*(2), 53–67.

Jones, P. S., Zhang, X. E., & Meleis, A. I. (1978). Transforming vulnerability. *Western Journal of Nursing Research, 25*(7), 835–853.

Kaas, M. J., Rousseau, G. K. (1983). Geriatric sexual conformity: Assessment and intervention. *Clinical Gerontologist, 2*(1), 31–44.

Laffrey, S. C., Meleis, A. I., Lipson, J. G., Solomon, M., & Omidian, P. A. (1989). Assessing Arab-American health care needs. *Social Science and Medicine, 29*(7), 877–883.

Lane, S. D., & Meleis, A. I. (1991). Roles, work, health perceptions, and health resources of women: A study in an Egyptian delta hamlet. *Social Science and Medicine, 33*(10), 1197–1208.

Lipson, J. G., & Meleis, A. I. (1983). Issues in health care of Middle Eastern patients. *Western Journal of Medicine, 139*(6), 854–861.

Lipson, J. G., & Meleis, A. I. (1985). Culturally appropriate care: The case of immigrants. *Topics in Clinical Nursing, 7*(3), 48–56.

Lipson, J. G., Reizian, A. E., & Meleis, A. I. (1987). Arab-American patients: A medical record review. *Social Science and Medicine, 24*(2), 101–107.

May, K. M., & Meleis, A. I. (1987). International nursing: guidelines for core content. *Nurse Educator, 12*(5), 36–40.

Meleis, A. I. (1975). Role insufficiency and role supplementation: A conceptual framework. *Nursing Research, 24*, 264–271.

Meleis, A. I. (1981). The Arab American in the health care system. *American Journal of Nursing, 81*(6), 1180–1183.

Meleis, A. I. (1997). *Theoretical nursing: Development and progress* (3rd ed.). Philadelphia, PA: Lippincott Williams & Wilkins.

Meleis, A. I. (2007). *Theoretical nursing: Development and progress* (4th ed.). Philadelphia, PA: Lippincott Williams & Wilkins.

Meleis, A. I. (2010). *Transitions theory: Middle-range and situation-specific theories in nursing research and practice.* New York, NY: Springer.

Meleis, A. I., Arruda, E. N., Lane, S., & Bernal, P. (1994). Veiled, voluminous, and devalued: Narrative stories about low-income women from Brazil, Egypt, and Colombia. *Advances in Nursing Science, 17*(2), 1–15.

Meleis, A. I., Douglas, M. K., Eribes, C., Shih, F., & Messias, D. K. (1996). Employed Mexican women as mothers and partners: Valued, empowered, and overloaded. *Journal of Advanced Nursing, 23*(1), 82–90.

Meleis, A. I., Kulig, J., Arruda, E. N., & Beckman, A. (1990). Maternal role of women in clerical jobs in southern Brazil: Stress and satisfaction. *Health Care for Women International, 11*(4), 369–382.

Meleis, A. I., & La Fever, C. W. (1984). The Arab American and psychiatric care. *Perspectives in Psychiatric Care, 22*(2), 72–76.

Meleis, A. I., Lipson, J., & Dallafar, A. (1998). The reluctant immigrant: Immigration experiences among Middle Eastern groups in Northern

California. In D. Baxter & R. Krulfeld (Eds.), *Selected papers on refugees and immigrants* (Vol. V, pp. 214–230). Arlington, VA: American Anthropological Association.

Meleis, A. I., Mahidal, V. T., Lin, J. Y., Minami, H., & Neves, E. P. (1987). International collaboration in research: Forces and constraints-by leaders from Thailand, People's Republic of China, Japan, and Brazil. *Western Journal of Nursing Research, 9*(3), 390–399.

Meleis, A. I., & Rogers, S. (1987). Women in transition: being vs. becoming or being and becoming. *Health Care for Women International, 8,* 199–217.

Meleis, A. I., Sawyer, L., Im, E., Schumacher, K., & Messias, D. (2000). Experiencing transitions: An emerging middle range theory. *Advances in Nursing Science, 23*(1), 12–28.

Meleis, A. I., & Sorrell, L. (1981). Bridging cultures. Arab American women and their birth experiences. *American Journal of Maternal and Child Nursing, 6*(3), 171–176.

Meleis, A. I., & Swendsen, L. (1978). Role supplementation: an empirical test of a nursing intervention. *Nursing Research, 27,* 11–18.

Meleis, A. I., Swendsen, L., & Jones, D. (1980). Preventive role supplementation: A grounded conceptual framework. In M. H. Miller & B. Flynn (Eds.), *Current perspectives in nursing: Social issues and trends* (Vol. 2, pp. 3–14). St. Louis, MO: Mosby.

Meleis, A. I., & Trangenstein, P. A. (1994). Facilitating transitions: Re-definition of the nursing mission. *Nursing Outlook, 42,* 255–259.

Schumacher, K. L., Dodd, M. J., & Paul, S. M. (1993). The stress process in family caregivers of persons receiving chemotherapy. *Research in Nursing & Health, 16,* 395–404.

Schumacher, K. L., Jones, P. S., & Meleis, A. I. (1999). Helping elderly persons in transition: A framework for research and practice. In L. Swanson & T. Tripp Reimer (Eds.), *Advances in gerontological nursing: Life transitions in the older adult* (Vol. 3, pp. 1–26). New York, NY: Springer.

Schumacher, K. L., & Meleis, A. I. (1994). Transitions: A central concept in nursing. *Image: Journal of Nursing Scholarship, 26*(2), 119–127.

Shaul, M. P. (1997). Transition in chronic illness: rheumatoid arthritis in women. *Rehabilitation Nursing, 22,* 199–205.

Shih, F. J., Meleis, A. I., Yu, P. J., Hu, W. Y., Lou, M. F., & Huang, G. S. (1998). Taiwanese patients' concerns and coping strategies: transitions to cardiac surgery. *Heart and Lung, 27*(2), 82–98.

Stevens, P. E., Hall, J. M., & Meleis, A. I. (1992). Examining vulnerability of women clerical workers from five ethnic/racial groups. *Western Journal of Nursing Research, 14*(6), 754–774.

Weiss, M. E., & Lokken, L. (2009). Predictors and outcomes of postpartum mothers' perceptions of readiness for discharge after birth. *Journal of Gyencological and Neonatal Nursing, 38*(4), 406–417.

Weiss, M. E., Piacentine, L. B., Lokken, L., Ancona, J., Archer, J., Gresser, S., ... Vega-Stromberg, T. (2007). Perceived readiness for hospital discharge in adult medical-surgical patients. *Clinical Nurse Specialist, 21*(1), 31–42.

12

Theory of Self-Reliance

John Lowe

Growing up Cherokee has everything to do with my understanding of self-reliance. Being one of 17 doctorally prepared Native American Indian nurses in the United States provides another perspective of who I am. The historical context of my people has shaped me and my scholarly work.

Cherokee historians, scholars, and tribal leaders have noted that the historical background and distinct culture of the Cherokee should be known in order to understand and respect the Cherokee today (Henson, J., personal communication, 2001; Mooney, 1975; Perdue, 1989). Historically, the Cherokee were the mountaineers of the South. They considered themselves inheritors of a dignity beyond their simple means and referred to themselves as the "principle people" (Ehle, 1988). The way of life and roles for them began to change under the new federal government of George Washington. Most of the land owned by the Cherokee was taken away through government treaties and force of arms. The federal government also established the Indian Boarding Schools where the language and practice of traditions were prohibited. This restriction was done in an attempt to strip the Native American Indian of his/her identity.

It is important to me that Cherokee identity shines through in this chapter on the middle range theory of self-reliance. The theory arose from Cherokee values and the work is being shared because I think these core values have meaning for the broader population of Native American Indian people as well as indigenous people throughout the world. In fact, the values that I learned as a Cherokee have the potential to affect health for populations beyond Native American Indians and indigenous people.

PURPOSE OF THE THEORY AND HOW IT WAS DEVELOPED

Self-reliance has been noted by Native American Indian leaders to be the mainstay and way of life that influence the health of Native American Indian people (Tyler, 1973). Additionally, self-reliance has been recognized as a key variable for keeping Cherokees in balance (Stuart, 1993). The history of the Cherokee has continued to affect the physical, emotional, psychosocial, economic, and spiritual well-being of the people. Formal and informal leaders and tribal members of Cherokee communities have expressed concern about the lack of self-reliance among their members. Historical events are viewed as undermining self-reliance, which in turn decreases well-being. The purpose of the middle range theory of self-reliance is to articulate a process for promoting well-being with attention to appreciation for one's culture.

Growing up Cherokee, I observed that Native American Indian people who became disconnected from the culture were plagued with health problems. These observations were the foundation of my commitment to make a difference for my people. My father, who stayed connected and grounded in Cherokee values, often said: "The Cherokee way is best." I later came to understand that self-reliance characterized the Cherokee way. Then, in my PhD program, I conducted an ethnographic study to understand the meaning of self-reliance for Cherokee people and how it was exhibited in daily life particularly by Cherokee men (Lowe, 2002a). The three concepts of the self-reliance theory, being responsible, disciplined, and confident, were the themes that emerged from the study. The self-reliance instrument was developed based on these concepts (Lowe, 2003).

Foundational Literature

The knowledge of the historical background and distinct culture of Native American Indians has been noted as important to increase the understanding of this group today (Henson, J., personal communication, 2001). Historically, the Cherokee inhabited the southeast region of the United States that now includes the states of Virginia, West Virginia, Tennessee, Kentucky, North Carolina, South Carolina, Georgia, and Alabama (Mooney, 1982). The way of life and roles of the Cherokee changed dramatically as a result of the dispossession of land and culture through government treaties and force of arms. The establishment of the Indian Boarding Schools was among the events that undermined self-reliance of the Cherokee. The traditional dress and speaking the tribal language were prohibited in an attempt to strip the

Cherokee of her/his identity. The physical, emotional, psychosocial, economic, and spiritual well-being of the Cherokee continue to be impacted today by prohibitions enforced decades ago.

Self-reliance is a concept within the Cherokee holistic worldview where all things are believed to come together to form a whole (Altman & Belt, 2008). Cherokee tribal leaders have noted self-reliance to be the mainstay and way of life that influences the health of the Cherokee people, helping them to find and keep balance (Henson, J., personal communication, 2001; Stuart, 1993).

Social change has been widespread in Native American Indian populations, challenging the traditional way of life, values, and relational systems. The Native American Indian family is changing rapidly as family members must now work outside the home, threatening the closeness of the family, in contrast to earlier years when families worked closely together to survive in a hostile environment (Frank, Moore, & Ames, 2000). Many Cherokee elders and tribal leaders report that the interdependence (Cherokee self-reliance) of the family, clan, and the tribe of earlier years has eroded (Lowe, 2002b), leading to stress-related health outcomes. Stress and coping processes have been reported to play an important role in physical and mental health outcomes among Native American Indians (Walters & Simoni, 2002). For instance, Native American Indian youth have significantly greater emotional distress than their White peers, and much of their distress is related to social and cultural factors (Bergstrom, Miller, & Peacock, 2003).

Assumptions

The cultural themes that constitute the assumptions of the theory are "being true to oneself" and "being connected." These assumptions cut across all the three concepts of self-reliance. The first assumption, "being true to oneself," refers to acknowledging one's heritage and living in keeping with the worldview of one's culture. The worldview of the Cherokee that provides the roots for this theory is considered to be circular and holistic where all things are believed to come together to form a whole (Altman & Belt, 2008). The second assumption, "being connected," refers to identifying and utilizing resources within creation. According to this dimension of the worldview, each person is a resource within the creation. The gifts and talents of each person will benefit not only the person but also the family, community, and cultural group. One identifies and utilizes his or her own gifts and talents and those of others. Figure 12.1 depicts the interrelatedness of the three concepts and assumptions of self-reliance.

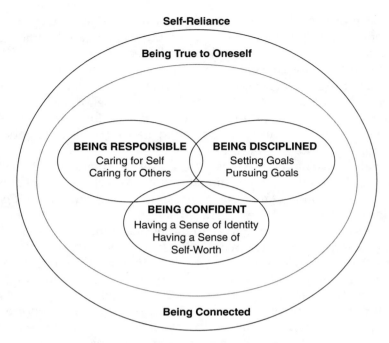

FIGURE 12.1   Self-Reliance
Source: Reprinted with permission from Lowe, J. (2003).
The Self-Reliance of the Cherokee Male Adolescent.
Journal of Addictions Nursing. 14, 209–214.

CONCEPTS OF THE THEORY

Self-reliance is being true-to-self and is lived by being responsible, disciplined, and confident while staying connected to one's cultural roots. The three concepts of self-reliance are (a) being responsible, (b) being disciplined, and (c) being confident.

Being responsible is being accountable to care for self and to care for others by getting assistance, respecting self, respecting others, and respecting the Creator. Respecting others occurs by being dependable and accountable. Honoring traditions, values, and language is a way to respect the Creator. The Creator in this context is the life force that grounds a sense of self.

Being disciplined is setting goals and pursuing goals by taking the initiative to make decisions and taking risks necessary to achieve goals. After decisions are made and goals are set, the pursuit of goals occurs by creating a plan, getting assistance, and redirecting one's effort.

Being confident refers to having a sense of identity and self-worth. Self-worth refers to knowing self within one's cultural heritage, being proud of one's heritage, and accepting cultural values and beliefs.

RELATIONSHIPS AMONG THE CONCEPTS: THE MODEL

The model of self-reliance (Figure 12.1) depicts a pattern of interrelating circles in keeping with a holistic world view. The three interlocking circles in the center of the model describe the interrelatedness through intertwining and interlacing of the concepts.

USE OF THE THEORY IN NURSING RESEARCH

Lowe began a program of research focused on substance abuse in Native American Indian communities while in graduate school at the master's level. His thesis research explored the social support that contributes to abstinence after substance-use treatment in the Native American Indian young adult. The research identified the overall concept of self-reliance as the mainstay and way of life that influences the health and well-being of Native American Indians. During his PhD studies, he continued to explore how the concept of self-reliance is defined by the Cherokee since self-reliance for the Cherokee had not been defined or researched previously. His PhD dissertation utilized the ethnographic method to identify how (a) self-reliance is conceptualized by the Cherokee; (b) the adult Cherokee perceives, achieves, and demonstrates self-reliance; and (c) nurses and health care professionals can incorporate the Cherokee concept of self-reliance in health care (Lowe, 2002a).

Dr. Lowe investigated the Cherokee adolescent's perception of self-reliance and its relationship to health (Lowe, 2003), finding that self-reliance was a way to keep the Cherokee from abusing drugs or alcohol. Participants in his studies reported a mentoring relationship, described as "being influenced," that is essential to enhance self-reliance (Lowe, 2005). The Cherokee self-reliance model that emerged from the findings of these studies was used to guide the development of a series of intervention studies. A Cherokee self-reliance instrument was developed and tested in the intervention studies. The instrument is a 24-item questionnaire with a 5-point Likert scale. A reliability coefficient alpha of 0.84 was documented for the instrument when it was used with Cherokee adolescents (Lowe, 2003).

In his intervention research, Dr. Lowe first conducted a pilot study funded by the Association of Nurses in AIDS Care/Biotech. The "Cherokee Teen Talking Circle" was evaluated for its effect on HIV/ AIDS knowledge and attitudes as well as protective behaviors. Cherokee self-reliance was also measured as a variable in this pilot study. The participants included 41 high school students who completed a 2-hour Talking Circle intervention. Pretest to posttest scores on HIV/AIDS knowledge and attitudes and protective behaviors were studied with paired t-tests. There were significant differences in knowledge (pretest mean: 4.44 + 0.92; posttest mean: 4.83 + 0.38) and attitudes (pretest mean: 9.88 + 0.38; posttest mean: 10.68 + 1.31). Cherokee self-reliance and HIV/AIDS knowledge, attitude, and protective behavior at posttest was significantly ($p < .01$) correlated [knowledge (0.499); attitude (0.421); behavior (0.254)] (Lowe, 2008). In addition, the Talking Circle was demonstrated to be a feasible cultural approach, resulting in meaningful participation with study participants.

In postdoctoral study funded by the National Institute on Alcohol Abuse and Alcoholism (NIAAA) Minority Supplement to R01 AA 10246-05 S1 Teen Intervention Project (TIP), Lowe conducted a Talking Circle intervention to help adolescents address alcohol and substance abuse problems. The parent TIP research was built on the standardized Student Assistance Program (SAP). The SAP involved a 10-session motivational, skills-building group intervention, developed for use with 8th through 12th graders (Wagner & Waldron, 2001; Wagner, Drinklage, Cudworth, & Vyse, 1999). This group intervention utilized a traditional group setting, approach, and process. Dr. Lowe merged the core ideas of the SAP with Cherokee values through the Talking Circle intervention to create the Teen Intervention Project—Cherokee (TIP-C) (Lowe, 2006).

Findings of the pilot TIP-C research revealed that the average Drug Use Screening Inventory-Revised (DUSI-R) score of the TIP-C participants ($N = 108$) reduced from 24.74 to 20.94 (t = −13.82, $p < .001$). The participants' average stress score also decreased from 43.60 at the baseline to 41.44 post intervention (t = −6.41, $p < .001$). By contrast, the participants' average Cherokee self-reliance score increased from 90.51 at baseline to 110.92 post intervention (t = 26.97, $p < .001$) (Lowe, 2006). During each follow-up assessment, TIP-C participants were encouraged to write about the impact of the intervention. One participant, who completed his 1-year follow-up assessment, had been diagnosed and was receiving treatment for cancer at the time of his written feedback. He said: "I am so thankful that I went through the TIP-C groups ... even though I have been very sick, this has been one of the best years of my life ... I have been clean and sober and I now know what it means to live the Cherokee way."

Dr. Lowe conducted another 3-year study "Community Partnership to Affect Keetoowah–Cherokee Adolescent Substance Abuse" funded by the National Institutes on Drug Abuse (NIDA) (1 R01 DA021714-030). A community-based participatory research approach was used to develop and test the culturally competent school-based intervention— Cherokee Talking Circle (CTC)—a revision of the TIP-C intervention. The difference in substance abuse, Cherokee self-reliance, and stress between Keetoowah–Cherokee adolescents who received the CTC prevention and those who received standard substance abuse education (SE) was evaluated. Findings revealed that higher self-reliance and less focus on self were related with the ability to express feelings, which was higher for those who scored higher on self-reliance. Substance abuse scores between the CTC and SE groups were significantly different (F = 13.14.10, $p < .001$) with the CTC group having lower substance abuse scores. There was also a significant interaction effect between time and group (F = 27.95, $p < .001$) with the greatest differences between the groups noted immediately after the intervention (t = −3.89, $p < .001$) and at the 3-month follow-up (t = −4.69, $p = .001$). At each time point, self-reliance was higher for the CTC group than the SE group and the difference between the groups increased over time (Lowe, Liang, Riggs, & Henson, 2012).

Dr. Lowe is currently conducting a 2-year NIDA (R34DA029724-01A1) funded study to examine the feasibility of using the CTC for Native American Indian 6th graders as they transition to middle school. In this study, preliminary results reveal a trend toward statistical significance. At 6-months postintervention, the CTC group had significantly lower substance involvement/interest scores than the SE control group. CTC substance abuse/use scores decreased from 2.3 to 1.3 (t (33) = 1.8, $p = .007$). Likewise, there was a significant increase in self-reliance, from 86.2 to 92.2 (t (43) = −2.6, $p = .007$).

A 5-year NIDA (R01DA029779-01A1) funded study is also being conducted by Dr. Lowe and colleagues that is guided by the self-reliance theory. This study is designed to develop and test a school-based, brief motivational intervention for substance abuse among Native American Indian high school students. Currently, there is no evidence from research concerning the use and effect of motivational interviewing (MI) among Native American Indian youth guided by a cultural specific theory such as the self-reliance theory.

Dr. Lowe has collaborated with researchers nationally and internationally, sharing the self-reliance work and the community-based participatory approach that he uses for his research. For instance, he collaborated with Native American Indian colleagues to expand the Cherokee self-reliance model so that it is appropriate for other tribes, renaming the model "Native Self-Reliance." The Native self-reliance model has been used to guide a study where the Talking Circle intervention was implemented with Plains tribal youth (Patchell, B., personal communication, 2011). From an international perspective, Dr. Lowe has begun work with indigenous people in Australia (Aboriginal and Torres Straight Islanders) and New Zealand (Maori) who are interested in his community-based approach to research, the self-reliance theory, and the process of using the Talking Circle. Australian and New Zealand colleagues recognize Dr. Lowe as a scholar who advocates for culturally competent health care of Native American Indians and indigenous people globally. When in Australia and New Zealand, Dr. Lowe meets with Australian and New Zealand indigenous nurses as well as Elders who seek his counsel.

USE OF THE THEORY IN NURSING PRACTICE

The Talking Circle is a meaningful approach to nursing practice. It is described here as it is lived in the Native American Indian tradition. It is used as the intervention in all of my studies. Nurses in practice are invited to consider how the Talking Circle may be used in other cultural traditions.

In the Native American Indian tradition, a Talking Circle is a coming-together and a place where stories are shared in a respectful manner and in a context of complete acceptance by participants. Native American Indians have long used the Circle to celebrate the sacred interrelationship that is shared with one another and with their world (Simpson, 2000). The idea of the Talking Circle permeates the traditions of Native American Indians to this day. It symbolizes an entire approach to life and to the universe in which each being participates in the Circle and each one serves an important and necessary function that is valued no more or no less than that of any other being.

By honoring the Circle, human beings honor the process of life and the process of growth that is an ever-flowing stream in the movement of life energy (Garrett & Carroll, 2000). Cherokees consider the whole greater than the sum of its parts and have always believed that healing and transformation should take place in the presence of the group since they are all related to one another in very basic ways (Reed, 1993). Through use of the Talking Circle, Cherokees can use the support and insight of their brothers and sisters to move away from something, such as substance abuse, and toward something else. In this way, the Talking Circle has served a very sacred function of healing or cleansing, while also serving as a way of bringing people together.

The traditional sense of belonging and comfort provides healing for all and the Circle reminds the Cherokee of life and their place in it (Ywahoo, 1987). Each person comes to the Circle as a human being with his or her own concerns, and together participants seek harmony and balance by sharing stories, praying, singing, talking, and sometimes even just sitting together in silence.

Use of the Theory in Nursing Education

Dr. Lowe has long-used the Talking Circle intervention in his work with nursing students. Every semester he takes a group of students to Cherokee tribal communities in Oklahoma to participate in a service learning cultural immersion experience where the Native American Indian culture and community become the classroom. Self-reliance is threaded throughout this learning experience. The Talking Circle became a powerful teaching approach that emerged from the self-reliance theory, offering opportunities for personal growth that extend beyond the community nursing content that is the focus for the course.

CONCLUSION

Although the Cherokee self-reliance model has been in existence for more than a decade, the middle range theory of self-reliance is being introduced for the first time in this chapter. The theory has its roots in Native American Indian culture and values. It has grown over time as a foundation guiding the Talking Circle intervention used in nursing research, practice, and education. The theory is strengthened by the existence of a psychometrically sound instrument that enables evaluation of self-reliance through self-report. Introduction of the middle range theory of self-reliance in this chapter is an expression of invitation to nurses who may choose to use the theory for practice, research, and education. Use of the theory will honor the Native American Indian people who cultivated self-reliance in the midst of unimaginable historical trauma. The theory is shared in a spirit of gratitude for the wisdom of ancestors and in a spirit of generosity, wishing to extend their wisdom to others who may benefit from the middle range theory of self-reliance.

REFERENCES

Altman, H. M., & Belt, T. N. (2008). Reading history: Cherokee history through a Cherokee lens. *Native South, 1*(1), 90–98.

Bergstrom, A., Miller, L., & Peacock, T. (2003). The seventh generation: Native students speak about finding the good path. Retrieved from ERIC database: ERIC ED472385.

Ehle J. (1988). Trail of tears: The rise and fall of Cherokee Nation. New York, NY: Doubleday.

Frank, J., Moore, R., & Ames, G. (2000). Historical and cultural roots of drinking problems among American Indians. *American Journal of Public Health, 90*(3), 344–350.

Garrett, M., & Carroll, J. (2000). Mending the broken circle: Treatment of substance dependence among Native Americans. *Journal of Counseling and Development, 78*(4), 379–388.

Lowe, J. (2002a). Cherokee self-reliance. *Journal of Transcultural Nursing, 13*(4), 287–295.

Lowe, J. (2002b). Balance and harmony through connectedness: The intentionality of Native American nurses. *Holistic Nursing Practice, 16*(4), 4–11.

Lowe, J. (2003). The self-reliance of the Cherokee adolescent male. *Journal of Addictions Nursing, 14*, 209–214.

Lowe, J. (2005). Being influenced: A Cherokee way of mentoring. *Journal of Cultural Diversity, 12*(2), 37–49.

Lowe, J. (2006). Teen intervention project – Cherokee (TIP-C). *Pediatric Nursing, 32*(5), 495–500.

Lowe, J. (2008). A cultural approach to conducting HIV/AIDS and HCV education among Native American adolescents. *Journal of School Nursing, 24*(4), 229–238.

Lowe, J., Liang, H., Riggs, C., & Henson, J. (2012). Community partnership to affect substance abuse among Native American adolescents. *The American Journal of Drug and Alcohol Abuse, 38*(5), 250–255.

Mooney, J. (1975). *Historical sketch of the Cherokee.* Chicago: Aldine Publishing Company.

Mooney, J. (1982). *Myths of the Cherokee and sacred formulas of the Cherokee.* Nashville, TN: Charles and Randy Elder Publishers.

Perdue, T. (1989). *The Cherokee.* New York, NY: Chelsea House Publishers. Prucha.

Reed, M. (1993). *Seven clans of the Cherokee society.* Cherokee, NC: Cherokee Publications.

Simpson, L. (2000). Stories, dreams, and ceremonies: Anishinaabe ways of learning. *Tribal College Journal of American Indian Higher Education, 11*(4), 26–29.

Stuart, D. (1993). *Letter of research support.* Tahlequah, OK: Cherokee Nation.

Tyler, S. L. (1973). *A history of Indian policy.* Washington, DC: U.S. Government Printing Office.

Wagner, E. F., Drinklage, S., Cudworth, C., & Vyse, J. (1999). A preliminary evaluation of the effectiveness of a standardized Student Assistance Program. *Substance Use and Misuse, 34*(11), 1571–1584.

Wagner, E., & Waldron, H. (Eds.). (2001). *Innovations in adolescent substance abuse intervention.* Oxford, UK: Pergamon.

Walters, K. L., & Simoni, J. M. (2002). Reconceptualizing Native women's health: An "indigenist" stress coping model. *American Journal of Public Health, 92*(4), 520–524.

Ywahoo, D. (1987). *Voices of our ancestors: Cherokee teachings from the wisdom fire.* Boston, MA: Shamabala.

13

Theory of Cultural Marginality

Heeseung Choi

*A*s transportation and communication technology advance, there is a complementary increase in contacts between culturally distinct populations. The number of immigrants has continued to grow; as of 2010, about 12.9% of the U.S. population was foreignborn (U.S. Census Bureau's American Community Survey, 2010). About 17% of the 40 million foreign-born immigrants in 2010 reported entry within the 6 years from 2005 to 2010 (Walters & Trevelyan, 2011). Although society is becoming more and more ethnically and culturally diverse, the lack of mutual understanding between health care providers and clients from different cultural backgrounds remains a barrier to progress in health care services for immigrants. The Theory of Cultural Marginality was developed to increase understanding of the unique experiences of individuals who are straddling distinct cultures and to offer direction for providing culturally relevant care.

PURPOSE OF THE THEORY AND HOW IT WAS DEVELOPED

While working with immigrant adolescents and living in the United States as an immigrant, I noticed unique circumstances that immigrant adolescents encountered as a result of the immigration process and the impact of the process on their mental health. A review of related theories and research on immigrant adolescents' mental health issues provided the foundation for developing a program of research that began with Korean American adolescents. In a community-based study, I discovered that Korean American adolescents demonstrated significantly lower levels of self-esteem, coping skills, and mastery in addition to higher levels of depression and somatic symptoms than American adolescents (Choi, Stafford, Meininger, Roberts, & Smith, 2002). The response pattern was more prominent among foreign-born

Koreans than U.S.-born Koreans. In a subsequent school-based study, compared with Whites, Asian and Hispanic American adolescents experienced higher levels of social stress and somatic symptoms and depression (Choi, Meininger, & Roberts, 2006). Among White, African, Hispanic, and Asian Americans, Asian American adolescents reported the lowest scores on self-esteem, coping, and family cohesiveness, and the highest score in family conflicts (Choi et al., 2006). These findings led to an exploration of the reasons for the adolescents' vulnerability and to examining the stress of the immigration process as a significant risk factor for mental distress. The next step in building my program of research required an extensive literature review searching for theories that contributed to understanding how distress was associated with immigration for Asian American adolescents.

Theories contributing to the development of the theory of cultural marginality were acculturation, acculturative stress, and marginality. Acculturation was first defined by the Social Science Research Council (SSRC) as "phenomena which result when groups of individuals having different cultures come into continuous first-hand contact, with subsequent changes in the original cultural patterns of either or both groups" (Redfield, Linton, & Herskovits, 1936, p. 149). Theories addressing acculturation have undergone many changes over time, expressed originally through unidimensional models to current expression as multidimensional and orthogonal models (Berry, Poortinga, Segall, & Dasen, 1992; Keefe & Padilla, 1987; Oetting & Beauvais, 1990–1991; Vega, Gil, & Wagner, 1998). The unidimensional bipolar model suggested that individuals inevitably lost their culture of origin as they became acculturated into a new culture (Redfield et al., 1936). Individuals were believed to have only two options: either they acculturated or they remained in their old culture. On the other hand, the multidimensional model focuses on the complex nature of acculturation and selective, or uneven, acculturation across domains of social life (Berry et al., 1992; Keefe & Padilla, 1987; Vega et al., 1998). The orthogonal model proposes biculturality and assumes that acculturating individuals could maintain two different cultural identities simultaneously (Oetting & Beauvais, 1990–1991). An individual may identify him- or herself as a member of both cultural groups, not necessarily choosing either cultural group. These two models opened a new era for theories of acculturation.

One of the popular approaches to acculturation is the fourfold theory of acculturation (Berry, 1995; Berry & Kim, 1988; Berry et al., 1992). The fourfold theory explains strategies that acculturating individuals use. Depending on the chosen culture of reference, strategies are categorized as assimilation, separation, integration, and marginalization.

In assimilation, individuals give up their cultural identity and are absorbed into the dominant, or new, culture. Separation, by contrast, is withdrawal from the dominant culture to reside within the old culture. Integration is regarded as the ideal response and involves "making the best of both worlds" (Berry et al., 1992, p. 279). In marginalization, individuals lose their cultural and psychological contacts with both cultures. Theories of acculturation are broad-ranging and complex, incorporating social, economic, and political components, as well as values, attitudes, self-identity, and behavior change components (Berry & Kim, 1988; Berry et al., 1992).

Acculturative stress—a second theory that contributed to cultural marginality—was developed to highlight the link between acculturation and mental health outcomes. Acculturative stress was defined by Vega et al. (1998) as "a by-product of acculturation that is specific to personal exposure to social situations and environments that challenge individuals to make adjustments in their social behavior or the way they think about themselves" (p. 125). Individuals experience acculturative stress during the acculturating process or as a result of discrimination or being different (Chavez, Moran, Reid, & Lopez, 1997). Acculturative stress has been associated with declining mental health status in acculturating immigrants (Gil, Wagner, & Vega, 2000; Hovey & Magana, 2002; Noh & Kaspar, 2003). The intensity of the relationship between acculturative stress and mental health outcomes is determined by a number of moderating factors including the nature of the dominant culture and the characteristics of the acculturating individuals and groups (Berry & Kim, 1988; Berry et al., 1992).

The third theory to contribute to the development of the theory of cultural marginality was the theory of marginality. The theory of marginality was first proposed by Park in 1928. Park introduced the "marginal man" concept with special attention to social context (Park, 1928, p. 893). He described the marginal man as experiencing conflicts of the divided self, the old and new self, a lack of integrity, spiritual instability, restlessness, malaise, and moral turmoil between at least two cultural lives. Stonequist (1935) further explored the nature, variations, social situations, and life cycle of the marginal man. By Stonequist's (1935) definition, life cycles consist of an introductory period of preparation, a crisis period, and an adjustment period that may provide opportunities and impetus for social and psychological growth. The theory of marginality has been applied to a wide range of situations, such as middle managers' experiences in the social hierarchy of the workplace (Ziller, 1973), student nurses' experiences (Andersson, 1995), and menopause experiences (Im & Lipson, 1997).

In nursing, Hall, Stevens, and Meleis (1994) defined marginality as the condition of being peripheralized from mainstream society or the center of the society based on identity, status, and experience. Marginalization and marginality were viewed from a sociopolitical perspective in relation to racial, gender, political, or economic oppression and were scrutinized along with inequities in economic, political, and social power and resources (Hall, 1999; Hall et al., 1994).

The broad perspective that characterizes the theories of acculturation, acculturative stress, and marginality has led to criticisms that cite vagueness and a lack of empirical support (Del Pilar & Udasco, 2004; Rudmin, 2003) as major weaknesses. Del Pilar and Udasco (2004) claimed that marginality contains so many different layers of experiences that it is impossible to explain it in a unified way. Keeping in mind the strengths as well as the limitations and criticisms of the previous theories, I began by defining cultural marginality. The first definition of cultural marginality was "situations and feelings of passive betweeness when people exist between two different cultures and do not yet perceive themselves as centrally belonging to either one" (Choi, 2001, p. 198). With continued contemplation of this definition, thoughtful ongoing review of literature, and research with immigrant adolescents, the theory of cultural marginality developed. Schwartz-Barcott and Kim (2000) emphasized the importance of an empirical component in the process of theory development. To validate the theory of cultural marginality with empirical data, I conducted a qualitative study exploring Korean American adolescents' and their parents' perceptions of being in between two different cultures. Twenty Korean American adolescents between the ages of 11 and 14 years and twenty-one parents were interviewed.

The qualitative study revealed that the main sources of stress for Korean American adolescents were managing a balanced peer relationship, discrimination, pressure to excel academically and to be successful, and lack of in-depth parent–child relationships. Parents experienced feeling uneasy and insecure about parenting children in the American culture, lacked a sense of belonging, felt ambivalent toward their children's ethnic identity, and found they were unable to advocate for children. Parents also reported struggling with a lack of depth in parent–child relationships (Choi & Dancy, 2009). As a result of these experiences, parents often felt inadequate, guilty, and regretful. The findings were integrated into the conceptual structure of the theory (Choi, Dancy, & Lee, in press). This process provides a strong empirical foundation for the theory of cultural marginality. I will introduce relevant quotes as I discuss the main concepts of the theory.

CONCEPTS OF THE THEORY

The major concepts of the theory of cultural marginality are cross-cultural conflict recognition, marginal living, and easing cultural tension. As an individual recognizes conflicts between cultures, he or she engages in marginal living and initiates adjustment responses to ease cultural tension. Therefore, cultural marginality is marginal living while recognizing cross-cultural conflicts and striving to ease cultural tension. An important dimension of cultural marginality, in addition to the major concepts, is contextual/personal influences that create the foundation for a person's experience of cultural marginality. Each of the major concepts of the theory as well as contextual/personal influences will be discussed. In describing the major concepts of the theory, quotes shared by parents and adolescents in my qualitative study will be shared.

Marginal Living

Marginal living—a major concept of the theory—is defined as passive betweeness in the pushing/pulling tension between two cultures while forging new relationships in the midst of old and living with simultaneous conflict/promise. In the theory of cultural marginality, marginal living is viewed as a process of being in between two cultures with emphasis on being in transition rather than being on the periphery of one culture.

Passive betweeness is the essential quality of marginal living. Park (1928) described the marginal experience as a situation that "condemned him to live in two worlds, in neither of which he ever quite belonged" (p. 893). Nobody chooses to be on the edge of two different cultures or to be in between. It is especially true for children who usually have no option when moving from one country to another (Guarnaccia & Lopez, 1998). They simply follow their parents' choice of new country for a better life. Even adults who decide to live in a new country really do not want to be in an "in between" position. Some people who have experienced marginality recalled the time as "a period when they stand with both feet in different boots" (Andersson, 1995, p. 131). The experience has been described as "trapped," "being betwixt and between," and "being located within a structure of double ambivalence" (Bennett, 1993, p. 113; Weisberger, 1992, p. 429). The following quotes capture the quality of passive betweeness. A mother said:

> I, myself, have to live a life of the crippled in this country ... I feel like I am floating in the air. I don't know if I will be able to stand on my feet before I die. I worry whether my children will grow up well ... I know

for sure that I came here for my children, but I was in agony because I thought I made a wrong decision … I am so worried about how to live my life as a mother.

An adolescent said:

I go crazy over … Korean pride and World Cup. But my friends are like, "Outside, you are Korean, but inside, you are White." So I feel like I'm part of them. Sometimes I'm like that and sometimes I'm not.

When people move to a new country or a different culture, they inevitably must become engaged in new relationships (Rogler, 1994). New relationships do not form in a single day, and building them is not as simple as taking off old clothes and changing into new ones. One of the qualities of marginal living is forging new relationships in the midst of old relationships. This quality is often more prominent among adolescents since forming new allegiances with peers and confirming their identities and values within the peer group are critical developmental tasks. Adolescents, who are eager to forge new relationships in the midst of old relationships, often encounter contradiction and conflicts. While moving forward to engage in new relationships, adolescents are concerned about losing connection with their old relationships. As adolescents actively forge new relationships while parents dwell in the past, the parent–child relationship gets untied. The following quote describes the experience of an adolescent who began to engage in new relationships in a new world:

We [mom and herself] will grow apart since we will be living in two different cultures, using different languages. I think she's already having a hard time … I wish you had a program to help her overcome such barriers so we may stay close.

Adolescents who are living "in between" face tension between two cultures. Parents encourage their children to mingle with new friends, to pursue further opportunities, so that they will be successful in the new society. This phenomenon is prominent especially among families who emigrated for better education and opportunities. However, parents feel threatened and become anxious about losing control over their children as their children blend into the new culture. The following quote illustrates the pushing/pulling quality of tension from the perspective of the father of a 12-year-old boy:

Many of their parents have double standards for them. They want their children to be successful in America as American citizens, yet they want them to remain Koreans at the same time. And that gives children an ambiguous message, which confuses them. … If you keep giving such contradicting messages to children, especially at a sensitive stage when they start questioning their parents' authority, they will surely get confused and it might lead to creating other problems. I think that is the real problem.

Complicating matters, the new society or dominant culture has similarly contradictory attitudes toward immigrants: It welcomes immigrants warmly and promises to provide them abundant opportunities and resources; however, in reality, what immigrants often face is overt and covert discrimination, as reported by both Korean American adolescents and their parents during the interviews. Korean American adolescents encountered teachers' insensitive attitudes toward different cultures, experienced limited opportunities, and got unfair grades and punishments. Korean American adolescents also reported that they had been teased or bullied because of their accent and physical appearance.

There is a demand for immigrants to make choices among contradicting norms, expectations, roles, and values. They often find themselves struggling in simultaneous conflict and promise. Conflict couched in promise is a quality of marginal living causing identity confusion, anxiety, ambivalence, feelings of alienation, loss, helplessness, worthlessness, a feeling of uncertainty, and apprehension about the future (Andersson, 1995; Berry et al., 1992; Fuertes & Westbrook, 1996; Scribner, 1995; Weisberger, 1992). However, conflict does not always create negative outcomes. Depending on how the individual perceives and manages conflict, it may offer possibility for change. In a previous article on the concept of cultural marginality (Choi, 2001), conflict and promise were categorized as two distinct attributes; however, subsequent research has indicated that promise is integral to conflict. Thus, for the theory of cultural marginality, conflict/promise is conceptualized as a single quality of marginal living. Hall and colleagues (Hall, 1999, p. 100; Hall et al., 1994) identified resilience and a "hope-positive view of the future" as well as vulnerabilities when marginalized people struggled to acquire their own survival strategies to protect themselves and enhance their sense of well-being. Marginal living presents both a conflict and a promise as well as a crisis and a turning point, thus providing an impetus for growth.

During the interviews, Korean American parents expressed hopes for their children's future even in the midst of feelings of alienation, powerlessness, worthlessness, and uncertainty. They expected their children to blend into mainstream society and move up the social ladder by obtaining high educational status, leading children to feel pressured to excel academically and to be successful. Integral to this experience of marginal living is the recognition of cross-cultural conflict, a second concept of the theory of cultural marginality.

Cross-Cultural Conflict Recognition

Cross-cultural conflict recognition is a beginning understanding of differences between two contradicting cultural values, customs, behaviors, and norms. Just as people feel and react to perceived temperature, not measured temperature, people feel and react to their recognition of differences while in between cultures. Conflict emerges as individuals face distinct value systems with accompanying expectations and are forced to make difficult choices. Korean American adolescents reported encountering two distinct cultural values and expectations between peers and their parents and between Korean and American friends.

Acknowledging cross-cultural conflict recognition as a concept of the theory of cultural marginality has significant implications for research and practice because it allows for individual differences in perception, responses, and mental health outcomes associated with cultural marginality. This is consistent with the theorizing of Lazarus (1997), who identified cognitive appraisal of cultural environment as one of the significant determinants of mental health outcomes. An adolescent said:

> You know how parents raise their kids based on how they were raised. … Well, if I compare my style with regular White friends, it's completely different. They are always out and my parents think you play too much or you do this too much but if you compare me with them, that's not really true. Well, I know it's best for me what they say but sometimes it's like that's how we live here in America.

Easing Cultural Tension

Easing cultural tension resolves cross-cultural conflict. Adjustment responses proposed in the theory of cultural marginality are adapted from Weisberger's work on marginality among German Jews (1992). Four responses, assimilation, reconstructed return, poise, and integration, are processes for easing cultural tension. The responses are not mutually exclusive; rather, they are mixed empirically (Weisberger, 1992) and will be referred to as response patterns to connote their contextual, situational, dynamic nature.

The first response pattern is assimilation. It is a process whereby individuals are absorbed into the dominant or new culture (Berry, 1995; Berry & Kim, 1988; Berry et al., 1992). This is usually the first response pattern exhibited by new immigrants, particularly when the dominant or new culture is unfavorable to the newcomers. Immigrants strive hard to acquire new language and customs and to mingle with people of the new society. It is a useful strategy for survival in the new culture; however, it may create self-denial, self-hatred, and feelings of guilt (Weisberger, 1992).

After encountering the new culture, individuals may return to their own culture, exhibiting the pattern of reconstructed return. They may choose to return as a result of resistance, obstacles, and conflicts with a new culture or as a result of reminiscence and longing for one's own culture. When they return, they do so with a new perspective toward their own culture as well as to the new culture since they cannot be free from the influences of the new culture (Anderson & Levy, 2003; Weisberger, 1992). Thus, every return is a reconstructed return. A typical characteristic of people who return to or remain in their culture is an overidentification with their own culture. Weisberger (1992, p. 442) describes the characteristics among the returning German Jews as "more Jewish than Jewish." The following quote is from a mother of a 14-year-old daughter who was referred by her teacher to a school counselor for her misbehavior at school:

> Even if she was born here [United States] and has never been to Korea, she always hangs out with Korean friends, particularly Korean kids who recently moved from Korea. She likes to have Korean clothes, accessories, phone, and stuff ... I think it is because [of] her longing for Korea and Korean culture.

Poise is a response pattern characterized by a tentative fit on the margin regardless of emotional conflict and struggle. Individuals who respond with poise may become free from obligation or attachment to a certain culture, but they have to be "homeless in a cultural sense" (Weisberger, 1992, p. 440). Even when responding with a pattern of poise, individuals will continue to experience emotional conflicts and a period of personal crisis continues. Accumulated effects of crisis may include stress and poor mental health outcomes such as personality changes, substance abuse, depression, and even suicidal ideation (Hovey & Magana, 2002; Park, 1928; Vega et al., 1998; Williams & Berry, 1991).

Integration is an adjustment response pattern where an individual creates a third culture by merging and integrating the old and new cultures. Through integration, individuals surpass cultural boundaries, contexts, and identities and acquire superior social functioning, gaining access to multiple cultural worlds (Guarnaccia & Lopez, 1998; Park, 1928; Weisberger, 1992) and easing cultural tension. They will experience a sense of cultural home, a sense of belonging, integration of identity, and psychological and cognitive growth (Bennett, 1993; Vivero & Jenkins, 1999). For them, the possibility of returning to the cultural tension of marginal living is minimized. When faced with another circumstance of cultural tension, it is likely that they will respond successfully. The level of ease experienced during the process will influence the mental health and well-being of the individual. A 14-year-old boy who used to struggle to fit in with peers due to language and cultural barriers now becomes comfortable with both American and Korean cultures and feels confident:

> I feel very special in a positive way. There are my friends who think I'm cool. They rather look UP to me ... I explain to my friends what Korean culture is. Like New Year's Day, they called me to go with them and watch fireworks. I was like, "I can't" and I explained to them what "Duk-gook" [Korean traditional food] is and "Sae-bae." Like I have to bow down and I get money. And they are like, "Can we come to your house and do 'Sae-bae' so we get money too?" I explained to them and they want to know more about it. One of my friends can actually count from 1 to like 25. They actually go to Web sites so they can learn, so they can talk to me. And I actually gave them Korean music, and he's like, can you type the lyrics in English? So they are more into Koreanness. They are more interested.

One adjustment response pattern may have more constructive impact on an individual's mental health than the others; however, there is no ideal or most useful pattern that works for everyone, nor is there one pattern that works for one person all of the time. For instance, integration may be a feasible adjustment response pattern for immigrant adolescents but not for immigrant elderly. For the elderly, remaining in contact with the old culture and returning to old-culture ways may make them more comfortable; the pattern of reconstructed return may be most useful for them. For health care providers working with immigrant populations, it is important to assess unique experiences and perceptions rather than to categorize individuals based on their adjustment response pattern. However, knowledge about the response patterns individuals use to ease cultural tension may enable understanding of the complex processes that are central to the struggle that many immigrants face.

Contextual/Personal Influences

Scholars of acculturation theory recognize nature or types of the dominant society and characteristics of acculturating individuals as significant factors in the acculturation process (Berry & Kim, 1988; Williams & Berry, 1991). In this theory of cultural marginality, the factors influencing the process of cross-cultural conflict recognition, marginal living, and easing cultural tensions are described as contextual/personal influences.

Contextual/personal influences identified in literature reviews and shared in interviews with Korean Americans are the nature of the dominant society, such as openness or tolerance to diversity, available social and health care resources for immigrants, racial and/or ethnic composition of school and neighborhood, support from teachers and peers, significant others' attitudes toward the dominant culture, knowledge about the dominant society, age at immigration, length of stay in the United States, educational backgrounds, socioeconomic status, language proficiency, ethnic identity, preimmigration experiences, reasons for immigration, loyalty to own culture, resilience or ability to endure the hardship, openness, parent–child relationships, and coping strategies (Berry, 1995; Berry & Kim, 1988; Berry et al., 1992; Trueba, 2002).

These influences govern not only the individuals who are in the midst of cultural marginality but also the dominant culture that is a source of interaction for immigrant people. Existing theories describing acculturation have been criticized for ignoring the influences of the acculturating individuals or groups to the dominant culture (Rudmin, 2003). The theories viewed acculturating individuals only as passive recipients. When two cultures clash, the interaction is reciprocal although the strength of the influence may not be comparable. Contextual/personal influences make the interaction between two cultures and the effect of one culture on another a mutual process.

RELATIONSHIPS AMONG THE CONCEPTS: THE MODEL

Figure 13.1 depicts the relationships among the major concepts of the theory. Marginal living begins with the recognition of a cross-cultural conflict. As individuals encounter marginal living, they strive to ease

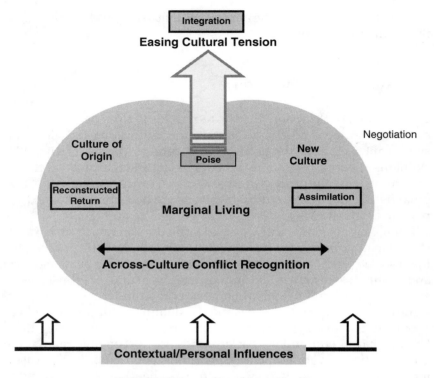

FIGURE 13.1   Cultural Marginality

cultural tension through adjustment response patterns. The four response patterns are assimilation, return, poise, and integration. Although not an explicit concept in the theory, the importance of contextual/personal influences is recognized by its inclusion as a foundation for the theory of cultural marginality.

USE OF THE THEORY IN NURSING RESEARCH

The idea of cultural marginality (Choi, 2001) has been cited in various areas of nursing research and practice. The concept was used to understand experiences of Mexican American families caring for children with serious chronic conditions (Rehm, 2003) and to study stress experienced by Pakistani Ismaili Muslim girls (Khuwaja, Selwyn, Kapadia, McCurdy, & Khuwaja, 2007).

Since the theory was introduced, it has been used to guide research and practice for people with marginal living. First, based on the social cognitive theory and cultural marginality theory, I developed an individually administered, computer-based mental health promotion program, **P**romoting **I**ntergenerational **D**ialogue on **E**motions (PRIDE). (Note: The program name was changed from "Be Connected" to PRIDE.) Using a two-group, repeated-measures, and controlled randomized study design, I tested the feasibility of PRIDE and compared the efficacy of PRIDE with an attention control (AC) group on parental knowledge, parental stress, parental self-efficacy, filial self-efficacy, parent–child (P–C) communication, P–C conflict, and P–C satisfaction. A total of 58 parents (28 fathers and 30 mothers) and 30 Korean American adolescents aged 11 to 14 years participated in the study (16 families in PRIDE and 14 families in AC group). PRIDE was found to be feasible for Korean American families and was favored by both parents and adolescents. Efficacy results of the study were also promising at 1 month postintervention. Particularly, fathers' parental knowledge ($d = 0.82$), mothers' parental knowledge ($d = 1.95$), fathers' report on P–C communication ($d = 0.61$), and Korean American adolescents report on conflicts with the father ($d = 0.44$) showed medium to large effects of PRIDE compared with an AC condition. As PRIDE is taken to a larger trial, this computer-based program may then be disseminated to multicity community settings.

Another area of research for the theory of cultural marginality is instrument development. Researchers have developed scales to measure levels of acculturation and acculturative stress and to explain the relationships between these concepts and mental health outcomes (Hovey & King, 1997; Padilla, Alvarez, & Lindholm, 1986; Phinney, 1992; Sam & Berry, 1995; Williams & Berry, 1991), but there is no scale specifically designed to measure cultural marginality.

The phenomenon of globalization is not limited to the United States. As of 2012, about 1.41 million foreigners reside in Korea and about 10.3 % of them (144,681) immigrated to Korea for marriage (Korean Immigration Service, 2012). Due to the heavy influx of immigrants into Korea over the last 10 years, more than 160,000 children are growing up in interracial families, and the numbers continue to grow steeply (Ministry of Public Administration and Security [MOPAS], 2012). To assess marginal living experiences of immigrant children living in South Korea, including biracial children, I recently developed the cultural marginality scale.

The items on this 13-item scale were derived from the qualitative descriptive study of Korean American adolescents and their parents and the existing acculturative stress scale, the Societal, Attitudinal, Familial, and Environmental Acculturative Stress Scale for Children (SAFE-C) (Chavez et al., 1997). Responses range from 0 = *hardly ever or never* to 3 = *almost always.* As the first step in enhancing reliability and validity of this newly developed instrument, I am currently conducting cognitive interviews with potential respondents.

The main purpose of the cognitive interview is to explore the cognitive processes that respondents use to answer the questions (i.e., how respondents understand, mentally process, and respond to the questions) (Knafl et al., 2007; Willis, 2005). The cognitive interview helps the researcher to clarify intention of questions and identify problems with wording, readability, item or section sequence, and lengths of the instrument. The cognitive interview is generally conducted with a small number of respondents (5–25 people) before field testing a newly developed instrument.

So far, I've conducted cognitive interviews with nine children aged 10 to 13. The cultural marginality scale will be refined based on findings from the cognitive interviews. The cultural marginality scale with items aligned according to the concepts of the theory would allow assessment of the structure of the associated concepts and of the extent to which cultural marginality influences health. Assessing the relationship between cultural marginality and mental health outcomes has significant implications for the health care of immigrants; it has particular relevance for preventive care, where nurses caring for immigrants develop approaches for recognizing those who are at risk for mental health problems.

Another ongoing research project guided by the theory of cultural marginality is the study titled *Cultural Competency Among Nursing Students.* One of the most critical contextual influences affecting an individual's experience of cultural marginality is the nurse's openness to diversity and competency in caring for patients from diverse sociocultural backgrounds. The specific aims of this mixed-method study are to (1) assess perceived levels of openness to diversity and cultural competence among Korean nursing students; and (2) explore Korean nursing students' needs for cultural competence education integrated into the nursing curriculum. The ultimate goal of the study is to develop a nursing curriculum that would prepare students for a culturally diverse patient population in Korea. So far, 448 undergraduate and graduate nursing students have completed the questionnaire and a total of 18 students participated in one of the three focus groups. The curriculum developed based on the findings from the study will equip nursing students with the knowledge and skills required for this culturally diverse society and finally contribute to creating a culturally sensitive health care environment for people with marginal living.

USE OF THE THEORY IN NURSING PRACTICE

Previously, the concept of cultural marginality has been used to discuss adherence issues of Mexican clients (Barron, Hunter, Mayo, & Willoughby, 2004) and to address the gap in health care provider–client relationships and its impact on health disparities (Cupertino, n.d.). The theory can also be applied to school nurse practice to foster awareness of culturally distinct adolescent needs (Labun, 2003).

Another example of use of the theory in nursing practice is the application of it to the case of a 23-year-old, English-speaking African refugee to the United States (Burke, 2011). At the age of 13, she experienced the most severe type of female genital mutilation (FGM) by an elder in Djibouti, Africa, and suffers from candidiasis and hematocolpos. In her article, Burke analyzed experiences of the patient using the concepts of the theory and discussed how the theory of cultural marginality can be used as a framework to guide culturally sensitive, evidence-based nursing care for women with FGM. Particularly, she emphasized the need for nurses to constantly assess contextual and personal influence factors, to serve as a significant contextual influence, to provide culturally relevant care, and to support patients' integration of cultures while assisting with health decisions.

Use of the theory in practice is limited; however, the aforementioned examples of research and practice demonstrate possible applications for the theory of cultural marginality. Possible areas include education or health promotion programs assessing and modifying an individual's personal influences, culturally sensitive therapeutic nurse–patient interactions, and development of cultural competence training for health care providers.

In this chapter, the theory of cultural marginality was described mainly in the context of immigrant adolescents' experiences; however, the theory is applicable to any immigrant who is encountering marginal living. The theory of cultural marginality can be used as a framework to explore unique experiences of diverse groups of immigrants and to provide care for them. Particularly, recognizing the influence of the contextual/personal factors has significant implications for health care providers. For instance, adjustment response patterns and health care needs among immigrants who came to a new country for freedom cannot be the same as those for people who immigrated for educational opportunities. By recognizing these influences and modifying them when appropriate, health care providers may ease the adjustment process, promote healthy development, and elicit desirable health outcomes.

CONCLUSION

What is it like to be caught between cultures? How does that experience impact one's health? How can health care providers ease the experience? These questions have inspired development of the theory of cultural marginality. The goal of the theory is to highlight the complexity of living between two cultures, emphasizing the challenge to immigrant well-being. The theory elucidates essences of marginal living, cross-cultural conflict recognition, and striving to ease cultural tension while recognizing the fundamental importance of contextual/personal influences. Understanding of the theory and the relationships among the concepts promises a framework for culturally relevant health care for immigrant people. Nowadays, health issues related to immigration affect many different countries. To better meet the needs of the increasingly diverse groups of people, the theory needs to continuously evolve and be refined through further research and practice for immigrant groups in and beyond the United States.

REFERENCES

Anderson, T. L., & Levy, J. A. (2003). Marginality among older injectors in today's illicit drug culture: Assessing the impact of ageing. *Addiction, 98,* 761–770.

Andersson, E. P. (1995). Marginality: Concept or reality in nursing education? *Journal of Advanced Nursing, 21,* 131–136.

Barron, F., Hunter, A., Mayo, R., & Willoughby, B. (2004). Acculturation and adherence: Issues for health care providers working with clients of Mexican origin. *Journal of Transcultural Nursing, 15,* 331–337.

Bennett, J. M. (1993). Cultural marginality: Identity issues in intercultural training. In R. M. Paise (Ed.), *Education for intercultural experience* (pp. 109–135). Yarmouth, ME: Intercultural Press.

Berry, J. W. (1995). Psychology of acculturation. In N. R. Goldberger & J. B. Veroff (Eds.), *The culture and psychology reader* (pp. 457–488). New York, NY: New York University.

Berry, J. W., & Kim, U. (1988). Acculturation and mental health. In P. R. Dasen, J. W. Berry, & N. Sartorius (Eds.), *Health and cross-cultural psychology: Toward applications* (pp. 207–236). Newbury Park: Sage.

Berry, J. W., Poortinga, Y. H., Segall, M. H., & Dasen, P. R. (1992). *Cross-cultural psychology: Research and applications.* New York, NY: Cambridge University.

Burke, E. (2011). Female genital mutilation: Applications of nursing theory for clinical care. *The Nurse Practitioner, 36,* 45–50.

Chavez, D. V., Moran, V. R., Reid, S. L., & Lopez, M. (1997). Acculturative stress in children: A modification of the SAFE Scale. *Hispanic Journal of Behavioral Sciences, 19,* 34–44.

Choi, H. (2001). Cultural marginality: A concept analysis with implications for immigrant adolescents. *Issues in Comprehensive Pediatric Nursing, 24,* 193–206.

Choi, H., & Dancy, B. L. (2009). Korean American adolescents' and their parents' perceptions of acculturative stress. *Journal of Child and Adolescent Psychiatric Nursing, 22,* 203–210.

Choi, H., Dancy, B. L., & Lee, J. (2012). Raising children in America: Korean parents' experiences. *Journal of Psychiatric and Mental Health Nursing.* Article first published online 1 FEB 2012. doi: 10.1111/j.1365-2850.2011.01864.x

Choi, H., Meininger, J. C., & Roberts, R. E. (2006). Ethnic differences in adolescents' mental distress, social stress, and resources. *Adolescence, 41*(162), 263–283.

Choi, H., Stafford, L., Meininger, J. C., Roberts, R. E., & Smith, D. P. (2002). Psychometric properties of the DSM Scale for Depression (DSD) with Korean American youths. *Issues in Mental Health Nursing, 23,* 735–756.

Cupertino, A. P. (n.d.). *Provider-patient relationship: Cultural competency and literacy.* Retrieved from http://www.minorityhealthks.org/download/Cultural_COmpetence.ppt

Del Pilar, J. A., & Udasco, J. O. (2004). Marginality theory: The lack of construct validity. *Hispanic Journal of Behavioral Sciences, 26,* 3–15.

Fuertes, J. N., & Westbrook, F. D. (1996). Using the Social, Attitudinal, Familial, and Environmental (S.A.F.E.) Acculturation stress scale to assess the adjustment needs of Hispanic college students. *Measurement and Evaluation in Counseling and Development, 29,* 67–76.

Gil, A. G., Wagner, E. F., & Vega, W. A. (2000). Acculturation, familism, and alcohol use among Latino adolescent males: Longitudinal relations. *Journal of Community Psychology, 28,* 443–458.

Guarnaccia, P. J., & Lopez, S. (1998). The mental health and adjustment of immigrant and refugee children. *The Child Psychiatrist in the Community, 7,* 537–553.

Hall, J. M. (1999). Marginalization revisited: Critical, postmodern, and liberation perspectives. *Advances in Nursing Science, 22*(2), 88–102.

Hall, J. M., Stevens, P. E., & Meleis, A. I. (1994). Marginalization: A guiding concept for valuing diversity in nursing knowledge development. *Advances in Nursing Science, 16*(4), 23–41.

Hovey, J. D., & King, C. A. (1997). Suicidality among acculturating Mexican Americans: Current knowledge and directions for research. *Suicide and Life-Threatening Behavior, 27,* 92–103.

Hovey, J. D., & Magana, C. G. (2002). Exploring the mental health Mexican migrant farm workers in the Midwest: Psychosocial predictors of psychological distress and suggestions for prevention and treatment. *Journal of Psychology, 136,* 493–513.

Im, E. O., & Lipson, J. G. (1997). Menopausal transition of Korean immigrant women: A literature review. *Health Care for Women International, 18,* 507–520.

Keefe, S. E., & Padilla, A. M. (1987). *Chicano ethnicity.* Albuquerque, NM: University of New Mexico Press.

Khuwaja, S. A., Selwyn, B. J., Kapadia, A., McCurdy, S., & Khuwaja, A. (2007). Pakistani Ismaili Muslim adolescent females living in the United States of America: Stresses associated with the process of adaptation to U.S. culture. *Journal of Immigrant Health, 9*, 35–42.

Knafl, K., Deatrick, J., Gallo, A., Holcombe, G., Bakitas, M., Dixon, J., & Grey, M. (2007). The analysis and interpretation of cognitive interviews for Instrument development. *Research in Nursing and Health, 30*, 224–234.

Korean Immigration Service. (2012). Immigration status by countries of origin and the annual status of international marriage migrant women. Retrieved from http://www.index.go.kr/egams/stts/jsp/potal/stts/PO_STTS_IdxMain.jsp?idx_cd=2819.

Labun, E. (2003). Working with a Vietnamese adolescent. *The Journal of School Nursing, 19*, 319–325.

Lazarus, R. S. (1997). Acculturation isn't everything. *Applied Psychology, 46*, 39–43.

Ministry of Public Administration and Security [MOPAS]. (2012). Statistics on children of multicultural families in 2012. Retrieved from http://www.mopas.go.kr/gpms/ns/mogaha/user/userlayout/bulletin/userBtView.action? userBtBean.bbsSeq=1039777&userBtBean.ctxCd=1258&userBtBean.ctxType=21010005.

Noh, S., & Kaspar, V. (2003). Perceived discrimination and depression: Moderating effects of coping, acculturation, and ethnic support. *American Journal of Public Health, 93*, 232–238.

Oetting, E. R., & Beauvais, F. (1990–1991). Orthogonal cultural identification theory: The cultural identification of minority adolescents. *The International Journal of the Addictions, 25*, 655–685.

Padilla, A. M., Alvarez, M., & Lindholm, K. J. (1986). Generational status and personality factors as predictors of stress in students. *Hispanic Journal of Behavioral Sciences, 8*, 275–288.

Park, R. E. (1928). Human migration and the marginal man. *The American Journal of Sociology, 33*, 881–893.

Phinney, J. S. (1992). The multigroup ethnic identity measure: A new scale for use with adolescents and youth adults from diverse groups. *Journal of Adolescent Research, 7*, 156–176.

Redfield, R., Linton, R., & Herskovits, M. J. (1936). Memorandum on the study of acculturation. *American Anthropologist, 38*, 149–152.

Rehm, R. S. (2003). Legal, financial, and ethical ambiguities for Mexican American families: Caring for children with chronic conditions. *Qualitative Health Research, 13*, 689–702.

Rogler, L. H. (1994). International migrations: A framework for directing research. *American Psychologist, 49*, 701–708.

Rudmin, F. W. (2003). Critical history of the acculturation psychology of assimilation, separation, integration, and marginalization. *Review of General Psychology, 7*, 3–37.

Sam, D. L., & Berry, J. W. (1995). Acculturative stress among young immigrants in Norway. *Scandinavian Journal of Psychology, 36*, 10–24.

Schwartz-Barcott, D., & Kim, H. S. (2000). An expansion and elaboration of the hybrid model of concept development. In B. L. Rodgers & K. A. Knafl (Eds.), *Concept development in nursing* (2nd ed., pp. 129–159). Philadelphia, PA: WB Saunders.

Scribner, A. P. (1995). Advocating for Hispanic high school students: Research-based educational practices. *The High School Journal, 78,* 206–214.

Stonequist, E. V. (1935). The problem of the marginal man. *The American Journal of Sociology, 41,* 1–12.

Trueba, H. T. (2002). Multiple ethnic, racial, and cultural identities in action: From marginality to a new cultural capital in modern society. *Journal of Latinos and Education, 1,* 7–28.

U.S. Census Bureau. (2010). U.S. Census Bureau's American Community Survey. Retrieved from http://www.migrationinformation.org/datahub/acscensus.cfm

Vega, W. A., Gil, A. G., & Wagner, E. (1998). Cultural adjustment and Hispanic adolescent drug use. In W. A. Vega & A. G. Gil (Eds.), *Drug use and ethnicity in early adolescence* (pp. 125–148). New York, NY: Plenum.

Vivero, V. N., & Jenkins, S. R. (1999). Existential hazards of the multicultural individual: Defining and understanding "cultural homelessness." *Cultural Diversity and Ethnic Minority Psychology, 5,* 6–26.

Walters, N. P., & Trevelyan, E. N. (2011). *The newly arrived foreign-born population of the United States: 2010.* Washington, DC: U.S. Department of Commerce. Economics and Statistics Administration. U.S. Census Bureau.

Weisberger, A. (1992). Marginality and its directions. *Sociological Forum, 7,* 425–446.

Williams, C. L., & Berry, J. W. (1991). Primary prevention of acculturative stress among refugees: Application of psychological theory and practice. *American Psychologist, 46,* 632–641.

Willis, G. B. (2005). *Cognitive interviewing.* Thousand Oaks, CA: Sage.

Ziller, R. C. (1973). *The social self.* New York, NY: Pergamon.

14

Theory of Caregiving Dynamics

Loretta A. Williams

Unpaid care provided by family, friends, or neighbors is a critical resource in today's health care system. The increasing value of caregiving in the United States in 2009 was estimated to be $450 billion, a rise of $75 billion in 2 years (Feinberg, Reinhard, Houser, & Choula, 2011). Although patients are the direct beneficiaries of care, paid care providers also benefit indirectly from the care provided by unpaid caregivers. Caregivers make possible the discharge of patients from inpatient facilities and often provide the link between ambulatory care facilities and patients. Just as nurses are the health care providers who have the most contact with patients, they also have the most contact with caregivers (U.S. Census Bureau, 2005). Because of the critical and frequent need to identify a caregiver for a patient and to have the patient and caregiver develop and sustain a caregiving relationship, understanding the dynamics of the caregiving relationship is especially important for nurses.

Family members, friends, or neighbors provide most of the day-to-day care for persons with health problems who are chronically ill, disabled, or aged (Thompson, 2004). This unpaid assistance often involves multiple tasks that may be physically, emotionally, socially, or financially demanding (Biegel, Sales, & Schulz, 1991). These caregivers are sometimes referred to as informal caregivers. The term *informal* is used to differentiate them from formal health care providers who receive pay for the care they provide. Informal caregivers are usually family, friends, or neighbors and are frequently key resources in the care of patients who would otherwise need institutional care (Pasacreta & McCorkle, 2000).

The dynamics of caregiving are the forces that motivate caregivers and care recipients to assume and continue the caregiving relationship. Although much caregiving inquiry has focused on the burden of caregiving, it is equally if not more important to understand the positive forces that move the caregiving relationship forward. In this middle range theory of caregiving dynamics, caregiving refers to the care given by family, friends, or neighbors.

PURPOSE OF THE THEORY AND HOW IT WAS DEVELOPED

The purpose of this middle range theory is to describe the positive forces that allow the caregiving relationship to change and grow. Recognition of these forces will enable nurses to identify methods for supporting the caregiving relationship. The theory began as a concept named "informal caregiving dynamics" (Williams, 2003). Informal caregiving dynamics was conceptualized as forces that stimulate and shape change in an informal caregiver–care recipient dyad.

As the concept has developed into a theory and has been presented and used, the decision was made to drop the term informal. Although informal caregiving is a recognized concept in health care and social science literature, those who are unfamiliar with the term sometimes misunderstand the word *informal* and think that it diminishes the importance of caregiving provided by family members, friends, and neighbors.

The clinical situation that stimulated the development of this theory was the need to identify strategies to ensure reliable caregivers for patients scheduled to undergo hematopoietic stem cell transplantation (HSCT). HSCT is an intensive—but potentially curative—therapy for patients with life-threatening illnesses (Horowitz, Loberiza, Bredeson, Rizzo, & Nugent, 2001). In 2002, approximately 40,000 HSCTs were performed worldwide, the majority for hematological cancers (Loberiza, 2003). Over the last 15 years, caregiving by family, friends, or neighbors has become an integral and essential aspect of the bone marrow transplant process (Grimm, Zawacki, Mock, Krumm, & Frink, 2000). Patients may even be denied the treatment option of HSCT if a caregiver cannot be identified (Frey et al., 2002).

A qualitative research study was conducted based on the experiences of caregivers of patients undergoing HSCT. Forty caregivers were invited to tell their caregiving stories in a one-on-one dialogue with the researcher. Story theory (Smith & Liehr, 2003) was the theoretical foundation for the interviews. The model emerging from the study provides the structure for the middle range theory of caregiving dynamics.

CONCEPTS OF THE THEORY

The major concepts of the theory of caregiving dynamics are commitment, expectation management, and role negotiation. Self-care, new insight, and role support are related concepts, each connected to one of the major concepts. Caregiving dynamics are interacting processes of commitment, expectation management, and role negotiation supported by self-care, new insight, and role support that move a caregiving relationship along an illness trajectory.

Commitment

Commitment is enduring caregiver responsibility that inspires life changes to make the patient a priority. Commitment calls caregivers to a supportive presence whether or not they were experiencing a self-affirming loving connection with the patient (Williams, 2007). There are four dimensions of commitment: enduring responsibility, making the patient a priority, supportive presence, and self-affirming loving connection. *Enduring responsibility* is caregiver determination to provide care despite difficulties for however long it takes. Enduring responsibility, based on obligation, reciprocity, or love, may begin long before the illness and continue after the illness resolves; it has both the connotation of being lasting and the connotation of bearing hardship without yielding (Williams, 2007). *Making the patient a priority* is placement of patient care needs before all other needs and wants because patient well-being is the most important goal. Significant and often difficult life changes are voluntarily made in the best interest of the patient (Williams, 2007). *Supportive presence* is remaining at the patient's side with comfort, encouragement, and a positive attitude when the caregiver can do nothing else to assist the patient. The senses of the caregiver are heightened to understand the patient experience completely so that patient emotional needs and wants are accurately identified and met with (Williams, 2007). *Self-affirming loving connection* is a feeling of open togetherness between the caregiver and the patient where meeting patient needs is emotionally satisfying for the caregiver (Williams, 2007).

When the caregiver and care recipient commit to the caregiving dyad, each brings with them past experiences, strengths, and weaknesses. The histories of the caregiver and care recipient—as well as their joint history—will influence the caregiving dyad (Phillips, Brewer, & Torres de Ardon, 2001). Caregivers and care recipients may bring technical knowledge and skills (Schumacher, Stewart, & Archbold, 1998), fears about caregiving (Ferrell, Cohen, Rhiner, & Rozek, 1991), physical or emotional deficits (Cohen et al., 1993; Hadjistavropoulos, Taylor, Tuokko, & Beattie, 1994; Ostwald, 1997), multiple other roles (Wuest, 2001), coping abilities (Folkman, 1997), previously developed support systems (Miller et al., 2001), and previous knowledge of the other member of the caregiving dyad (Phillips et al., 2001). The caregiving dyad will be influenced by these unique qualities and experiences that the caregiver and care recipient bring to the caregiving situation.

Self-Care

Self-care is a concept related to commitment. Self-care is acting to maintain health by cultivating healthy habits while letting out the feelings and frustrations of caregiving and getting away from caregiving demands when necessary. There are four dimensions of self-care: supportive physical environment, cultivating healthy habits, letting it out, and getting away from it. *Supportive physical environment* refers to accommodations, food, and other amenities that are comfortable and convenient for the caregiver and the patient. *Cultivating healthy habits* is taking action to maintain or improve health necessary for caregiving. The caregiver and the patient support and encourage each other to follow health-improving habits such as eating well and exercising. *Letting it out* is finding ways to express feelings and frustrations associated with caregiving. Caregivers may communicate intentionally with others to share their feelings or may disclose their thoughts and feelings through writing or other methods of expression that may not necessarily be shared with others. *Getting away from it* is finding physical or mental space to experience temporarily ordinary life separate from the demands of illness, treatment, and caregiving. Caregivers sometimes find the need to be physically away from the caregiving situation, but at other times merely leaving the situation mentally provides adequate respite. Caregivers may report feeling guilty in leaving the care recipient.

Caregivers of patients with dementia have reported using exercise to maintain their own health (Connell, 1994), whereas caregivers of patients with multiple sclerosis frequently seek interpersonal support to maintain their health (O'Brien, 1993). Caregivers of frail elders reported using a variety of behaviors to maintain their health, but most behaviors addressed physical health (McDonald, Fink, & Wykle, 1999). Caregivers of cancer survivors practice a high number of health maintenance activities (Bowman, Rose, & Deimling, 2005). Regardless of the population, self-care is a critical dimension of committing to a caregiving relationship over time.

Expectation Management

Expectation management is envisioning the future and yearning to return to normal. It includes taking one day at a time when the future is uncertain, gauging behavior from past experiences with the patient, and reconciling actual to anticipated treatment twists and turns (Williams, 2007). There are five dimensions of expectation management: envisioning tomorrow, getting back to normal, taking one day at a time, gauging behavior, and reconciling treatment twists and turns. *Envisioning tomorrow* is grappling with an ambiguous future with hope, fear, or both. Images of the future span a continuum from very certain and specific to very vague and general. Imagining a hopeful future provides caregivers with goals to strive for and a reason to endure difficulties, whereas imagining a fearful future allows caregivers to minimize losses and prepare for future disappointments (Williams, 2007). *Getting back to normal* is seeing light at the end of the tunnel and anticipating going back to an ordinary life of health that was lost in the demands of illness and treatment (Williams, 2007). *Taking one day at a time* is focusing in the present as a means of dealing with an uncertain future that cannot or will not be envisioned. As perspectives and priorities change with a present orientation, attempts may be made to slow down and make the most of the present rather than rushing to an uncertain future. Caregivers sometimes avoid the future because they fear what it might hold, but at other times they savor the positive aspects of the present (Williams, 2007). *Gauging behavior* is explaining, predicting, or reacting to actions or statements of the patient based on prior knowledge of and experience with the patient. Expectations developed from gauging behavior allow caregivers to react positively to even difficult patient behaviors (Williams, 2007). *Reconciling treatment twists and turns* is comparing actual to anticipated patient outcomes to confirm, explain, and eventually accept the reality of the actual outcomes (Williams, 2007).

The caregiver and care recipient naturally bring expectations to the caregiving situation. Expectations are the anticipation or looking forward to the coming or occurrence of something. Expectations consider an occurrence probable, certain, reasonable, due, necessary, or bound by duty or obligation (Merriam-Webster OnLine, 2007). Expectations may also be the strong belief that something will happen in the future, or that someone will or should achieve something (Jewell & Abate, 2001). Realistic and congruent expectations on the part of the caregiver and care recipient improve the functioning of the caregiving dyad (Kylma, Vehviläinen-Julkunen, & Lähdevirta, 2001). Expectations may involve the behavior of the other member of the caregiving dyad, the caregiving relationship, the roles that will exist in the caregiving dyad, and the illness trajectory (Boyle et al., 2000; Speice et al., 2000). The illness trajectory is the path, progression, or line of development of the care recipient's illness (Merriam-Webster OnLine, 2007). The trajectory will be expected in the future until it occurs in the present and becomes part of the past (Padilla, Mishel, & Grant, 1992). As the trajectory becomes known, the expectation of the trajectory may need to be changed (Boyle et al., 2000). Changes in expectations are some of the transitions in caregiving (Seltzer & Li, 2000). Understanding the illness trajectory and managing to have realistic expectations is an area of caregiving dynamics where nurses and other health care professionals can make an impact (Speice et al., 2000).

New Insight

New insight is a concept related to expectation management. New insight is changing awareness through experiencing personal growth, believing that a higher power controls the situation, and recognizing positive treatment outcomes. There are three dimensions of new insight: experiencing personal growth, leaning on the Lord, and recognizing positive outcomes. *Experiencing personal growth* is finding unexpected benefits of new perspectives, knowledge, and skills in the caregiving experience. Caregivers gain new appreciation of the importance of relationships in their lives and develop a new confidence and sense of worth in themselves because of the care they are able to provide. Experiencing personal growth often reframes the caregiving experience and allows the discovery of positive meaning in events and outcomes that may not have been anticipated or desired in the past. *Leaning on the Lord* is finding comfort in the belief that a higher power has control of the situation and will see that the final outcome will be what is best for the patient. Prayer is often used to ensure that the best outcome is achieved. Belief that a higher power has control and is acting in the best interest of the care recipient may allow acceptance of outcomes that on the surface seem negative. *Recognizing positive outcomes* is being uplifted by events pointing to improved health for the patient. These may or may not be outcomes that the caregiver originally envisioned and yet are recognized by the caregiver as part of the process of recovery.

The caregiving relationship is constantly evolving, and caregivers gain new perspectives that help them deal with caregiving challenges and consider the illness trajectory in realistic ways. These perspectives primarily assist caregivers to reframe caregiving outcomes and maintain a positive view of the caregiving situation. Caregiver perception has long been understood as one of the most important factors influencing caregiving outcomes (Zarit, Reever, & Bach-Peterson, 1980). New insights are especially helpful as the illness process moves forward, and caregivers strive to manage expectations successfully.

Role Negotiation

Role negotiation is defined as appropriate pushing by the caregiver toward patient recovery and independence after getting a handle on complex care that demands shared responsibilities. Role negotiation happens as caregivers determine action with attention to patient voice and vigilantly bridge communication between patients and the health care system. There are five dimensions of role negotiation: appropriate pushing, getting a handle on it, sharing responsibilities, attending to patient voice, and vigilant bridging. *Appropriate pushing* is caregiver responsibility to see that rules for recovery set by the health care providers are followed. The caregiver may encourage the patient to follow the rules independently, may develop individualized, innovative methods to support the patient in following rules, or may carry out the rules if the patient is deemed unable to meet rule requirements (Williams, 2007). *Getting a handle on it* is the struggle to come to grips with the reality of and changes demanded by illness and treatment. Strategies are identified and routines organized to meet caregiving role demands (Williams, 2007). *Sharing responsibilities* is determining illness and treatment needs, identifying the appropriate person to meet each need, and accepting the division of duties. Sharing is done among the caregiver, the patient, other family, friends, and health care providers (Williams, 2007). *Attending to patient voice* is careful listening and consideration of patient perspective by the caregiver before crafting a response or deciding on a course of action. Caregivers did not always accede to patients' wishes, but they considered patients' points-of-view in relation to situations before making decisions in the patients' best interests (Williams, 2007). *Vigilant bridging* is caregiver communication with the health care system to support the best interests of the patient. Messages from the health care system are critically evaluated by the caregiver to determine if they require action or should be relayed to the patient. Caregiver knowledge and assessments of the patient are relayed to the health care system to generate action and support for the patient (Williams, 2007).

Committing on the part of the caregiver and care recipient to the caregiving relationship starts a series of ongoing negotiations to define and redefine roles in the caregiving dyad (Shyu, 2000). With negotiation, the caregiving dyad becomes a dynamic whole, where the roles of caregiver and care recipient ebb and flow reciprocally in constant adjustment to achieve a balance that is most acceptable to both the caregiver and care recipient (Schumacher, 1996). Care recipients have been found to negotiate role functions, when possible, to maintain autonomy and relieve caregivers of tasks to protect the caregiver and the caregiving dyad (Russell, Bunting, & Gregory, 1997; Schumacher, 1996). Likewise, some caregivers will negotiate role functions to encourage care recipient autonomy (Bunting, 2001; Wrubel, Richards, Folkman, & Acree, 2001). When the outcome of the negotiation is acceptable to the caregiver and care recipient, there is a strengthening of the caregiving dyad (Schumacher, 1996).

Role Support

Role support is a concept related to role negotiation. Role support is knowing that others care by encountering competent compassionate care, finding support for other responsibilities, and receiving helpful information. Others may also provide help in meeting financial obligations or the caregiver may discover creative ways of meeting the financial obligations. There are five dimensions of role support: encountering competent, compassionate care; finding support for other responsibilities; knowing others care; meeting financial responsibilities; and receiving helpful information. *Encountering competent, compassionate care* is finding health care providers and workers who determine the needs of the patient and family caregiver and meet those needs in a proficient and timely way. *Finding support for other responsibilities* is accessing assistance from others in meeting responsibilities not directly related to illness and treatment caregiving. These responsibilities may be present before the need for illness caregiving. Finding support for other responsibilities involves finding others to assume roles that the caregiver relinquishes to provide care. *Knowing others care* is experiencing emotional support from family, friends, and acquaintances. Contact with supportive others may occur over long distances and keeps the caregiver in touch with familiar people and events. Knowing others care gives the caregiver a sense of personal value and worth. *Meeting financial obligations* is finding ways to pay for added expenses of treatment while normal income is decreased. Help may be received from family, friends, or employers, or decisions may be made to reassign financial resources to other uses. *Receiving helpful information* is gaining knowledge that is necessary and useful for performing the caregiver role. Caregivers may feel overwhelmed by some of the responsibilities they assume as part of caregiving. Being given information or knowing that information resources are accessible if needed helps with caregiving. Role support enables caregiver negotiation within the health care system to optimize care recipient movement along the illness trajectory.

There are numerous reports of resources that caregivers use to support role functions. For instance, caregivers of patients at the end of life are less stressed when they experience open communication with health care professionals and experience continuity of care (Jo, Brazil, Lohfeld, & Willison, 2007). Swanberg (2006) found that caregivers of patients with cancer were supported in the workplace by coworkers who provided help by filling in job responsibilities, contributing money to help with medical expenses, and listening when caregivers needed someone in whom to confide. Caregivers of patients with cancer use knowledge to improve their caregiving skills and decrease feelings of burden (Aranda & Peerson, 2001; Pasacreta, Barg, Nuamah, & McCorkle, 2000; Rose, 1999; Schumacher, Beidler, Beeber, & Gambino, 2006; Soothill et al., 2001). Information also provides caregivers of patients at the end of life with a sense of power and connectedness (McGrath, 2001; Mok, Chan, Chan, & Yeung, 2002; Wilkes, White, & O'Riordan, 2000).

RELATIONSHIPS AMONG THE CONCEPTS: THE MODEL

Caregiving dynamics are interacting processes of commitment, expectation management, and role negotiation supported by self-care, new insight, and role support that move the caregiving relationship along an illness trajectory (Figure 14.1). The circles in the model represent the relationship of the caregiver and care recipient in the past, present, and future. The present relationship is most prominent, but it is continuous with the past and the future. Commitment, expectation management, and role negotiation connect the caregiver and patient and provide the

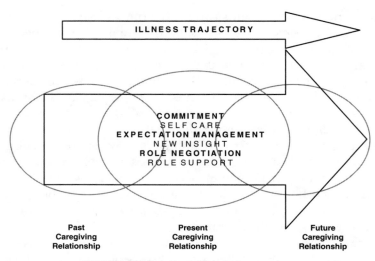

FIGURE 14.1   Caregiving Dynamics

force to move the caregiving relationship through time. Self-care, new insights, and role support ground the concepts of commitment, expectation management, and role negotiation, respectively. Through self-care, caregivers maintain their commitment to care recipients. When physically and emotionally healthy, caregivers can continue to focus attention on the care recipients' needs. New insight comes with support for managing expectations. New understandings and ways of framing the caregiving experience help caregivers make sense of illness outcomes. Role support offers caregivers tools to fulfill care demands for the care recipient successfully. The illness trajectory overlays the caregiving relationship, moves forward through time in parallel with the relationship, and influences the relationship (Williams, 2003).

USE OF THE THEORY IN NURSING RESEARCH

The theory was initially tested and refined in a qualitative research study of 40 caregivers of patients undergoing HSCT (Williams, 2007). Although the care recipients had potentially fatal malignancies, HSCT was performed with the intent to cure or provide extended remission from disease. The caregivers were asked to tell their caregiving story approximately 3 to 4 weeks after the HSCT.

Stories were collected using the story path method (Liehr & Smith, 2000) where the storyteller begins with the present, then goes to the past, and finally moves to the future by talking about hopes and dreams. Data were content analyzed using standard descriptive exploratory methods. Based on a review of literature that identified forces that motivated caregivers, expressions of commitment, expectations, and negotiation were first identified and organized into themes. The data were then searched for other forces that motivated caregivers. The caregiver stories confirmed the importance of commitment and contributed to a more precise understanding of expectation and negotiation. Expectation was renamed expectation management and negotiation was renamed role negotiation (Williams, 2007). The study concluded that (a) commitment, expectation management, and role negotiation sustain caregivers in their role; and (b) self-care, new insight, and role support were energy sources critical to caregiving dynamics.

Although many of the caregivers in the study reported that they had been providing care for many months or years, possibly from the time that the patient was diagnosed with cancer, the HSCT therapy was a new experience for many caregivers and represented a chance for a possible cure. At the time these caregivers were interviewed, the care recipients were recovering from the initial effects of the HSCT. The care recipients had just come through a critical period and were doing well. The caregivers had reason to be hopeful when they told their stories and to feel that their efforts at caregiving, even if difficult at times, might contribute to a cure for the care recipient. There was concern that a theory based on the experiences of these caregivers at this stage of an illness trajectory might not apply to caregiving for patients with incurable, moribund illnesses.

A second researcher has studied caregivers of patients with primary brain tumors to determine if the theory describes their experience (Whisenant, 2011). This qualitative study of 20 caregivers used a single dialogue based on story theory (Smith & Liehr, 2003) to explore the caregiving experience. These caregivers confirmed that the six concepts in the theory were the forces that propelled their caregiving forward. No additional forces were identified.

Caregivers of patients with brain tumors attached different meaning and made different use of the forces than did caregivers of patients undergoing HSCT. Whisenant (2011) suggested that this may be due to differences in the illness trajectories and outcomes for patients with brain cancer compared with patients undergoing HSCT. Although HSCT is often a curative therapy for a disease that had been previously treated (Horowitz et al., 2001), patients with primary brain tumors usually experience a sudden onset of disease with rapid personality changes and cognitive decline that leads to death (Whisenant, 2011). Caregivers of patients with brain tumors described more negative experiences in their caregiving stories than did the caregivers of patients undergoing HSCT. This may be due to the fact that caregivers of patients undergoing HSCT see hope for eventual patient recovery after difficult therapy, whereas caregivers of patients with primary brain tumors see loss of the person they love followed by death (Whisenant, 2011).

Caregivers of patients with brain tumors described being able to *endure the responsibility* of care by *envisioning future* patient needs as behavioral and cognitive declines continued and being able to *get a handle on* how to provide the care demanded by these changes. Caregivers looked to health care providers to allow the caregivers to *let out their frustrations* with caregiving and to *meet the caregivers' needs* for affirmation as an important part of the health care team (Whisenant, 2011).

Whisenant's (2011) work confirmed the generalizability and comprehensiveness of the concepts of the theory. By testing the theoretical structure with a population of caregivers of cancer patients with very different disease and treatment trajectories than those originally studied by Williams (2007), Whisenant (2011) opened the door for use with other caregiver populations, such as caregivers for people with Alzheimer's disease and congestive heart failure or caregivers of children with traumatic brain injury. At this time, most of the work related to the theory has been done with caregivers of cancer patients and, more specifically, HSCT patients.

Authors have compared the results of the initial theory development with other samples of HSCT caregivers. Wilson, Eilers, Heermann, and Million (2009) report that this group of caregivers *commit to doing whatever it takes, take one day at a time* to handle uncertainty, and use *vigilant bridging* to communicate the patients' needs to the health care system. Stajduhar, Nickel, Martin, and Funk (2008) found that *receiving helpful information* helped caregivers *navigate the role* more easily and effectively. Bevans and Sternberg (2012) recommend caregiver education in *self-care* before HSCT to relieve the stress that *making the patient priority* might cause. Chow and Coyle (2011) suggest that health care providers acknowledge the *commitment* of caregivers during HSCT as one method of decreasing feelings of burden from caregiving. Gemmill, Cooke, Williams, and Grant (2011) endorsed the importance of the theory components of *self-care*, *letting it out*, and *new insights* for caregivers in managing the extended trajectory of HSCT. Grundy and Ghazi (2009) supported the theory concepts of *receiving helpful information* and *knowing others care* as crucial caregiver needs during HSCT. Stenberg, Ruland, and Miaskowski (2010) supported the need to *receive helpful information* for caregivers of patients with cancer in general, including those whose patients are undergoing HSCT.

Commitment, self-care, and *receiving helpful information* are the dimensions of the theory most consistently endorsed in samples of caregivers of patients receiving HSCT. These may be priority areas for testing interventions to support caregivers of these patients.

Acknowledgment by health care professionals of the caregiver's commitment is an intervention that deserves further exploration. Caregivers in a variety of situations have reported feeling ignored and devalued by health care professionals (Andershed & Ternestedt, 2000; Stetz, McDonald, & Compton, 1996). How best to acknowledge caregivers, and the amount of acknowledgment necessary to affect outcomes, require further exploration. Story theory (Smith & Liehr, 2003) produced an effective method of data collection among caregivers. Providing caregivers with an opportunity to tell their caregiving stories to attentive listeners or to write their stories may be methods of acknowledging and memorializing their contributions.

Health maintenance and promotion as part of self-care is another potential area for intervention research suggested by the theory. Health promotion among caregivers has been studied, but most research has been descriptive (Acton, 2002; Chen, 1999; Matthews, Dunbar-Jacob, Sereika, Schulz, & McDowell, 2004; McDonald, et al., 1999; O'Brien, 1993; Sisk, 2000). The caregivers of HSCT patients found exercise and eating healthy meals to be helpful in sustaining their caregiving. Interventions to encourage health promotion and make health promotion activities accessible to caregivers even when they are busy or away from home warrant further study.

Studies describing helpful information for caregivers are needed. The types of information needed, how best to present the information, and when to present it all deserve additional exploration. Innovative methods of information delivery that meet individual learning needs and styles would be especially useful. This becomes increasingly important because caregivers are being asked to assume increased responsibilities as care moves from inpatient to outpatient settings (Geiger, Heermann, & Eilers, 2005).

Further research is also needed to test the theory and define its application in caregivers of patients with other cancers receiving other types of care and in caregivers of patients with other illnesses. The majority of the caregivers in the two studies that have tested the theory were White, non-Hispanic. Additional research is needed to test the applicability and appropriateness of the concepts of the theory for other cultural and ethnic groups.

Because the theory considers the dyad of caregiver and care recipient, research is also needed to explore the experience of the care recipient. Although research on the experience of being a caregiver is becoming more prevalent, there is little research on the experience of being a care recipient. The care recipient—as a member of the caregiving dyad—is a vital part of caregiving dynamics. It is possible that there are additional forces that move caregiving along the illness trajectory for care recipients. As further research expands understanding of the experience of caregivers and care recipients, additional modifications of the theory may be needed.

USE OF THE THEORY IN NURSING PRACTICE

The HSCT inpatient and outpatient units at the University of Texas MD Anderson Cancer Center (Houston) have used the theory to develop a comprehensive program to support caregivers of patients undergoing HSCT (Adornetto-Garcia et al., 2008). The program consists of three components: (1) a comprehensive caregiver manual, (2) expressive arts materials, and (3) caregiver appreciation programs.

The comprehensive manual was developed by a multidisciplinary committee of HSCT personnel at MD Anderson Cancer Center. Development of the manual included conducting focus groups with caregivers of patients at various stages in the HSCT trajectory who were receiving both autologous and allogeneic HSCTs. These focus groups discussed specific and critical information needs of the caregivers during the HSCT trajectory. The manual contains both educational information and lists of caregiver resources (Adornetto-Garcia et al., 2008).

Expressive arts materials include journals, photo albums, and scrapbooks. Caregivers are offered these resources at the start of the HSCT therapy. Classes on journaling and scrapbooking are also conducted periodically. For caregivers who choose to use them, these creative outlets may be helpful in promoting a sense of well-being and comfort and decreasing anxiety (Adornetto-Garcia et al., 2008).

Caregiver Appreciation Weeks are conducted quarterly on both the inpatient and outpatient HSCT units. Banners are hung announcing the event and thanking caregivers for the important work they do in supporting patients. Activities are conducted to show the value that the professional staff places on the work of the caregivers. Activities include refreshments, classes in creative arts, massage sessions, games, and social networking. Field trips to sites of interest near the HSCT center are also planned. At the end of each Caregiver Appreciation Week, caregivers are asked to complete an evaluation to help guide planning for future Caregiver Appreciation Weeks.

Other opportunities to support caregivers by providing positive forces to move caregiving forward are suggested by the theory of caregiving dynamics. Specific applications of the theory will vary among different caregiver and care recipient populations. Important considerations in deciding how best to support caregivers will include age, gender, and ethnicity of the caregiver and care recipient; the illness, treatment, and illness trajectory; and the site of caregiving. It is expected that use of the theory in practice will result in evaluation of outcomes, which serve as evidence of the usefulness of interventions suggested by the theory.

CONCLUSION

Caregiving by family members, friends, and neighbors is a crucial component of care in the current health system. Although the burden of caregiving has been investigated, little attention has been paid to the forces that drive caregiving forward. The middle range theory of caregiving dynamics was developed to help understand these forces so that caregiving might be strengthened. The literature-derived model was tested, refined, and proposed as a middle range theory 5 years ago (Williams, 2008). Further research is needed to confirm the applicability and appropriateness of the theory to care recipients, to caregivers in other situations, and to caregiving dyads of various cultural and ethnic backgrounds. Interventions suggested by the theory also need investigation. Use of the theory in practice is just beginning. As more experience is gained with the theory, it will be modified to better describe the caregiving experience and to better guide nursing practice and research. Use of the theory to date has shown that it describes the caregiving situation from the perspective of the caregiver and is useful in suggesting interventions to support caregiving.

REFERENCES

Acton, G. J. (2002). Health-promoting self-care in family caregivers. *Western Journal of Nursing Research, 24,* 73–86.

Adornetto-Garcia, D. L., Williams, L. A., Jackson, A., Norman, L., Lederleitner, C., & Mir, M. (2008). Stem cell transplantation patient family caregivers: A program focused on "caring for the caregiver." *Biology of Blood and Marrow Transplantation, 14*(Suppl 2), 155.

Andershed, B., & Ternestedt, B. M. (2000). Being a close relative of a dying person: Development of the concepts "involvement in the light and in the dark." *Cancer Nursing, 23,* 151–159.

Aranda, S., & Peerson, A. (2001). Global exchange. Caregiving in advanced cancer: Lay decision making. *Journal of Palliative Care, 17*(4), 270–276.

Bevans, M., & Sternberg, E. M. (2012). Caregiving burden, stress, and health effects among family caregivers of adult cancer patients. *Journal of the American Medical Association, 307,* 398–403.

Biegel, D., Sales, E., & Schulz, R. (1991). *Family caregiving in chronic illness: Heart disease, cancer, stroke, Alzheimer's disease, and chronic mental illness.* Newbury Park, CA: Sage.

Bowman, K. F., Rose, J. H., & Deimling, G. T. (2005). Families of long-term cancer survivors: Health maintenance advocacy and practice. *Psychooncology, 14,* 1008–1017.

Boyle, D., Blodgett, L., Gnesdiloff, S., White, J. R., Bamford, A. M., Sheridan, M., & Beveridge, R. (2000). Caregiver quality of life after autologous bone marrow transplantation. *Cancer Nursing, 23,* 193–203.

Bunting, S. M. (2001). Sustaining the relationship: Women's caregiving in the context of HIV disease. *Health Care for Women International, 22,* 131–148.

Chen, M. Y. (1999). The effectiveness of health promotion counseling to family caregivers. *Public Health Nursing, 16,* 125–132.

Chow, K., & Coyle, N. (2011). Providing palliative care to family caregivers throughout the bone marrow transplantation trajectory. *Journal of Hospice and Palliative Nursing, 13,* 7–13.

Cohen, C. A., Gold, D. P., Shulman, K. I., Wortley, J. T., McDonald, G., & Wargon, M. (1993). Factors determining the decision to institutionalize dementing individuals: A prospective study. *The Gerontologist, 33,* 714–720.

Connell, C. (1994). Impact of spouse caregiving on health behaviors and physical and mental health status. *American Journal of Alzeheimer's Care and Related Disorders and Research, 9,* 26–36.

Feinberg, L., Reinhard, S. C., Houser, A., & Choula, R. (2011). *Valuing the invaluable: 2011 update, the growing contributions and costs of family caregiving.* Retrieved from AARP Public Policy Institute website: http://assets.aarp. org/rgcenter/ppi/ltc/i51-caregiving.pdf

Ferrell, B. R., Cohen, M. Z., Rhiner, M., & Rozek, A. (1991). Pain as a metaphor for illness. Part II: Family caregivers' management of pain. *Oncology Nursing Forum, 18,* 1315–1321.

Folkman, S. (1997). Positive psychological states and coping with severe stress. *Social Science and Medicine, 45,* 1207–1221.

Frey, P., Stinson, T., Siston, A., Knight, S. J., Ferdman, E., Traynor, A., … Winter, J. N. (2002). Lack of caregivers limits the use of outpatient hematopoietic stem cell transplant program. *Bone Marrow Transplantation, 30,* 741–748.

Geiger, D. L., Heermann, J. A., & Eilers, J. (2005). Identification and validation of competencies for use in objective structured clinical examinations for lay caregivers. *Cancer Nursing, 28,* 54–61.

Gemmill, R., Cooke, L., Williams, A. C., & Grant, M. (2011). Informal caregivers of hematopoietic cell transplant patients: A review and recommendations for interventions and research. *Cancer Nursing, 34,* E13–E21.

Grimm, P. M., Zawacki, K. L., Mock, V., Krumm, S., & Frink, B. B. (2000). Caregiver responses and needs. An ambulatory bone marrow transplant model. *Cancer Practice, 8,* 120–128.

Grundy, M., & Ghazi, F. (2009). Research priorities in haemato-oncology nursing: Results of a literature review and Delphi study. *European Journal of Oncology Nursing, 13,* 235–249.

Hadjistavropoulos, T., Taylor, S., Tuokko, H., & Beattie, B. L. (1994). Neuropsychological deficits, caregivers' perception of deficits and caregiver burden. *Journal of the American Geriatrics Society, 42,* 308–314.

Horowitz, M. M., Loberiza, F. R., Bredeson, C. N., Rizzo, J. D., & Nugent, M. L. (2001). Transplant registries: Guiding clinical decisions and improving outcomes. *Oncology, 15,* 649–659, 663–664, 666.

Jewell, E. J., & Abate, F. (Eds.). (2001). *The new Oxford American dictionary.* New York, NY: Oxford University Press.

Jo, S., Brazil, K., Lohfeld, L., & Willison, K. (2007). Caregiving at the end of life: Perspectives from spousal caregivers and care recipients. *Palliative and Supportive Care, 5,* 11–17.

Kylma, J., Vehviläinen-Julkunen, K., & Lähdevirta, J. (2001). Dynamically fluctuating hope, despair and hopelessness along the HIV/AIDS continuum as described by caregivers in voluntary organizations in Finland. *Issues in Mental Health Nursing, 22,* 353–377.

Liehr, P., & Smith, M. J. (2000). Using story theory to guide nursing practice. *International Journal of Human Caring, 4,* 13–18.

Loberiza, F., Jr. (2003). Summary slides 2003. *IBMTR/ABMTR Newsletter, 10*(1), 1, 7–10.

Matthews, J. T., Dunbar-Jacob, J., Sereika, S., Schulz, R., & McDowell, B. J. (2004). Preventive health practices: Comparison of family caregivers 50 and older. *Journal of Gerontological Nursing, 30*(2), 46–54.

McDonald, P. E., Fink, S. V., & Wykle, M. L. (1999). Self-reported health-promoting behaviors of black and white caregivers. *Western Journal of Nursing Research, 21,* 538–548.

McGrath, P. (2001). Caregivers' insights in the dying trajectory in hematology oncology. *Cancer Nursing, 24,* 413–421.

Merriam-Webster OnLine. (2007). *Merriam-Webster's Collegiate Dictionary* [Web site]. Retrieved from http://www.m-w.com/dictionary

Miller, B., Townsend, A., Carpenter, E., Montgomery, R. V., Stull, D., & Young, R. F. (2001). Social support and caregiver distress: A replication analysis. *Journal of Gerontology Series B: Psychological Science and Social Science, 56,* S249–S256.

Mok, E., Chan, F., Chan, V., & Yeung, E. (2002). Perception of empowerment by family caregivers of patients with a terminal illness in Hong Kong. *International Journal of Palliative Nursing, 8,* 137–145.

O'Brien, M. T. (1993). Multiple sclerosis: Health-promoting behaviors of spousal caregivers. *Journal of Neuroscience Nursing, 25,* 105–112.

Ostwald, S. K. (1997). Caregiver exhaustion: Caring for the hidden patients. *Advanced Practice Nursing Quarterly, 3*(2), 29–35.

Padilla, G. V., Mishel, M. H., & Grant, M. M. (1992). Uncertainty, appraisal and quality of life. *Quality of Life Research, 1,* 155–165.

Pasacreta, J. V., Barg, F., Nuamah, I., & McCorkle, R. (2000). Participant characteristics before and 4 months after attendance at a family caregiver cancer education program. *Cancer Nursing, 23,* 295–303.

Pasacreta, J. V., & McCorkle, R. (2000). Cancer care: Impact of interventions on caregiver outcomes. *Annual Review of Nursing Research, 18,* 127–148.

Phillips, L. R., Brewer, B. B., & Torres de Ardon, E. (2001). The elder image scale: A method for indexing history and emotion in family caregiving. *Journal of Nursing Measurement, 9,* 23–47.

Rose, K. E. (1999). A qualitative analysis of the information needs of informal carers of terminally ill cancer patients. *Journal of Clinical Nursing, 8,* 81–88.

Russell, C. K., Bunting, S. M., & Gregory, D. M. (1997). Protective care-receiving: The active role of care-recipients. *Journal of Advanced Nursing, 25,* 532–540.

Schumacher, K. L. (1996). Reconceptualizing family caregiving: Family-based illness care during chemotherapy. *Research in Nursing and Health, 19,* 261–271.

Schumacher, K. L., Beidler, S. M., Beeber, A. S., & Gambino, P. (2006). A transactional model of cancer family caregiving skill. *Advances in Nursing Science, 29,* 271–286.

Schumacher, K. L., Stewart, B. J., & Archbold, P. G. (1998). Conceptualization and measurement of doing family caregiving well. *Image: Journal of Nursing Scholarship, 30,* 63–69.

Seltzer, M. M., & Li, L. W. (2000). The dynamics of caregiving: Transitions during a three-year prospective study. *Gerontologist, 40,* 165–178.

Shyu, Y. I. (2000). Role tuning between caregiver and care receiver during discharge transition: An illustration of role function mode in Roy's adaptation theory. *Nursing Science Quarterly, 13,* 323–331.

Sisk, R. J. (2000). Caregiver burden and health promotion. *International Journal of Nursing Studies, 37,* 37–43.

Smith, M. J., & Liehr, P. (2003). The theory of attentively embracing story. In M. J. Smith & P. R. Liehr (Eds.), *Middle range theory for nursing* (pp. 167–187). New York, NY: Springer Publishing.

Soothill, K., Morris, S. M., Harman, J. C., Francis, B., Thomas, C., & McIllmurray, M. B. (2001). Informal carers of cancer patients: What are their unmet psychosocial needs? *Health and Social Care in the Community, 9,* 464–475.

Speice, J., Harkness, J., Laneri, H., Frankel, R., Roter, D., Kornblith, A. B., ... Holland, J. C. (2000). Involving family members in cancer care: Focus group considerations of patients and oncological providers. *Psycho-Oncology, 9,* 101–112.

Stajduhar, K. I., Nickel, D. D., Martin, W. L., & Funk, L. (2008). Situated/being situated: Client and co-worker roles of family caregivers in hospice palliative care. *Social Science & Medicine, 67,* 1789–1797.

Stenberg, U., Ruland, C. M., & Miaskowski, C. (2010). Review of the literature on the effects of caring for a patient with cancer. *Psycho-Oncology, 19*(10), 1013–1025.

Stetz, K. M., McDonald, J. C., & Compton, K. (1996). Needs and experiences of family caregivers during marrow transplantation. *Oncology Nursing Forum, 23,* 1422–1427.

Swanberg, J. E. (2006). Making it work: Informal caregiving, cancer, and employment. *Journal of Psychosocial Oncology, 24*(3), 1–18.

Thompson, L. (2004). *Long-term care: Support for family caregivers* [Issue Brief]. Washington, DC: Georgetown University. Retrieved from http://ltc.georgetown.edu/pdfs/caregivers.pdf

U.S. Census Bureau. (2005, April 29). Facts for features: Special addition: National nurses week (May 6–12) and national hospital week (May 8–14). Retrieved from http://www.census.gov/Press-Release/www/releases/archives/cb05-ffse.02.pdf

Whisenant, M. (2011). Informal caregiving in patients with brain tumors. *Oncology Nursing Forum, 38*(5), 373–381.

Wilkes, L., White, K., & O'Riordan, L. (2000). Empowerment through information: Supporting rural families of oncology patients in palliative care. *Australian Journal of Rural Health, 8,* 41–46.

Williams, L. A. (2003). Informal caregiving dynamics with a case study in blood and marrow transplantation. *Oncology Nursing Forum, 30,* 679–688.

Williams, L. A. (2007). Whatever it takes: Informal caregiving dynamics in blood and marrow transplantation. *Oncology Nursing Forum, 34,* 379–387.

Williams, L. A. (2008). Theory of caregiving dynamics. In M. J. Smith & P. Liehr (Eds.), *Middle range theory for nursing* (2nd Ed., pp. 261–276). New York, NY: Springer Publishing.

Wilson, M. E., Eilers, J., Heermann, J. A., & Million, R. (2009). The experience of spouses as caregivers for recipients of hematopoietic stem cell transplants. *Cancer Nursing, 32,* E15–E23.

Wrubel, J., Richards, T. A., Folkman, S., & Acree, M. C. (2001). Tacit definitions of informal caregiving. *Journal of Advanced Nursing, 33,* 175–181.

Wuest, J. (2001). Precarious ordering: Toward a formal theory of women's caring. *Health Care for Women International, 22,* 167–193.

Zarit, S. H., Reever, K. E., & Bach-Peterson, J. (1980). Relatives of the impaired elderly: Correlates of feelings of burden. *Gerontologist, 20,* 649–655.

15

Theory of Moral Reckoning

Alvita Nathaniel

Today's health care environment—with its spiraling technology, longer life spans, power imbalance, and budget restraints—engenders an atmosphere with moral problems of ever-increasing complexity—problems for which the most basic moral beliefs about life, death, right, and wrong are challenged. An increasing number of researchers have examined nurses' responses to these types of stressors and their impact on patient care, often determining that nurses experience moral distress in many such situations. The Theory of Moral Reckoning began with an interest in this compelling concept.

PURPOSE OF THE THEORY AND HOW IT WAS DEVELOPED

Andrew Jameton, a philosopher and ethicist, first described moral distress in nursing. When Jameton asked nurses to talk about moral dilemmas, he noticed that their stories failed to meet the definition of dilemma (Jameton, 1984, pp. 335–336). A moral dilemma forces one to choose between two undesirable, mutually exclusive alternatives—the correct choice is unclear, since all alternatives have nearly equal moral weight and none are more right or wrong than others. The nurses' stories did not fit the definition of moral dilemma. Relating their personal stories, nurses consistently talked to Jameton about situations in which they believed they knew the morally right actions to take, yet they felt constrained from following their convictions (Jameton, 1993). Jameton concluded that nurses were compelled to tell these stories because of their profound suffering and their belief about the importance of the situations. Mentioning this concept only briefly, Jameton proposed that "moral distress arises when one knows the right thing to do, but institutional constraints make it nearly impossible to pursue the right course of action" (Jameton, 1984, p. 6). Jameton also stipulated that nurses who participate in an action that they have judged to be morally wrong experience moral distress (Jameton, 1993). Building upon Jameton's definition, Wilkinson defined moral distress as "the psychological disequilibrium and negative feeling state experienced when a person makes a moral decision but does not follow through by performing the moral behavior indicated by that decision" (Wilkinson, 1987, p. 16). In the intervening years, there has been increasing interest in moral distress. Most subsequent nursing sources rely on Jameton's or Wilkinson's definition of moral distress.

For many years, I taught a nursing ethics course and later coauthored an ethics textbook (Burkhardt & Nathaniel, 2008). The concept of moral distress caught my imagination. I wondered, for example, if we in the profession claim that nurses are autonomous professionals, why do so many nurses violate their own moral codes when faced with constraints to action? How can institutional pressure override an individual's moral values formed over a lifetime? Why do highly educated professionals view themselves as powerless in morally troubling situations? How does moral distress affect nurses, patients, and the health care system as a whole?

Even though the early literature offered emotionally charged descriptions of nurses' moral distress, the knowledge was limited in four essential ways. First, there were few studies, with few informants, so even though many nurses had written about moral distress, we really knew very little about it. Second, only a handful of published studies identified moral distress in their purpose statements. In addition, most published studies were rudimentary and exploratory in nature. Third, theoretical foundations did not adequately explain moral distress. Fourth, there were gaps in the literature in terms of the impact of moral distress on nursing care and patients' health outcomes.

Awareness of these limitations compelled me to try to learn more about the process. I began conducting interviews with nurses who reported that they had experienced morally troubling patient care situations. My purpose was to address gaps in knowledge by seeking answers to one basic research question: What transpires in morally laden situations in which nurses experience distress? Using the inductive approach of classic grounded theory (Glaser, 1965, 1978, 1998; Glaser & Strauss, 1967), I soon recognized that more was going on in these situations than could be explained adequately by the concept of moral distress. Distinct patterns and processes emerged from the data, making it clear that nurses' experiences followed a relatively predictable pattern as each nurse made important choices before, during, and after becoming entangled in a morally significant situational bind.

As required by the classic grounded theory method, I laid aside preconceived notions, logical elaborations, and ideas gleaned from the extant literature. New concepts, processes, and tentative hypotheses began to emerge from the empirical data through careful investigation, inductive reasoning, and analysis. Early in the data-gathering phase, I noticed that nurses vividly recalled important junctures in their professional lives that included morally troubling patient care situations yet seemed to be part of a much bigger process. Extant research focusing on moral distress remained pertinent and was subsequently interwoven into the larger, more explanatory and predictive process of moral reckoning, adding depth and complexity to the resultant theory.

The theory of moral reckoning emerged through the inductive process of the classic grounded theory method. I recorded the interviews as field notes immediately after each interview. Analysis began with the first episode of data gathering and was simultaneous with other steps of the process. Using constant comparison as suggested by Glaser (1965), data were analyzed sentence by sentence as they were coded. Data were organized into concepts and further into categories. I composed conceptual-level memos as concepts became evident. As the research continued, social psychological processes began to surface. Moral reckoning emerged as the theory to which all other concepts related. Identification of moral reckoning enabled subsequent selective theoretical sampling, coding, and memoing. Theoretical sampling began when concepts seemed to require more refinement or areas needed more depth. Memos consisted of the emerging concepts and categories (highly abstract concepts). When it became clear that the indicators were saturated, I began sorting and organizing the memos.

The larger process of moral reckoning overlaps moral distress as described in the extant literature. Both moral reckoning and moral distress include a situational bind (unnamed in moral distress literature) and short- and long-term consequences for nurses. Because it explicates choices and actions and includes precursor conditions and long-term consequences, the substantive and more comprehensive and explanatory theory of moral reckoning effectively synthesizes, organizes, and transcends what was previously known about moral distress.

Moral reckoning captures the culmination of the process as nurses critically and emotionally reflect on motivations, choices, actions, and consequences entangled in a particularly troubling patient care situation. They are alone with their experiences, wrestling with something they have difficulty communicating. According to Strauss (1959), critical events occur in which there is a temporary gap between events and the person's understanding of them. The person is aware of this gap. Under certain social conditions, such as with moral reckoning, a person will undergo so many or such critical experiences for which conventional explanations seem inadequate that the person begins to question large segments of what was previously learned. Subsequently, there is an internal rhetorical battle. The person cannot question what was learned in the past without questioning internal purposes. If the person rejects the explanations once believed, then there will be a type of alienation—a perception of a world lost. The person may feel spiritually dispossessed as he or she embraces a set of counter explanations to recreate a worldview (Strauss, 1959).

The term *reckon* is especially suitable to describe the name of the theory. To reckon is to enumerate serially or separately; to name or mention one after another in due order; to go over or through (a series) in this manner; to recount, relate, narrate, and tell; to mention; to allege; to calculate, work out, decide the nature or value of; to consider, judge, or estimate by, or as the result of calculation; to consider, think, suppose, be of opinion; to speak or discourse of something; to render or give an account (of one's conduct, etc.); and to regard in a certain light (Simpson & Weiner, 1989, pp. 335–336).

Reckoning is "the action of rendering to another an account of one's self or one's conduct; an account, statement of something" (Simpson & Weiner, 1989, p. 336).

CONCEPTS OF THE THEORY

Concepts in the middle range theory of moral reckoning include ease, situational binds, resolution, and reflection. The named concepts of the theory are processes that comprise the stages of moral reckoning that occur over time. The second concept, situational bind, is an event that interrupts the stage of ease.

Ease

Ease is a state of naturalness, a sense of comfort. Ease assumes a certain measure of freedom from constraint, worry, hardship, and agitation. Ease also denotes readiness and skillfulness. Nurses who experience ease are comfortable. They have technical skills and feel rewarded to practice within the boundaries of self, profession, and institution. They know their patients and witness their suffering, making the implicit promise that they have skill and knowledge to relieve suffering. These nurses are competent and confident. They know what others expect of them and experience a sense of flow and at-homeness. When at ease, nurses have high standards and are proud of their technical abilities and skill at communicating with patients and others. As long as the work of nursing fulfills the nurse and the nurse experiences a sense of comfort with the integration of core beliefs and professional and institutional norms, then ease continues.

Situational Binds

Situational binds are serious and complex conflicts within individuals and tacit or overt conflicts between nurses and others—all having moral overtones. The concept *situational bind* was discussed by Strauss (1959), who theorized that when situational binds occur the person questions his or her central purpose, asking to what, for what, or to whom he or she is committed. The person experiences turmoil and inner dialogue that leads to a decision.

Situational binds lead to life turning points. These incidents transform identity and force a person to recognize that "I am not the same as I was, as I used to be" (Strauss, 1959, p. 93). Critical incidents lead to "surprise, shock, chagrin, anxiety, tension, bafflement, self-questioning—and also the need to try out the new self, to explore and validate the new and often exciting or fearful conceptions" (Strauss, 1959, p. 93). Situational binds lead to decisions that ultimately change people's lives.

Resolution

Resolution is a move to set things right, to resolve the turmoil, and to relieve the tension. Resolution occurs when a person terminates the intolerable condition by finding a solution to the problem, deciding on a course of action, and bringing a situation to a conclusion. The person might make a declaration or carry out a plan. Resolution tends to disentangle one from a situational bind.

Reflection

Reflection is contemplating, pondering, and thinking about past events. Having made and acted upon a decision, a person reflects as he or she reckons past behavior and actions. The person carefully considers the events and generates opinions. Reflection raises questions about previous judgments, particular acts, and the essential self. Reflection may extend over a lifetime.

RELATIONSHIPS AMONG THE CONCEPTS: THE MODEL

Moral reckoning consists of a three-stage process and critical juncture as nurses reflect on motivations, choices, actions, and consequences of a morally troubling patient care situation (Nathaniel, 2004, 2006). The relationship among the stages is depicted in Figure 15.1. In the middle range theory of moral reckoning, the stage of ease is disrupted by a situational bind and then followed by the processes of resolution and reflection.

The Stage of Ease

After the initial novice phase, nurses experience a stage of ease in which they enjoy a sense of satisfaction and at-homeness in the workplace. They feel comfortable with their knowledge and skills. Properties central to the stage of ease include becoming, professionalizing, institutionalizing, and working. There is a fragile balance among the properties during the stage of ease such that each property is related to the other, creating a feeling of comfort.

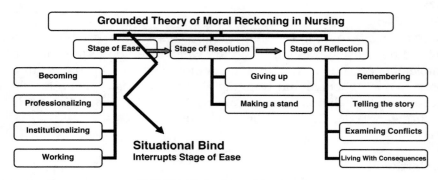

FIGURE 15.1   Moral Reckoning
Source: Reprinted from: Nathaniel, A. K. (2006). Moral reckoning in nursing. *Western Journal of Nursing Research, 28*(4), 419–438.

Becoming

As Strauss once wrote, "The human experience of time is one of process: the present is always a becoming" (Strauss, 1959, p. 31). Through the process of becoming every person evolves a set of core beliefs and values, which are a product of lifelong learning about what is important and how to behave in society. Core beliefs evolve through experience, from the testimony of authority, and from the modeling of parents, teachers, ministers, peers, and others. Integration and consistency of core values produce moral integrity (Beauchamp & Childress, 2001). Through the lifelong process of becoming, nurses develop core beliefs and values.

Professionalizing

The process of becoming a nurse includes inculcation of certain cultural norms learned in nursing school and early practice. Professional norms are conceptual ideals that contribute to the nurse's idea of what a good nurse should be or do. Explicitly, nurses learn that they have unique relationships with patients and are responsible to keep promises, which are sometimes implicit in the relationship. Penticuff identified moral goals that are part of nursing's common perspective, such as "the protection and enhancement of human dignity, the alleviation of vulnerability, the promotion of growth and health, and the enhancement of coping and comfort in the face of hardship" (Penticuff, 1997, p. 51). Likewise, nurses honor the common professional norms of knowing patients as persons, listening to their needs and preferences, supporting their everyday choices through advocacy, and maintaining their dignity (Doutrich, Wros, & Izumi, 2001).

Professionalizing is supported by the theoretical work of Strauss (1959) and Glaser (1998). Strauss suggested that to become a member of a group, a person must invest in the goals of the group. Investment in a group occurs through the transmission of ideas and signifies shared meanings. Insofar as the person thinks of himself or herself as an integral part of the group, he or she embraces its goals. The person, then, has dual commitment to the group and to self. Strauss also suggested that a person may be so heavily identified with the group that "he is no longer quite himself" (Strauss, 1959, p. 37). Validation by the group is so important that the person reinterprets activity and meaning. Thus, as can be seen in moral reckoning, the person's core values may be either supported or challenged by the values of the group as the person becomes professionalized. Similarly, Glaser (1998) proposed that personal identities may merge with properties of a profession so that members find it difficult to break through the boundaries (Glaser, 1998). In this situation, the unit identity becomes the person's self-image. Professional norms sometimes lead nurses to act according to role-set behavior, governed by blind adherence to professional norms and by their perception of the expectations of others.

Institutionalizing

The third property rests on the premise that the nurse works in an institutional setting with both implicit and explicit institutional norms. This is corroborated by the studies of Liaschenko (1995) and Ehrenreich and Ehrenreich (1990), who propose that institutionalized medicine is a complex interconnected tangle of practice patterns, cultural beliefs, and values in which the practice of nursing takes place. Institutional health care delivery norms constitute basic social structural processes within which the practice of nursing takes place. Explicit institutional norms include completing a job according to institutional standards and respecting lines of authority. Implicit institutional norms include such concepts as ensuring that the business makes a profit, following orders, and handling crises without making waves.

Working

The work of nursing is varied, challenging, and rewarding. Nurses attend to the most personal and private needs and learn much about patients' hopes, fears, and desires (Penticuff, 1997). They get to know patients who stay on their unit for extended periods or return many times. Doing the work of nursing includes knowing patients intimately, witnessing their suffering, accepting the responsibility to care, desiring to do the work well, and knowing what to do.

Situational Binds

Sometimes troubling events occur that challenge the integration of core beliefs, professional norms, and institutional norms. When this happens, nurses find themselves in *situational binds* that force them into a critical juncture in their professional lives (Nathaniel, 2004, 2006).

A situational bind terminates the stage of ease and throws the nurse into turmoil when core beliefs and other claims conflict. Three types of situational binds include conflicts between core values and professional or institutional norms, moral disagreement among decision makers in the face of power imbalance, and workplace deficiencies that cause real or potential harm to patients (Nathaniel, 2004, 2006). These binds produce dramatic consequences for nurses when they must choose one value or belief over another—forcing a turning point in their professional lives.

Situational binds in nursing involve an intricate interweaving of many factors including professional relationships, divergent values, workplace demands, and other implications with moral overtones. Situational binds vary in their complexity, context, and particulars but are similar in terms of their immediate and long-term effects. When situational binds occur, nurses must make critical decisions—choosing one value or belief over another. Specific types of binds include conflict between the nurse's core beliefs and professional or institutional norms, power imbalance complicated by differences in beliefs and values, conflicting loyalty, and serious workplace deficiencies (Nathaniel, 2004, 2006). Types of cases most frequently mentioned in the extant literature included causing needless suffering by prolonging the life of dying patients or performing unnecessary tests and treatments, especially on terminal patients; lying to patients; incompetent or inadequate treatment by a physician; and coercing consent from poorly informed patients (Cavaliere, Daly, Dowling, & Montgomery, 2010; Corley, 1995; Cummings, 2011; Deady & McCarthy, 2010; Dewitte, Piers, Steeman, & Nele, 2010; Dunwoody, 2011; Gaeta & Price, 2010; Hall, Brinchmann, & Aagaard, 2012; Halpern, 2011; Huffman & Rittenmeyer, 2012; McArthur, 2010; Mueller, Ottenberg, Hayes, & Koenig, 2011; Piers et al., 2011, 2012; Rodney, 1988; Wilkinson, 1987).

The disruption of ease that nurses experience during situational binds results from a number of dynamic internal and external tensions (Nathaniel, 2004, 2006). For example, the ability to act on moral decisions may be constrained by socialization to follow orders, self-doubt, lack of courage, and conflicting loyalty. Penticuff (1997) also found that nurses struggle with conflicting loyalties to patients, nursing peers, physicians, and institutions. Asymmetrical power relationships and powerlessness often lead to situational binds. Nurses may have insight into the problem at hand yet believe they cannot participate in the decision-making process. They sense a moral responsibility, want the best outcome for patients, know what is needed, and yet believe they are powerless to get it done. In some instances, nurses experience distress when they know the professional and institutional norms, and yet are unable to uphold them because of workplace deficiencies. Workplace deficiencies include such factors as chronic staff shortage, unreasonable institutional expectations, and equipment inadequacy (Nathaniel, 2004, 2006). Situational binds force nurses to make difficult decisions in the midst of crises characterized by intolerable internal conflict. Something must be done to rectify the situation: One must make a choice.

In the midst of the situational bind or soon after, nurses experience consequences such as profound emotions, reactive behaviors, and physical manifestations. Nurses may experience feelings of guilt, anger, powerlessness, conflict, depression, outrage, betrayal, and devastation. Physical manifestations such as lightheadedness, crying, sleeplessness, and vomiting may also occur.

During the time of or after situational binds, nursing care is affected—sometimes negatively and sometimes positively. Some nurses are unable to care for the patient or to even return to the unit after a troubling incident. Some nurses make up for what they consider to be wrongdoing by giving more compassionate care—even to the point of sacrificing personal time. For others, care improves in the long term because of lessons learned in the process.

The Stage of Resolution

Situational binds constitute crises of intolerable internal conflict. The nurse seeks to resolve the problem and set things right. This signifies the beginning of the stage of resolution. This stage often alters one's professional trajectory. There are two properties of the stage of resolution: making a stand and giving up. These properties are not mutually exclusive. In fact, a nurse might give up, reconsider, and make a stand.

Making a Stand

In the midst of a situational bind, some nurses choose to make a stand. Making a stand takes a variety forms—all of which include professional risk. Nurses may even make a stand by stepping beyond the proscribed boundaries of the profession to do what, to them, seems to be the morally correct action. Nurses may make a stand by refusing to follow physicians' orders, initiating negotiations, breaking rules, whistle blowing, and so forth. Making a stand is rarely successful in the short term. Not a single informant in Liaschenko's (1995) study reported an instance where treatment was stopped on his/her testimony. Nevertheless, making a stand may occasionally improve the overall situation in the long term.

Giving Up

Sometimes nurses resolve a morally troubling situation by giving up. Giving up may overlap with making a stand in some instances. Nurses often give up because they recognize the futility of making an overt stand. They are simply not willing to sacrifice for no purpose. They may give up to protect themselves or to seek a way or find a place where they can better integrate core beliefs, professional norms, and institutional norms. Giving up includes participating (with regret) in an activity they consider to be morally wrong, such as leaving the unit, the institution, or the profession altogether. Sometimes nurses seem to give up in the short term but move toward more advanced autonomous roles or toward leadership positions—all of which prepare them to make a stand in the future.

The Stage of Reflection

During the stage of reflection, the nurse thoughtfully examines beliefs, values, and actions. Properties of the stage of reflection include remembering, telling the story, examining conflicts, and living with the consequences. During this stage, which may last a lifetime, nurses reflect on the moral problem and their response. Nurses recall vivid mental pictures and evoked emotions such as feelings of guilt and self-blame, lingering sadness, anger, and anxiety. Moral reckoning continues over time as nurses remember, tell the story, examine conflicts, and live with the consequences.

Remembering

One of the more intriguing properties of moral reckoning is the manner in which nurses remember critical events. After particularly troubling situations, nurses retain vivid mental pictures, which tend to evoke emotions many years later. Nurses remember sensual particulars of the incident—the sights, sounds, and smells. Even after many years, the images are seared into their minds. Remembering evokes emotions including feelings of guilt and self-blame, lingering sadness, anger, and anxiety. Lingering emotional effects may be profound for many.

Strauss (1959) proposed that a remembered act is never finished. As a person recalls the act, he or she selectively reconstructs it, remembering certain aspects and dropping others. The person reassesses acts many times, seeking new perspectives or new facts. Thus, learning leads to revision of concepts that, in turn, leads to reorganization of behavior. Strauss further proposed that the process of continual learning and revision results in a new identity. This reflection raises challenges and the discovery of new values through which transformation takes place.

Telling the Story

Nurses want to tell the story to sympathetic others. They may tell a friend or family member immediately after an incident occurs or meet with other nurses to discuss the event. Nurses rely upon others to hear the story and to understand it from their perspective. A listening, nonjudgmental person allows the nurse to tell the story as he or she attempts to seek meaning and to reckon belief and action. Nurses continue the process over time—telling and re-telling the story as they try to make sense of it. Smith and Liehr (2008) address story gathering in the chapter describing Story Theory. They contend that engaging in dialogue about unique human experience catalyzes the beginning of a process of personal change. Through following the story path as recollected, one begins a process of discovery, self-revelation, and reckoning. As the story unfolds, the person attempts to understand the meaning of experiences and gain new perspectives and wisdom. The person goes into the depths of the story to find unique meanings and reconstruct a story that has a beginning, middle, and end. Consistent with the theory of moral reckoning, Smith and Liehr propose that as the person tells the story, he or she gains a full-dimensional, reflective awareness of bodily experiences, thoughts, feelings, emotions, and values. Patterns are discerned, made explicit, and named. Telling the story relieves pain and creates possibilities for human development.

Examining Conflicts

As nurses tell their stories, they begin to examine conflicts in the troubling situation. They examine their values and ask questions about what actually happened, who was to blame, and how they can avoid similar situations in the future. As they thoughtfully examine the conflicts, some intellectualize their participation, some set limits, and some gain strength to make a stand and accept the consequences in future situations.

Nurses continue to struggle with conflicts between personal values and professional ideals. They want to be able to identify themselves as good nurses. Similarly, Kelly (1998) reported that some nurses have a painful awareness of the discrepancy between who they aspired to be and what they have become. These nurses suffer the loss of their own professional self-concept, their vision of the kind of nurses they wanted to be, and their image of nursing as they believed it was.

As nurses think about their roles in what they consider past moral wrongdoing, some set limits or make pronouncements about their future actions. Some identify a point beyond which they will not again be willing to go. Others vow to step outside their boundaries to help a patient in the future, fully aware and willing to accept the consequences of their future actions. Thus, the nurse's ethical practice evolves through the iterative process of experience and reflection.

Living With the Consequences

Nurses live with the consequences of morally troubling situations for a prolonged period of time. Consequences other than those already mentioned include fractured professional relationships and a change in one's life trajectory. Following a situational bind in which the nurse believes another person committed moral wrongdoing, he or she may be unable to work collaboratively with that person or others who were unsupportive. They lose faith in the person's integrity and respect for them as practitioners. Since they are no longer comfortable in the original workplace and have fractured professional relationships, many nurses change their work setting following a situational bind. They may change employers or specialties and are likely to seek further education intending to correct the type of moral wrongs they experienced in the past.

USE OF THE THEORY IN NURSING RESEARCH

The theory calls for programs of research that will further explore and more fully develop the concepts, begin to identify causes, and make comparisons and predictions. Vigorous theoretical sampling is needed to (a) allow a more thorough and useful understanding of the concepts of ease, situational bind, resolution, and reflection; (b) provide a better understanding of core values as they intersect with professional and institutional norms; and (c) modify the theory to include different levels of nursing practice.

In addition, nursing ethics research is needed to shed light on what nurses understand about nursing ethics, the depth of this understanding, how the understanding factors into everyday decision making, and what kind of learning leads to empowered, patient-centered, ethical decision making. Further qualitative and quantitative research is needed to determine the characteristics of nurses who experience moral distress and moral reckoning versus those who do not, including the quality of patient care provided by each group. Correlational research is needed to identify nurses who leave the bedside and those who stay, particularly in relation to whether or not they have experienced situational binds. In the face of the nursing shortage, this has implications for nurse recruiting and retention. If caring and sensitive nurses leave the bedside, it is important to identify strategies to retain them.

Research on moral reckoning should not be limited to the profession of nursing. Investigators have an opportunity to use the theory with a wide variety of populations. For instance, people who live through disasters such as September 11, 2001, or Hurricane Katrina may experience moral reckoning. Significant losses, such as the death of a child or the loss of a family-sustaining job, create a context for moral reckoning. In addition, the obvious use of the theory with other disciplines deserves consideration, particularly as related to nursing practice and patient outcomes.

USE OF THE THEORY IN NURSING PRACTICE

Interest in the theory of moral reckoning and moral distress has become intense within the nursing profession in the last several years. The literature reveals that these phenomena are problems for other professions and other cultures as well. The theory of moral reckoning has been cited in nearly 60 publications worldwide. Literature focusing on nurses, nursing students, bioethicists, physicians, podiatrists, educators, pharmacists, and police has cited the theory of moral reckoning. Moral distress has even been documented among veterinarians. Recent research and/or publication about moral reckoning originated from ten countries including the United States, Spain, Canada, Uganda, New Zealand, Chile, China, Poland, South Africa, and the UK.

Implications for Nursing Ethics Development

Moral reckoning points to a chasm between the ethical practice of nurses and formal ethics theory. This may indicate what MacIntyre (1988) terms an "epistemological crisis" in nursing: a crisis that occurs when events bring into question ideals and convictions of a tradition and when previous methods of inquiry, conceptualization, and principles fall into question. MacIntyre suggests that an epistemological crisis can be resolved successfully through innovations that meet three requirements: (1) New concepts and new theory must furnish a systematic and rational solution to a previously unmanageable problem; (2) innovations must explain what it was that made the tradition ineffective; and (3) the new tradition must carry out tasks in a way that exhibits some fundamental continuity of new conceptual and theoretical structures with shared beliefs (MacIntyre, 1988). Such ethics will allow for consideration of the uniqueness and particularity of patient situations, while acknowledging diverse moral perspectives. As MacIntyre (1988) suggests, nurses should come to understand rival perspectives as different, yet comprising complementary understandings of reality.

Implications for Nursing Educators

The middle range theory of moral reckoning brings forth several implications for nursing education. Recommendations include strengthening nursing ethics education, teaching strategies to improve nurses' empowerment, and helping students learn effective ways to establish intra- and interprofessional relationships. Nurse educators teach students to be ethically self-aware and provide opportunities for them to learn about normative ethics. Educators can closely examine implicit messages transmitted to students, particularly traditions of the discipline that inhibit meaningful dialogue and sustain conflict and power imbalance. In this manner, they help students learn strategies and language that prepare them to enter into ethical dialogue with other professionals and to prepare students for the realities of practice.

Specifically, the middle range theory of moral reckoning uncovers a basic social process that educators should discuss with students. Nurse educators help to prepare novice nurses through curricula that include recognition of the conditions of the stage of ease—becoming, professionalizing, and institutionalizing. To help prepare students for the real world, educators can facilitate dialogue that uncovers sources of conflict between core beliefs, professional traditions, and institutional expectations. They can acknowledge the unique relationship between nurses and patients, recognizing special elements of the relationship such as knowing intimately and witnessing suffering.

Nurse educators can also prepare students for situational binds related to asymmetrical power relationships, loyalty conflicts, and workplace deficiencies. When students practice dealing with these problems in simulated educational circumstances, they may find better ways to deal with situational binds before encountering them in the workplace. Educators might also prepare students for the stage of resolution and the properties of giving up and making a stand in order to be better prepared to follow integrity-preserving courses of action.

Nurse educators must return to a clear focus on nursing codes of ethics. When nurses internalize professional ethics, they may be less likely to waver when faced with situational binds. Ongoing research of moral reckoning is being conducted utilizing a sample of professionals from other disciplines. Preliminary findings seem to indicate that professionals from disciplines in which educators clearly focus on a code of professional ethics are less likely to experience moral reckoning.

Implications for Practicing Nurses

Practicing nurses should internalize their code of professional ethics and claim their professional autonomy. Preliminary findings of the research, mentioned above, also seem to indicate that professionals who acknowledge their own autonomy are less likely to experience moral reckoning. When situational binds occur, they may be more likely to act according to their own values, rather than feel compelled to violate them.

Avoiding situational binds and searching for integrity-saving compromise in morally troubling situations may help practicing nurses engaged in morally troubling situations. A structured discussion of the process of moral reckoning may lead to an increase of satisfaction with nursing care. In these discussion groups, nurses can purposely examine core values and their relationship to professional and institutional norms.

CONCLUSION

This middle range theory of moral reckoning encompasses moral distress yet reaches further—identifying a life event experienced through disruption of ease as one confronts a situational bind demanding resolution and reflection. The concepts of the theory—ease, situational bind, resolution, and reflection—name the stages of the basic social process of moral reckoning. The theory has been developed in the context of the discipline of nursing, but its use in other contexts promises meaningful guidance and ongoing development.

REFERENCES

Beauchamp, T. L., & Childress, J. F. (2001). *Principles of biomedical ethics* (5th ed.). New York, NY: Oxford University Press.

Burkhardt, M. A., & Nathaniel, A. K. (2008). *Ethics & issues in contemporary nursing* (3rd ed.). New York, NY: Delmar.

Cavaliere, T. A., Daly, B., Dowling, D., & Montgomery, K. (2010). Moral distress in neonatal intensive care unit RNs. *Advances in Neonatal Care, 10*(3), 145–156.

Corley, M. C. (1995). Moral distress of critical care nurses. *American Journal of Critical Care, 4*(4), 280–285.

Cummings, C. L. (2011). What factors affect nursing retention in the acute care setting? *Journal of Research in Nursing, 16*(6), 489–500.

Deady, R., & McCarthy, J. (2010). A study of the situations, features, and coping mechanisms experienced by Irish psychiatric nurses experiencing moral distress. *Perspectives in Psychiatric Care, 46*(3), 209–220.

Dewitte, M., Piers, R., Steeman, E., & Nele. (2010). Moral distress and burn-out in nurses on acute geriatric wards. Fourth European Nursing Congress. *Journal of Clinical Nursing, 19*, 19–20.

Doutrich, D., Wros, P., & Izumi, S. (2001). Relief of suffering and regard for personhood: Nurses' ethical concerns in Japan and the USA. *Nursing Ethics, 8*(5), 448–458.

Dunwoody, D. (2011). Nurses' level of moral distress and perception of futile care in the critical care environment. *Dynamics, 22*(2), 22–24.

Ehrenreich, B., & Ehrenreich, J. (1990). The system behind the chaos. In N. F. McKenzie (Ed.), *The crisis in health care: Ethical issues* (pp. 50–69). New York, NY: Meridian.

Gaeta, S., & Price, K. J. (2010). End-of-life issues in critically ill cancer patients. *Critical Care Clinics, 26*(1), 219–227.

Glaser, B. G. (1965). The constant comparative method of qualitative analysis. *Social Problems, 12*, 10.

Glaser, B. G. (1978). *Theoretical sensitivity: Advances in the methodology of grounded theory*. Mill Valley, CA: Sociology Press.

Glaser, B. G. (1998). *Doing grounded theory: Issues and discussion*. Mill Valley, CA: Sociology Press.

Glaser, B. G., & Strauss, A. L. (1967). *The discovery of grounded theory: Strategies for qualitative research*. Chicago, IL: Aldine.

Hall, E. O. C., Brinchmann, B. S., & Aagaard, H. (2012). The challenge of integrating justice and care in neonatal nursing. *Nursing Ethics, 19*(1), 80–90.

Halpern, S. D. (2011). Perceived inappropriateness of care in the ICU: What to make of the clinician's perspective? *JAMA: Journal of the American Medical Association, 306*(24), 2725–2726.

Huffman, D. M., & Rittenmeyer, L. (2012). How professional nurses working in hospital environments experience moral distress: A systematic review. *Critical Care Nursing Clinics of North America, 24*(1), 91–100.

Jameton, A. (1984). *Nursing practice: The ethical issues*. Englewood Cliffs, NJ: Prentice-Hall.

Jameton, A. (1993). Dilemmas of moral distress: Moral responsibility and nursing practice. *Clinical Issues in Perinatal and Women's Health Nursing, 4*(4), 542–551.

Kelly, B. (1998). Preserving moral integrity: A follow-up study with new graduate nurses. *Journal of Advanced Nursing, 28*(5), 1134–1145.

Liaschenko, J. (1995). Artificial personhood: Nursing ethics in a medical world. *Nursing Ethics, 2*(3), 185–196.

MacIntyre, A. C. (1988). *Whose justice? Which rationality?* Notre Dame, IN: University of Notre Dame Press.

McArthur, A. (2010). How professional nurses working in hospital environments experience moral distress: A systematic review. *Journal of Advanced Nursing, 66*(5), 962–963.

Mueller, P. S., Ottenberg, A. L., Hayes, D. L., & Koenig, B. A. (2011). "I felt like the angel of death": Role conflicts and moral distress among allied professionals employed by the US cardiovascular implantable electronic device industry. *Journal of Interventional Cardiac Electrophysiology: An International Journal of Arrhythmias and Pacing, 32*(3), 253–261.

Nathaniel, A. K. (2004). A grounded theory of moral reckoning in nursing. *Grounded Theory Review, 4*(1), 43–58.

Nathaniel, A. K. (2006). Moral reckoning in nursing. *Western Journal of Nursing Research, 28*(4), 419–438; discussion 439–448.

Piers, R. D., Azoulay, E., Ricou, B., Dekeyser, G. F., Decruyenaere, J., Max, A., ... Benoit, D. D. (2011). Perceptions of appropriateness of care among European and Israeli intensive care unit nurses and physicians. *JAMA: The Journal of The American Medical Association, 306*(24), 2694–2703.

Piers, R. D., Van den Eynde, M., Steeman, E., Vlerick, P., Benoit, D. D., & Van den Noortgate, N. J. (2012). End-of-Life Care of the Geriatric Patient and Nurses' Moral Distress. *Journal of the American Medical Directors Association, 13*(1), 80.e7–80.e13.

Penticuff, J. H. (1997). Nursing perspectives in bioethics. In K. Hoshino (Ed.), *Japanese and western bioethics* (pp. 49–60). The Dordrecht: Kluwer Academic Publishers.

Rodney, P. (1988). Moral distress in critical care nursing. *Canadian Critical Care Nursing Journal, 5*(2), 9–11.

Simpson, J. A., & Weiner, E. S. C. (1989). *The oxford English dictionary* (2nd ed., Vol. XIII). New York, NY: Oxford University Press.

Smith, M. J., & Liehr, P. (2008). The theory of attentively embracing story. In M. J. Smith & P. Liehr (Eds.), *Middle range theory for nursing* (pp. 205–224). New York, NY: Springer Publishing.

Strauss, A. L. (1959). *Mirrors and masks: The search for identity.* Glencoe, IL: Free Press.

Wilkinson, J. M. (1987). Moral distress in nursing practice: Experience and effect. *Nursing Forum, 23*(1), 16–29.

Section Three

Concept Building for Research—Through the Lens of Middle Range Theory

This section includes a beginning chapter that describes a rigorous concept building process that moves the scholar from a practice story to a conceptual foundation that can be used for research. This concept building process identifies 10 phases: (1) writing a meaningful practice story; (2) naming the central phenomenon of the practice story—the emerging concept; (3) identifying a theoretical lens for the emerging concept; (4) linking the emerging concept to existing literature; (5) gathering a story from a person who has experienced the central phenomenon of the emerging concept; (6) writing a reconstructed story (from the story collected in phase 5) and a mini-saga, that captures the message of the reconstructed story; (7) identifying core qualities of the emerging concept; (8) formulating a definition that integrates core qualities—the working concept; (9) drawing a model that depicts relationships between core qualities of the working concept; and (10) creating a mini-synthesis that integrates the working concept definition with a population to suggest a research direction. The concept building process described in the first chapter sets the stage for the next two chapters, where the process is presented by doctoral students who have developed the concepts of "yearning for sleep while enduring distress" and "reconceptualizing normal." The reader will notice that each doctoral student scholar has embraced the concept building process in a unique way so that the phases of the process are represented in a way that makes sense for the scholar. The concept building processes—as described in these two chapters—are exemplars showing intellectual discipline and a respect for the logical connection essential for creating meaningful conceptual structures to guide research. The last two chapters show how evolution of a concept that was developed using the 10-phase process has blossomed into a proposal for dissertation research.

16

Concept Building for Research

Patricia R. Liehr and Mary Jane Smith

S ince we first wrote about the 10-phase concept building approach 5 years ago (Liehr & Smith, 2008), our experience has shaped our thinking and contributed to our critique and refinement of the approach (Smith & Liehr, 2012). In this chapter, we describe the most recent refinement of the process for concept building.

Building concepts for research is a critical thought process central and necessary to becoming a researcher. Critical thought processes include understanding of levels of abstraction, abduction/induction/deduction, analysis/synthesis, and appreciation for tacit/explicit knowing. We begin with a focus on the ladder of abstraction (Chapter 2), teaching students to agilely move up and down the ladder rungs from philosophical to theoretical to empirical perspectives. Discoursing at differing levels of abstraction is a logical endeavor of connecting ideas in a way that makes sense, is coherent, and can be understood by the use of reason. Dimensions of logical reasoning essential for developing concepts for research include abduction, induction, and deduction. These logic dimensions are not separate but move back and forth in an iterative way. Abduction is an interpretative reconstruction and a logic of discovery (Wirth, 2004). Adbuctive reasoning begins with an incomplete set of observations such as a practice story and moves toward naming the emerging concept that surfaces in the practice story. Abductive reasoning is inventive; it demands the ability to synthesize. Inductive reasoning takes empirical information such as observations and comments noted while gathering a practice story and moves to a more general or theoretical perspective. Deduction moves from a general or theoretical perspective to specifics. Learning to respect all levels of abstraction in the logical progression of analysis/synthesis is the rigorous foundation essential for building a concept for research.

Analysis/synthesis shines through the phases of the concept building process. For instance, identifying core qualities of a concept demands analysis to distill defining elements in the literature and the empirical evidence from practice stories; and synthesis demands coherent organized expression that makes sense to others. Inherent in this expression is tacit and explicit knowing. Polanyi (1958, 1966) describes tacit knowing as intuitive and inexpressible ... beyond what can be made explicit. In contrast, explicit knowing is expressed as full description with details that paint a picture. As students become aware of what they tacitly know, for instance through nursing practice experience, they attempt to make what is tacit, explicit. This is an important critical thought process that proceeds with the understanding that some dimension of knowing will always remain tacit.

Each of these critical thinking processes is intertwined with the other, challenging the student to stay with concept building, revisiting and revising as views that are cloudy become clear, incorporating other dimensions and requiring another cycle of revisiting and revising ... patient presence with an idea to bring it to a place that enables guidance for practice and research. Smith (1988) has described "wallowing while waiting" as a critical skill for students who are growing their ideas for research. She describes wallowing as dwelling with the obscure and says: "In coming through the obscurity, sudden insights illuminate the connections. These insights are moments of coherence, flashes of unity, as though suddenly the fog lifts and clarity prevails. These moments of coherence push one beyond to deepened levels of understanding" (p. 3).

Although we consistently refer to "students" throughout this chapter, we have used this term to indicate any scholar who is building a concept to guide research. The chapter offers guidance to graduate students and to faculty teaching courses where students are working to build concepts that will guide research. The chapter may also be helpful to practitioners and junior nursing faculty who are actively engaged in developing their ideas for research. The systematic approach to be described in this chapter includes 10-phases: (1) write a meaningful practice story, (2) name the central phenomenon in the practice story—it is your emerging concept, (3) identify the theoretical lens for viewing the emerging concept, (4) link the emerging concept to existing literature, (5) gather a story from a person who has experienced the central idea of the emerging concept, (6) write a reconstructed story using what was shared in phase 5 and create a mini-saga that captures the message of the reconstructed story, (7) identify core qualities of the emerging concept, (8) formulate a definition that integrates the core qualities—it is your working concept, (9) draw a model that depicts relationships between the core qualities of the working concept, and (10) create a mini-synthesis that integrates the working concept definition with a population to suggest a research direction. This process is not meant to be linear, where the student completes one phase and then goes on to the next. Rather, the process begins and then touches back to previous phases, always creating a work in progress with care to maintain correspondence among the phases and ongoing clarification of the defining core qualities.

It is important to note that the student is building a concept rather than building a theory. Sometimes conceptual structures advance through research to become theories (Choi, 2008; Nathaniel, 2008; Williams, 2008) but such development is not the focus of this chapter. The two chapters that follow by Shapiro (Chapter 17) and Greif (Chapter 18) are provided as exemplars of the concept-building process; this chapter will reference those to allow the reader to consider ways that the 10-phase process comes to life in the work of doctoral students.

PRACTICE STORY

The first phase begins with evidence from a practice story. The practice story addresses a critical incident in nursing practice related to caring in the human health experience that stirs the students' interest. Before writing the story, students are engaged in a discussion about their research interest and then requested to think about a practice situation. Sometimes, students who are clear about their research interests write a story that is closely tied to that interest. Sometimes, if a student is unclear about research interests, a detailed practice story that captures caring in the human health experience will help to uncover an interest that can be pursued for research.

Writing the story can take place in class or as an assignment. Students are invited to bring the practice situation into focus, place themselves in a quiet place where they can stay with their focus, and begin writing. They are instructed to begin by describing their first encounter and writing the story event by event, ending with how the situation came to a close. The practice story has a beginning, middle, and end and is centered on a nurse–person situation. Students are told not to worry about grammar or spelling but just to write the story as it comes to them. They then set the story aside and attend to details about the situation that come to them in their everyday coming and going.

After a few days, they can edit their story for sentence mechanics and add detail. Discussion with colleagues often leads to clarification of confusing story elements. These discussions—which can occur during face-to-face or Internet discussion board dialogue—help the students to craft the final version of the practice story.

There is a range of ways that stories about caring in the human health experience are recounted. Sometimes, as in the case of Greif (Chapter 18), the story comes from pressing issues that arise in current practice. Sometimes, the story comes from an indirect source, as in the case of Shapiro (Chapter 17), where the practice story emerges from her role as a clinical instructor for students caring for the patient she describes. Sometimes the story is the composite of more than one patient; it is created to address observations essential for caring in the human health experience. The practice story is retrospective. It is a recounting of an event that has happened in the past that sticks with the student, calling for attention as a focus for research. The focus for research is an issue that the student wants to "do something about" and the practice story will be a nurse–patient situation that highlights the issue demanding attention … it is the central phenomenon of the story.

CENTRAL PHENOMENON

The central phenomenon is a human health experience. For Greif (Chapter 18), the central phenomenon was "reconceptualizing normal," which eventually became her concept for research. For Shapiro (Chapter 17), the central phenomenon was "yearning for sleep while enduring distress." "Reconceptualizing normal" and "yearning for sleep while enduring distress" are both human health experiences that can be applied to many populations across a broad range of age groups. For instance, although "reconceptualizing normal" was identified as experienced by families whose child had experienced a traumatic brain injury, the phenomenon has applicability for newly diagnosed cancer patients, parents who are experiencing an "empty nest," or persons recently admitted to a nursing home. Likewise, who hasn't experienced "yearning for sleep while enduring distress?" The broad range of applicability for these phenomena highlight their place at the middle range level of abstraction, not too high so that they can't readily translate for use in practice and research and not too low so that they apply to only one population.

The phenomenon begins to emerge as the practice story is analyzed in relation to a student's area of research interest. Analysis requires that the student draw inferences about what is going on in the story that evokes passion. Story analysis can be a group endeavor led by a faculty mentor where all participants in a seminar receive a copy of the practice story to establish a foundation for dialogue, or it can occur through an Internet discussion board. Once the phenomenon is identified, it must be named.

Naming the phenomenon requires considerable scrutiny and deliberation. It is an arduous process aimed at addressing a substantive area for study. Usually, several names are considered before settling on a name to move on with concept building. At this point, when a name is selected, we recognize that it is a snapshot of a work in progress and therefore may be fine-tuned as the concept building work continues. Maximum flexibility is attained when the phenomenon is named at a middle range level of abstraction. A common mistake made by beginners is that a diagnosis, like congestive heart failure, is named instead of a human health experience. In this situation, students are called to focus on the human health experience, such as persistent tiredness, instead of the diagnosis. When the phenomenon has been named, the student has identified an emerging concept.

THEORETICAL LENS

The theoretical lens is a perspective for viewing the emerging concept. This perspective can come from a grand theory or from a middle range theory. The perspective shapes the meaning of the emerging concept. For instance, persistent tiredness will be described differently if one is looking through the lens of human becoming theory (Parse, 1992), as compared with the theory of unpleasant symptoms (Lenz & Pugh, 2008). If viewing persistent tiredness through the lens of human becoming grand theory, the meaning of the emerging concept might reflect multidimensional co-creation of the reality of tiredness through recognition of the value placed on feeling energetic. If viewing through the middle range theory of unpleasant symptoms, the meaning of the phenomenon could include physiological, psychological, and situational factors influencing persistent tiredness and symptoms that interact and accentuate tiredness.

Paley (1996) argues for the importance of the theoretical niche when clarifying concepts: "The meaning of a term is made specific when it becomes part of a specific theory" (p. 577). He advocates locating concepts within a theoretical niche so that the meaning is specified by the overall structure of the theory. From this perspective, students are guided to develop a solid understanding of a theory and its related methodologies, acknowledging the niche for their emerging concept.

For an emerging concept named at a middle range level of abstraction, a middle range theory can create a contextual niche with a strong logical connection. A stronger logical connection enhances clarity of the emerging concept supported through coherence with the theory ontology, epistemology, and methodology. As examples, Greif selected the middle range theory of uncertainty for "reconceptualizing normal" and Shapiro selected the theory of symptom management for the emerging concept, "yearning for sleep while enduring distress." The reader will recognize the glove-like fit for these concepts with their theoretical niches when they read Chapters 17 and 18. The tightness of this fit contributes significantly to ongoing development of the emerging concept.

In the appendix of this book, there is a table of middle range theories published over the last few decades. Theories in this table were identified through a Cumulative Index of Nursing and Health Literature (CINAHL) search using the search terms "middle range theory," "mid-range theory," and "midrange theory." The editors selected these theory citations as ones that: were published in English; focused on theory development and/or presentation; and clearly identified the theory by name. Also, none of the citations in the table were the culmination of a concept analysis process. Students could use this table to identify a theoretical lens that "fits like a glove" with their emerging concept. Once the theory is identified, it is important to come to know it so that the nuances of the theory can be fully embraced as a comfortable space for growing the ideas central to the emerging concept.

RELATED LITERATURE

The related literature is the existing body of knowledge associated with the emerging concept. The question guiding the literature review is: What core qualities describe the essence of the emerging concept? Three approaches for beginning exploration of related literature are described: theoretical, population-based, and linguistic. While all three are recommended, the order for using the three approaches is not dictated by the concept building process.

One approach for viewing the emerging concept is to explore the foundational literature supporting the theoretical perspective. Oftentimes, if the fit between the theory and the emerging concept is tight, the literature supporting the theory will provide insights that will guide reflective analysis of the emerging concept.

A second approach is population based. Oftentimes, the population that was the context for the human health experience described in the practice story will provide a literature source. For instance, if the practice story described persistent tiredness in a population with congestive heart failure, the literature related to heart failure symptoms will provide direction about the core qualities of the emerging concept. However, persistent tiredness affects other populations besides those with congestive heart failure. People undergoing chemotherapy may describe persistent tiredness as may pregnant women. In this approach to analyzing related literature, the student reviews the literature from multiple population perspectives, seeking to find the reoccurring descriptors for the emerging concept.

A third approach is to explore the literature associated with the emerging concept name, the linguistic approach. For instance, for persistent tiredness, tiredness and fatigue would be search terms that would be explored. If the emerging concept is more abstract, such as cultural belonging, then exploring the literature on social support to identify descriptors of belonging would be helpful. Even literature about gangs might provide insight about the meaning of belonging. There is an element of creative vision in exploring the literature related to the emerging concept. The student is challenged to stay with the concept as it is grounded in familiar literature and move beyond familiar literature to access perspectives that may extend understanding. For instance, if a student has not encountered the literature from other disciplines while seeking to identify core qualities, it is important to intentionally seek out such literature to consider the emerging concept through those scholarly writings.

Some students have found that a structured approach to analysis/synthesis of the literature enhances the concept-building process. One method helpful in reviewing the literature on the emerging concept is a literature matrix set forth on a spreadsheet with rows and columns (Garrard, 2011). Column topics are based on the question guiding the literature search, emphasizing topics that will inform identification of core qualities. Selection of information to insert in the matrix is a process of analysis that includes both critical reading and thinking to select literature that fits with the column topic and has relevance for the emerging concept. For instance, when exploring the theoretical literature, column headings could be author, title, journal, year, purpose, and theoretical perspective. The columns labeled "purpose" and "theoretical perspective" demand discernment to select appropriate content for the matrix. Shapiro's matrix (Chapter 17) provides an example of theoretical literature and literature foundational to the core qualities. She chose column headings of author, year, journal, title, core quality, substantive nursing foundation, and key words. Organizing the literature in this manner provided a base for synthesizing relevant information in the related literature.

At the completion of this phase, students will have a rudimentary list of core qualities for their emerging concept that is rooted in the literature. Core qualities are the defining properties of the concept. At this point, before moving to the next phase, the student is encouraged to consider the list of core qualities and use an inductive approach to group and name like qualities so that at least two and no more than four core qualities are identified for further exploration.

GATHER A STORY

We have found that students can use guidance regarding story gathering. For the purpose of concept building, we are advocating two phases of story gathering. In the first phase, the student will query the human health experience designated by the emerging concept, and in the second phase, the student will query each of the core qualities identified from the literature.

In the first phase, if the emerging concept is persistent tiredness, the student might ask the person to describe a time when tiredness lasted an unusually long time. Sometimes it is useful to begin by asking about tiredness now, about when it started, how it progressed until now, and what hopes are held regarding the experience of tiredness in the future. This present, past, and future perspective has been described as a story-path approach (Liehr & Smith, 2008). The intent of this first phase of story gathering is to come to know the unbiased thoughts and feelings about the emerging concept.

One of the lessons regarding story gathering is related to languaging the question for the person sharing the story. For instance, Greif (Chapter 18) was interested in "reconceptualizing normal" for families whose child suffered a traumatic brain injury. It would not be appropriate to ask family members how they reconceptualized normal. This question is likely to have little meaning if asked directly. Rather, the student might pose a series of statements/questions such as: I would like to know what is normal, everyday living for you now; how is that different since your son's/daughter's traumatic brain injury?; let's talk about what has happened between the time of the injury and now. This approach to engaging will allow the student to gather a story that captures what matters most about reconceptualizing normal.

In the second phase of story gathering, the student will specifically query the core qualities identified through analysis/synthesis of relevant literature. This phase will be prefaced with an explanation indicating that literature sources have suggested these qualities and the intention of the dialogue is to verify or bring into question each of the qualities noted from the literature. In this case, the person sharing the story is an expert who knows the emerging concept as an embodied experience. This way of knowing contributes powerful evidence to expand the student's understanding.

After gathering a story from someone who knows the emerging concept through experience, it may be necessary to return to the literature to seek out a core quality that arose in the dialogue but was not evident in the original literature search. Another reason to go back to the literature is to re-examine a literature-based core quality that was not confirmed in the story-gathering dialogue. When gathering a story to inform concept building, it is important to conduct the story gathering as the phases direct, so that questions about the core qualities are introduced after an open unbiased discussion about the human health experience. Sometimes a core quality will be introduced in the first-phase open discussion. When that happens, the student should take note and re-introduce the core quality in phase two so that further development and enhanced understanding can be pursued.

RECONSTRUCT STORY AND MINI-SAGA

In writing the reconstructed story, the student creates a beginning, middle, and end that highlight the core qualities situated in the human health experience described by the storyteller in the previous phase. The reconstructed story incorporates the personal knowing of the nurse but strives to present a whole story about the emerging concept as shared by the storyteller. This writing asks that the nurse "get into the shoes" of the other to bring to life the emerging concept.

The mini-saga is a short story that synthesizes the reconstructed story. According to Pink (2005), "Mini-sagas are *extremely* short stories—just fifty words long ... no more, no less" (p. 117). Like the reconstructed story, there is a beginning, middle, and end. The mini-saga captures the core meaning of the storyteller, so that anyone hearing it has a sense of the importance of the emerging concept as it is lived. The purpose of the mini-saga is to crystallize the essence of the emerging concept so that it can be readily shared with others. Writing the mini-saga is hard work and requires dialogue with peers and mentors that can be structured through either face-to-face seminars or Internet discussion boards.

DEFINE THE CORE QUALITIES

The core qualities are the defining properties of the emerging concept. The student has been formulating the core qualities throughout the phases of this process, and at this phase of concept building, there is enhanced clarity about the nature of the qualities, enabling an explicit definition of each of the two to four core qualities. Each core quality definition will cite the associated literature essential to the definition. The student is asked to stay with the identified core qualities at each phase of the continuing process. At this point, the concept is on the brink of moving from emerging to working.

DEFINE THE WORKING CONCEPT

Once the definition is expressed, the working concept is established for use. The definition is a sentence that begins with the name of the concept followed by "is" (e.g., Persistent tiredness is ...). The rest of the sentence arranges the core qualities as related to each other to describe the working concept. Although this seems straightforward, it is often difficult to create this defining sentence so that the core qualities are arranged in a meaningful way. Oftentimes, there is much attention to the connecting words, such as *through, to,* or *from.* Repositioning of core qualities and alternate choices of connecting words can create very different definitions. For instance, Greif (Chapter 18) defined reconceptualizing normal: Reconceptualizing normal is willing openness to know anew through intentional flexibility and unconditional love. Shapiro (Chapter 17) defined yearning for sleep while enduring distress as: Yearning for sleep while enduring distress is suffering yet longing for comfort. In both of these examples, there is a lead core quality: willing openness to know anew for Greif and suffering for Shapiro. If the lead core quality was shifted so that, for instance, unconditional love was the lead core quality for Greif, the definition could convey a very different meaning that would affect the structure of the ensuing model. The concept definition is an original contribution of the student. It requires that the student take a stand and make a unique contribution.

MODEL

The model is a structural representation of the definition, depicting the relationships between the core qualities of the working concept. It is expected that there is congruence between the definition and the model. That is, the core qualities that appear in the definition will appear in the model. It is understood that the model is situated in a theoretical niche, and the student will be able to discuss the link among the theoretical perspective, concept definition, and model.

MINI-SYNTHESIS

The mini-synthesis is a three-sentence creation that pulls together the concept building process. The first sentence addresses the significance of the phenomenon in the context of a particular population. The second sentence is the definition of the working concept. The third sentence suggests an approach for moving toward a research question.

Although described as a linear process, concept building is iterative and creative with every opportunity to circle back and bring new knowledge to an already accomplished phase. The entire 10-phase process simply brings the student to the doorstep of further development through research. In Chapters 19 and 20, Ramsey and Wands take the reader onto the next step of their PhD journey by sharing how their working concepts provided guidance for their dissertation research proposals.

REFERENCES

Choi, H. (2008). Theory of cultural marginality. In M. J. Smith & P. R. Liehr (Eds.), *Middle range theory for nursing.* New York, NY: Springer Publishing.

Garrard, J. (2011). *Health sciences literature review made easy.* Sudbury, MA: Jones & Bartlett Learning.

Lenz, E. R., & Pugh, L. C. (2008). Theory of unpleasant symptoms. In M. J. Smith & P. R. Liehr (Eds.), *Middle range theory for nursing.* New York, NY: Springer Publishing.

Liehr, P. R. & Smith, M. J. (2008). Building structures for research. In M. J. Smith & P. R. Liehr (Eds.). *Middle range theory for nursing.* New York, NY: Springer Publishing.

Nathaniel, A. (2008). Theory of moral reckoning. In M. J. Smith & P. R. Liehr (Eds.), *Middle range theory for nursing.* New York, NY: Springer Publishing.

Paley, J. (1996). How not to clarify concepts in nursing. *Journal of Advanced Nursing, 24,* 572–578.

Parse, R. R. (1992). Human becoming: Parse's theory of nursing. *Nursing Science Quarterly, 5*(1), 35–42.

Pink, D. H. (2005). *A whole new mind: Moving from the information age to the conceptual age.* New York, NY: Penguin Group.

Polanyi, M. (1958). *The study of man.* Chicago, IL: University of Chicago Press.

Polanyi, M. (1966). *The tacit dimension.* London, UK: Routledge & Kegan Paul Ltd.

Smith, M. J. (1988). Theoretical dilemmas: Wallowing while waiting. *Nursing Science Quarterly, 1*(1), 3.

Smith, M. J. & Liehr, P. R. (2012). Concept building: Applying rigor to conceptualize phenomena for nursing research. *Applied Nursing Research, 25,* 65–67.

Williams, L. (2008). Theory of caregiving dynamics. In M. J. Smith & P. R. Liehr (Eds.), *Middle range theory for nursing* (2nd ed., pp. 261–276). New York, NY: Springer Publishing.

Wirth, U. (2004). What is abductive inference. Retrieved from http://user.uni-frankfurt.de/~with/inference.htm

17

Yearning for Sleep While Enduring Distress: A Concept for Nursing Research

April Lynne Shapiro

Nursing science evolves as phenomena for research are generated. Phenomena stem from nursing practice and explicate the meaning of caring in the human health experience (Newman, Sime, & Corcoran-Perry, 1991). The peeling out of concepts and theories is derived from the abductive method of inquiry and inferences are made in the conceptual leap from practice to phenomena for study (Reed, 1995).

The purpose of this chapter is to describe and discuss a phenomenon for further study and the iterative process by which it was developed. Each step of the phenomenon-building process is described, followed by the sequential unfolding of the structure. A neomodernist approach to inquiry is presented, with emphasis on practice-based epistemology (Reed, 1995).

Sleep pattern disturbance is prevalent globally; this is evident in nursing practice and described in the literature. Poor sleep plagues the individual with a multitude of distressing physical and emotional symptoms that permeate every aspect of an individual's daily life, affecting intimate, family, social, and work relationships (Rakel, 2009; Reishtein et al., 2006). The need for further inquiry into this human health experience led to the development of the phenomenon yearning for sleep while enduring distress.

PHENOMENON DEVELOPMENT: THE JOURNEY

This phenomenon was developed based on the systematic, 10-step process for building structures for research (Liehr & Smith, 2008). This process walks the budding scholar through the phases of concept building to develop a phenomenon of interest—from the writing of a practice story that addresses a human health experience significant to the scholar, to the creation of a mini-synthesis that summarizes the process (Liehr & Smith, 2008). However, these steps are not linear; they only serve to guide the scholar through the necessary phases of the phenomenon-building process.

THE BEGINNING: A PRACTICE STORY AND THE PHENOMENON

The researcher begins the process of inquiry by writing a practice story about a significant human health experience encountered in practice (Liehr & Smith, 2008). This practice theorizing—as proposed by Reed (2006)—assists the scholar in making the link between empirical and conceptual knowledge. The practice story—in the developmental context—provides a meta-narrative foil to which the researcher evaluates his or her phenomenon. In this phase, the researcher asks three questions: "Does this phenomenon demonstrate human developmental potential? Does it demonstrate a transcendent capacity for health and healing? Does the phenomenon recognize the individual's history in its developmental context?" (Reed, 1995). From a careful analysis of the practice story, the phenomenon of interest unfolds.

The development of the phenomenon—yearning for sleep while enduring distress—began with the writing of the practice story about Mark, a 47-year-old man with sleep apnea.

PRACTICE STORY EXEMPLAR

Mark is 47 years old and appears much older. His 5-foot-7-inch frame carries around 375 pounds every moment of every day. His weight did not come on overnight; he has been gaining pounds steadily since he was a teen. He has struggled with the teasing and taunting of being overweight, as he refers to it, all of his life.

Mark doesn't sleep well. In fact, he says he wakes up many mornings feeling like he hadn't even slept a wink, navigating through life in a 24/7 fog. He tosses and turns all night long, as reflected in the 11 to 7 nurse's notes throughout his chart. His loud snoring and intermittent gasps resonate down the long hall to the nurse's station, usually waking up many residents along the way, especially the three men sharing a room with him.

Mark is often caught dozing during his day-to-day activities, even during his favorite Bingo and Pokeno games. His daytime sleepiness interferes with even the simplest socialization. He falls asleep in the middle of a conversation with peers and nursing staff, sometimes at mid-sentence. When my students and I are in the room assisting with his hygiene or giving him his medications, he cannot stay awake for more than 10 or 15 minutes at a time. Consequently, when he is able to stay awake, he complains about how tired he is and how much of a struggle it is just to get to the bedside commode or into his wheelchair.

Mark often complains of headache, for which he takes acetaminophen or ibuprofen to no avail. He says that headache wakes him up in the morning and put him to sleep at night. He tells me he has developed a high pain tolerance and, thus, has learned to cope with these nuisances. He accepts them as a part of his everyday life, just as he does eating and breathing.

As a result of his obesity, Mark has developed type 2 diabetes. This is another area where obstructive sleep apnea (OSA) makes its presence known; sleep apnea has been demonstrated to contribute to poor blood sugar control. Before meals and at bedtime, Mark gets his finger stuck to check his glucose level to see whether he will need yet another needle-stick of insulin. In most cases (especially before lunch), his sugars are high, and therefore, he gets the additional sticks he so dreads. He often complains about all this poking and prodding, especially on laboratory days when the phlebotomist comes in to draw his blood for more tests.

Through the years, my students and I talked to Mark about OSA, its effects on his body, and the benefits of treatment with continuous positive airway pressure. He always told me, "I don't want to have to wear that mask. I sleep with a fan on my nightstand; that's enough. It helps me breathe." I sense he has accepted living in this hypercapnic world he has created; he wants no part of any changes we suggest. These experiences define Mark's everyday existence.

This past spring, I brought a new group of students to the nursing home. Mark was still there, but with a new chapter of his life story to share with me. Last winter, he suffered a heart attack and had been in the intensive care unit on a ventilator. They had much difficulty weaning him from the ventilator due to the thick size of his neck and poor oxygenation status. As I listened to Mark, I noticed the tracheostomy at almost the exact same time he pointed to it. "They had to put in a trach," he said. I asked him about how he was coping with all this, including the heart attack, the long hospital stay, being on a ventilator, and now living with a permanent trach. Again, I heard the familiar echoes, "I've just learned to live with it," he said, as he pulled off the purple speaking valve to show me. He let one of the nursing students do his trach care that morning; predictably, he slept through every moment of it after the initial coughing with the inner cannula change. I realized, in that moment, that the trach had become part of him and not just in the literal sense. Without planning for or realizing it, Mark did get treatment for his sleep apnea in the form of the trach.

I often reflect on Mark's life before that winter and before the heart attack and trach, and ask myself some all-too-familiar questions as I have with other patients like him. What would Mark's life have been like if he could just sleep? What if Mark had had good sleep during the night with no tossing, turning, snoring, or gasping? A life with no headache? A life without the fog? If he didn't have sleep apnea, I wonder, would he be who he is today?

Based on the author's personal nursing practice and themes that emerged from Mark's story, the need to explore the phenomenon of yearning for sleep emerged. This specific phenomenon addresses a substantive area for study based on human health experience and reflects the middle range level of abstraction (Liehr & Smith, 2008).

THEORETICAL UNDERPINNINGS AND THE PARADIGMATIC PERSPECTIVE: FINDING THE NICHE

The researcher extrapolates the meaning of the phenomenon of study by examining it through a theoretical lens, a niche that bridges the connection between the ontology, epistemology, and methodology (Liehr & Smith, 2008). The theoretical niche provides a conceptual link to ground the phenomenon in nursing theory (Paley, 1996). On the ladder of abstraction, the theoretical connection emerges most logically from a middle range theory but may also make the leap to grand theory or paradigm (Liehr & Smith, 2008). Moving the phenomenon to the theoretical literature is a step in conceptualization and begins the structure building for a theoretical concept.

Middle Range Theory: Symptom Management Theory

The phenomenon—yearning to sleep while enduring distress—is directly linked to the middle range theory of symptom management (SMT) (Dodd et al., 2001; Humphreys et al., 2008). This theory provides a framework that ties the concept to nursing science and research. SMT is composed of three essential concepts: symptom experience, symptom management strategies, and symptom status outcomes. These concepts are framed within the nursing science dimensions of person, environment, and health and illness (Dodd et al., 2001; Humphreys et al., 2008).

Defining a Symptom

A symptom is a subjective phenomenon regarded by an individual as a deviation from that which is normal in the aspects of function, sensation, or appearance (Rhodes & Watson, 1987). Several different types of symptoms have been described in the literature, including physical, psychophysical, emotional, and cognitive; these symptoms negatively impact a person's health perception, ability to function, and overall quality of life (Wilson & Cleary, 1995). The distress caused by these symptoms may also involve physical and emotional suffering and anguish (Rhodes & Watson, 1987). Rarely does a symptom occur in isolation; discussion of symptom clusters is emerging in symptom theory development (Brant, Beck, & Miaskowski, 2009).

An individual with a sleep disturbance is plagued by a myriad of distressing physical, psychological, and emotional symptoms. These symptoms affect not only the individual but also those within his or her family and social networks. This symptom distress, over time, may lead to decreased self-esteem, dependence, and a sense of powerlessness. "Symptom distress has particular importance in nursing practice, education, and research to detect disease, promote the speed of recovery, maintain health, and enhance the quality of life" (Rhodes & Watson, 1987, p. 242).

Symptom Experience

The symptom experience is the individual's perception, evaluation, and response to a symptom (Humphreys et al., 2008). A person with a sleep disturbance experiences a multitude of distressing psychological and physical symptoms, both night and day. These symptoms range from mild to severe and include feelings of anxiety and depression, excessive sleepiness and fatigue, impaired memory and concentration, and pain related to headache. The individual suffers from the effect of these symptoms that varies in relation to the number and severity of symptoms endured.

Symptom Management Strategies

Symptom management strategies are actions taken by the individual or others to reduce, minimize, or relieve the symptom. More responsibility is shifted to the individual; in essence, he or she becomes the primary caregiver. The individual longs for relief from the multitude of symptoms endured. However, nonadherence may occur if the individual deems the strategies too demanding (Humphreys et al., 2008). For a person yearning for sleep, self-management may involve lifestyle modifications, such as weight loss, environment manipulation, and sleep position changes. If these strategies are not effective or the individual has more severe symptoms, more aggressive intervention may be necessary.

Symptom Status Outcomes

Symptom status outcomes are assessment parameters used to measure the success of the strategies (Humphreys et al., 2008). Improved symptom status may lead to a sense of improved mental and physical functioning and quality of life, as well as improved treatment adherence. This results in an overall feeling of comfort for the individual and can be measured with quality of life (Flemons & Reimer, 1998; Weaver et al., 1997) and psychological outcomes instruments (Beck, Epstein, Brown, & Steer, 1988; Spielberger, 1983; Zigmond & Snaith, 1983).

A person yearning for sleep struggles to find relief from the symptoms endured. He or she suffers from distressing sequelae, including daytime sleepiness and fatigue, impaired concentration and memory, and feelings of anxiety and depression. The individual is forced to integrate these symptoms into daily living and adapt to each day's challenges. The person is more than the symptoms, but becomes overwhelmed by them and the impact they have on existence. The person's suffering is perceived subjectively, and it permeates extensively into all aspects of his or her world. The person longs for change and comfort in the form of rest and sleep.

RELATED LITERATURE: GROUNDING THE CONCEPT IN NURSING SCIENCE

Related literature that explores the existing knowledge base within the concept is then gathered (Liehr & Smith, 2008). The literature search begins with the exploring of the foundational concepts and theories, then shifts to establish the population of interest and the core qualities. This detailed synthesis of the literature roots the new concept in the existing knowledge base of nursing science.

A search of CINAHL, MEDLINE, PsycINFO, and PsycARTICLES— with the key words sleep, suffering, yearning, longing, and comfort— was conducted to explore this concept. The results yielded qualitative studies, conceptual analyses, and discussion papers related to the core qualities and middle range theory. These writings help to align the concept with the established literature and further define the concept's core qualities. The literature findings were organized chronologically onto a review matrix using The Matrix Method (Garrard, 2011; see Table 17.1).

TABLE 17.1
Literature Matrix

Author	Year	Journal	Title	Core quality	Definition	Nursing substantive foundation	Key words
Cassell, E. J.	1982	*The New England Journal of Medicine*	The nature of suffering and the goals of medicine	Suffering	State of severe distress associated with events that threaten intactness of person; can actually grow from suffering, so suffering can be good for people Paradox: suffering is often caused by treatment	Experienced by persons, not merely by bodies; can include pain but not limited to it; personal matter; "the only way to learn what damage is sufficient to cause suffering, or whether suffering is present, is to ask the sufferer" (p. 643; temporal [time] dimension)	None
Rhodes, V. A. & Watson, P. M.	1987	*Seminars in Oncology Nursing*	Symptom distress—the concept: past and present	Middle range theory	Need to alter (restrain or produce) actions in response to a subjective indication of disease or illness	Also defined as physical or mental anguish that results from experience of symptom occurrence and/or perception	None
Costello, R. B. (Ed.)	1991	*Webster's College Dictionary*	N/A	Definitions: Longing Comfort Suffering	See phenomenon	None	N/A
Newman, M. A., Sime, A. M., and Corcoran-Perry, S. A.	1991	*Advances in Nursing Science*	The focus of the discipline of nursing	Unitary trans-formative paradigm	Unitary, self-organizing field embedded in a larger self-organizing field; identified by pattern and interaction with larger whole; interpenetration of fields; unidirectional, unpredictable change	Knowledge is personal, involves pattern recognition, and is a function of both viewer and the phenomenon viewed; from this perspective, caring in the human health experience would be studied as a process of mutuality and creative unfolding	None

(continued)

TABLE 17.1

Literature Matrix (*continued*)

Author	Year	Journal	Title	Core quality	Definition	Nursing substantive foundation	Key words
Palaian, S. K.	1993	Dissertation	The experience of longing: a phenomenological investigation	Longing	Existential part of one's being; ever changing experience yet has an enduring and permanent quality; component of excitement and anticipation of a perfect existence in the future	Five core themes of longing; the concept of longing lives on the continuum of human motivation	None
Morse, J., Bottorf, J. L., & Hutchinson, S.	1994	*Journal of Advanced Nursing*	The phenomenology of comfort	Comfort	State of embodiment that is beyond awareness; best recognized when patient first leaves state of discomfort	Nine themes/states of discomfort: diseased, disobedient, vulnerable, violated, enduring, resigned, deceiving, betraying body, and betraying mind	None
Wilson, I. B. & Cleary, P. D.	1995	*Journal of the American Medical Association*	Linking clinical variables with health-related quality of life	Symptom management	Types of symptoms; health perception, functioning, and quality of life affected by symptoms	Presents a conceptual model of symptoms and health-related quality of life (p. 60)	None
Holm, O.	1999	*The Journal of Psychology*	Analyses of longing: origins, levels, and dimensions	Longing	Blend of primary emotions of love/happiness and sadness/depression; need for something without which one's life does not feel complete	Describes longing in three models; also as secondary emotion, different levels, kinds, and different dimensions of longing; if person feels he or she can do something for him/herself, the feelings of being a helpless/victim get reduced	None

Author	Year	Journal	Title		Description	Model/Process	Concepts/constructs
Dodd et al.	2001	*Journal of Advanced Nursing*	Advancing the science of symptom management	Middle range theory	Symptom defined as subjective experience reflecting changes in biopsychosocial functioning, sensations, or cognition of an individual	Symptom experience, management strategies, and outcomes; person, environment, and health/illness domains; intervention strategies too demanding associated with increased risk; nonadherence	Concepts/constructs related to health, symptom management model, symptom management theory
Fredriksson, L. & Eriksson, K.	2001	*Scandinavian Journal of Caring Science*	The patient's narrative of suffering: apath to health?	Suffering	Suffering and health viewed as two sides of human life; suffering compatible with health if experienced as bearable. Suffering is a "drama" with two acts: confirmation of suffering, and becoming in suffering	Model process: 1. Telling stories (understanding) 2. Making up narrative of suffering (interpretation) 3. Reconnecting to the life history (creation of meaning)	Caring, communication, conversation, narratives, qualitative research synthesis
Morse, J.	2001	*Advances in Nursing Science*	Toward a praxis theory of suffering	Suffering	Emotional suppression (enduring) and emotional suffering; enduring is inward and suffering is outward	Model of suffering (p. 54) Enduring is emotional suppression and suffering is emotional releasing; we move back and forth	Enduring, pain, suffering, theory
Malinowski, A. & Stamler, L. L.	2002	*Journal of Advanced Nursing*	Comfort: exploration of the concept in nursing	Comfort	Outcome of nursing, function of nursing, basic human need, a process	Watson's theory of human caring is discussed	Comfort, Watson, Leininger, nursing theory, caring, health promotion

(continued)

TABLE 17.1

Literature Matrix (*continued*)

Author	Year	Journal	Title	Core quality	Definition	Nursing substantive foundation	Key words
Edwards, S. D.	2003	*Medicine, Health Care, and Philosophy*	Three concepts of suffering	Suffering	Critical assessment of two rivals of suffering: Cassell and van Hooft; sketch a more plausible concept and further scientific understanding of suffering	Good overview of Cassell's and van Hooft's definitions of suffering	Cassell, scientific understanding, suffering, van Hooft
Ohman, M., Soderberg, S., & Lundman, B.	2003	*Qualitative Health Research*	Hovering between suffering and enduring: The meaning of living with serious chronic illness	Suffering	Hover between an escape from the emotional suffering pain of illness and emotionless state of enduring	Feelings presented in three major themes: experiencing body as hindrance, being alone in illness, and struggling for normalcy	Chronic serious illness, lived experience, phenomenological hermeneutic, enduring, suffering, reformulated self
Tutton, E. & Seers K.	2003	*Journal of Clinical Nursing*	An exploration of the concept of comfort	Comfort	State linked to outcomes such as ease, well-being, and satisfaction	Lack of clarity regarding use of the term "comfort"	Caring, comfort, conceptual evaluation, conceptual frameworks, nursing as therapy
Ferrell, B. R. & Coyle, N.	2008	*Oncology Nursing Forum*	The nature of suffering and the goals of nursing	Suffering	Cassell's definition of suffering—it is experienced by persons, not merely by bodies, and has its source in challenges that threaten intactness of person as a complex social and psychologic entity; may include pain, but not limited to it	Suffering is associated with loss, intense emotions, spiritual distress, and inability to express those experiences Ten tenets of suffering	None

Author(s)	Year	Source	Title	Concept	Description	Key Points	Keywords
Mayser, S., Scheibe, S., & Riediger, M.	2008	*European Psychologist*	(Un)Reachable? An empirical differentiation of goals and life longings	Longing	Intense desire for something remote or unattainable; involves sense of incompleteness, personal utopias, symbolism, ambivalent emotional quality, evokes life reflections, evaluations, and ontogenetic tritime phenomenon (past, present, and future)	Sehnsucht (life longing) Life longings more ambivalent, long-term oriented, strongly related to the past, involving a stronger sense of incompleteness than goals	Personal goals, Sehnsucht, life longings, self-regulation
Liehr, P. R. & Smith, M. J.	2008	*Book: Middle Range Theory for Nursing, 2nd ed., Springer, Smith, M. J. & Liehr, P. R., eds.*	Chapter 3: Building Structures for Research	Phenomenon and middle range theory	Ten-step process for building research structure	All levels of phenomenon building process; ladder of abstraction	None
Brant, J. M., Beck, S., and Miaskowski, C.	2009	*Journal of Advanced Nursing*	Building dynamic models and theories to advance the science of symptom management research	Middle range theory	Compares Symptom Management Theory with Theory of Unpleasant Symptoms, symptoms experience model and symptoms experience in time model	Need to build more expansive, dynamic symptom management model paralleling advances in symptom research and practice; need to include symptom clusters, interactions, and changes over time; model (p. 237)	Models, nursing, science, symptom management, theories
Carnevale, F.	2009	*Nursing Ethics*	A conceptual and moral analysis of suffering	Suffering	Suffering is not pain, can only be understood in terms of how it is subjectively experienced by a person; suffering is an emotion, conventionally implied to be "bad"	Suffering is regarded as morally wrong that needs to be made right by health care; paradigm shift: suffering better understood through empathic attunement; What is suffering? Can one's suffering be assessed by another? What is moral significance?	Emotions, empathy, epistemology, moral, pain, suffering

(continued)

TABLE 17.1
Literature Matrix (*continued*)

Author	Year	Journal	Title	Core quality	Definition	Nursing substantive foundation	Key words
Foss, B. & Naden, D.	2009	*Nordic Journal of Nursing Research and Clinical Studies*	Janice Morse' theory of suffering: A discussion in a caring science perspective	Suffering	Emotional response to phenomenon that have previously been endured and suppressed	Comparison of Morse's and Eriksson's theories of suffering; Morse in contextual area and Eriksson in ontological area	Morse, theory, suffering, caring science
Bruce, A., Schreiber, R., Petrovskaya, O., & Boston, P.	2011	*BMC Nursing*	Longing for ground in a ground (less) world: A qualitative inquiry of existential suffering	Longing and suffering	Suffering—concerns related to hopelessness, futility, meaninglessness, disappointment, remorse, death anxiety, disruption of personal identity	To be fully human means to suffer; engage groundlessness, take refuge, and live in between; existential concerns inherent in being human; acknowledge complexity of fear and anxiety, uniquely dynamic nature of these processes for each person	None

A RECONSTRUCTED STORY: THE THEORETICAL NICHE (PAST), CONCEPT (PRESENT), AND POPULATION (FUTURE)

A reconstructed story is gathered from an individual living the concept; this activity further clarifies the concept and the theoretical perspective (Liehr & Smith, 2008). The story is gathered from an individual who has lived the concept to affirm or disaffirm the significance of the concept and its core qualities. The scholar synthesizes the information that was shared as a reconstructed story. The reconstructed story serves to provide empirical evidence for the concept.

Reconstructed Story

Jenny is a 32-year-old woman who has dealt with chronic insomnia since age 16. She was evaluated medically—with both daytime and overnight sleep studies—and was told she has no indications of sleep apnea or narcolepsy. In the past, she took several prescription hypnotics, such as Ambien, Lunesta, and trazodone, but says they did not help her in the long term. She said currently she takes Tylenol PM, with some relief. Here is her story.

Jenny told me that sleep problems are something she has dealt with for half her life, so it is something she just accepts. "I call it 'the counting.' Each night, I watch the clock and think to myself, 'Okay, if I fall asleep within the next 20 minutes, I'll have 5 hours of sleep.' A half hour later, I'm still awake, and I think, 'Okay, if I fall asleep now, I'll have 4 and a half hours of sleep.' I worry about not falling asleep, and that interferes with my falling asleep. This is every night for me; it affects me constantly."

She described her typical evening. "I finish my homework around 9 (I work part time and go to school part time). I wind down, watch television with my roommate, take my Tylenol PM around 11:30, lie down, and wait. I do 'the counting' for sometimes 3 or 4 hours; then I finally fall asleep. When my alarm goes off, I know I need to get up, and I tell myself it's time to get up, but my body doesn't want to, I am tired. I drink coffee, Coke, or Mountain Dew for the caffeine; it helps at first, but then I feel more tired later as the caffeine wears off. This is my every day."

She described the chronic problems she deals with as a result of lack of sleep—both physically and mentally—and the impact they have on her quality of life. "I feel so anxious about it during the day. Sometimes, I even Google 'lack of sleep'! I worry. What if I fall asleep at the wheel, or at work, or at school? And if I am this sleepy going to work or school, how will I feel on the way home?" She notices a decline in her focus and concentration. "I'll be at work or school; I especially notice it at school. My teacher asks a question, and I'll think to myself, 'I know that.' The problem is I can't think of the answer fast enough. When someone else says it, I think, 'Yeah, that's it; I knew that.' I feel groggy. My mind isn't clear. I'm not as sharp."

Jenny described her feelings of desperation for sleep and frustration from the effects on her school, work performance, and socialization skills. "After work or class, my friends say, 'Let's go get dinner.' I don't even have the energy to do that. It's like I just want to do what I have to do and go home, because I'm so tired. I'm so tired throughout the day." She shares how distressing not sleeping well is for her. "Am I ever going to sleep like a normal person? If I could just sleep well, I know I would have better moods, more energy, and better concentration, and would probably lose weight. I also worry about dependence on sleeping pills."

When I asked Jenny how she finds comfort, she shrugged her shoulders. "It's really not that big of a deal to me. I've had this problem so long, I just accept it. I am thankful for the sleep I do get. I do sleep; I just don't sleep well. I've had the sleep studies and tried all the pills, but nothing seems to work. When I was younger, I would try to be busier in the day, like by being more active or doing more things to exert myself, and that would help me sleep better at night; now that doesn't help at all. I talk about it; that helps my anxiety somewhat. My mom says maybe if I wouldn't nap during the day, I would sleep better at night. I think it's the opposite—I nap because I don't sleep well at night. Regardless of whether I nap or not, I still fall asleep at the same time!" Jenny says she has adapted to her lack of sleep, for now.

The Mini-Saga: Crystallizing the Essence of the Concept

The reconstructed story of Jenny highlights the core qualities and captures the essence of this concept of interest. Jenny's plight with sleep disturbance exemplifies the human health experience of an individual plagued with its life-changing ramifications. Like Mark, she is yearning for sleep while enduring distress, suffering daily as a result, and longing for comfort.

The mini-saga synthesizes the reconstructed story and captures its essence and meaning (Liehr & Smith, 2008). A mini-saga is an extremely short story with 50 words (no more, no less) and, like all stories, has a beginning, middle, and end (Pink, 2005). This short story captures the meaning conveyed by the storyteller using creative, yet concise, verbiage.

The essence of Jenny's story is captured in the following mini-saga:
Half her life, she has endured sleep problems. Night after night she
watches the clock, desperately counting the hours, waiting for sleep.
Anxious and frustrated, the lack of sleep permeates school, work,
social life, and health. Testing and treatment have brought no relief.
She yearns for a good night's sleep.

Core Qualities: Defining and Clarifying the Concept

Core qualities are the defining properties of the concept (Liehr &
Smith, 2008). These core qualities make up the definition of the concept
and especially for the connections between the core qualities (Liehr &
Smith, 2008). The core qualities ground the concept in nursing science
and highlight the significance and potential unique contribution of
the concept.

The core qualities of the concept—yearning for sleep while enduring distress—are longing, comfort, and suffering. Yearning for sleep
while enduring distress is suffering, yet longing for comfort. This
definition bridges the core qualities (longing, comfort, and suffering)
to the concept (yearning for sleep while enduring distress). Each core
quality will be described with pertinent literature.

Suffering

Suffering is defined as enduring or settling for and adapting to physical and emotional deterioration, including pain, distress, injury, loss,
or harm (Costello, 1991). Suffering and ease can be viewed as two
sides of human life (Fredriksson & Eriksson, 2001). There are many
dimensions to suffering, including physical, psychological, and spiritual. Suffering is experienced by the individual person, not merely
by the body, and can only be fully understood by the unique person
experiencing it. "The only way to learn what damage is sufficient to
cause suffering, or whether suffering is present, is to ask the sufferer"
(Cassell, 1982, p. 643). It is a subjective phenomenon that only the individual can experience and feel, not something that can be seen in an
objective way (Carnevale, 2009; Edwards, 2003).

A suffering individual is said to move back and forth between
enduring (emotional suppression) and suffering (emotional releasing)
(Morse, 2001) and may even adapt to chronic suffering just as he or she
would to a chronic illness (Cassell, 1982). Cassell (1982) discusses the
paradox that even medical treatment—which is supposed to comfort

a patient—can actually contribute to or even cause suffering. Morse (2001) describes another paradox in suffering: "The paradox is that whereas its public nature enables others to assist in alleviating the suffering, its public nature also demands the emotional suffering be a private behavior" (p. 55). In this sense, suffering can actually mute the voice of the sufferer (Fredriksson & Eriksson, 2001).

Suffering involves loss, but not necessarily pain (Edwards, 2003; Ferrell & Coyle, 2008). The sufferer focuses on the present, allowing him or her to begin to cope with the situation and its circumstances (Morse, 2001). A suffering individual struggles with uncertainty and a sense of groundlessness and "... must continuously renegotiate and reconfigure what is normal ..." (Bruce, Schreiber, Petrovskaya, & Boston, 2011). Suffering is draining to the body and the mind (Morse, 2001); for an individual with a sleep disturbance, this compounds an already distressing existence. A suffering body then becomes a hindrance, a barrier forcing the afflicted individual to live a restricted, dependent life. This has health outcomes, such as feelings of powerlessness and despair, and leaves the individual hovering between the states of suffering and enduring (Ohman, Soderberg, & Lundman, 2003). However, many argue that suffering is actually necessary for healing and recovery and that from suffering comes growth and a reformulated sense of self (Foss & Nåden, 2009; Morse, 2001). "In every setting, across diseases, and in people of all ages, suffering is part of being human, often intensified when being human also involves being ill" (Ferrell & Coyle, 2008, p. 244). An individual with a sleep disturbance longs for relief from the suffering, yet, in many instances, resolves to endure the distress imposed upon the body by it.

Longing

Longing, by definition, is strong, persistent desiring, especially for something unattainable or distant (Costello, 1991). It is a frequent human experience, involving a sense of life incompleteness, ambivalence, and life evaluation and reflection in the past, present, and future (Mayser, Scheibe, & Riediger, 2008). Longing is an existential part of one's being, characterized by excitement and anticipation of a perfect existence in the future, and contributing to human motivation (Palaian, 1993).

Longing forms in childhood, as the child learns attachment (Holm, 1999). It has been regarded as a secondary emotion with different dimensions, mainly a blend of love and happiness with sadness and depression (Holm, 1999). It is dynamic and is not experienced in the same way by every person, every time. "Longing is a complete and utter mystery to its experiencers. It is suffering and it is pleasure. It is inside yet it is outside. It is permanent and ever-present, yet it changes so quickly, often and in many ways" (Palaian, 1993, p. 94). There are various kinds and levels of longing, "for example, longing for something positive to come or for something that is lost forever" (Holm, 1999, p. 623).

Longing can be detrimental to the person psychologically, developmentally, and socially (Holm, 1999). Many persons who are longing are suffering; this can lead to decreased self-confidence and hopelessness (Holm, 1999). These feelings of helplessness and victimization may be lessened if the individual feels empowered to do something for himself or herself (Holm, 1999). For an individual who cannot sleep, these longings persist night into day, causing suffering that can only be ameliorated by comfort and rest.

Comfort

Derived from the Latin word *confortare*, the word "comfort" is described in many ways throughout the literature. According to Costello (1991), comfort is the state of bodily ease and satisfaction, resulting in a feeling of physical and mental rest. It is something one yearns for from birth, the most basic of needs (Malinowski & Stamler, 2002). Comfort is linked to outcomes of well-being and satisfaction (Tutton & Seers, 2003). "Things that provide comfort are familiar, often provide warmth, they help us feel safe, snug, sheltered, protected, and to feel less vulnerable or exposed" (Morse, Bottorff, & Hutchinson, 1994, p. 194). Comfort is an embodied state beyond awareness, best recognized when a person first leaves the state of discomfort (Morse et al., 1994). The concept of comfort can be viewed in the context of sleeplessness; the human health experience involves a constant state of discomfort from which the sufferer yearns to escape.

THE MODEL: A VISUAL REPRESENTATION OF THE CONCEPT AND CORE QUALITIES

In the research structure-building process, a model is created to depict the core qualities and their representation of the concept (Liehr & Smith, 2008). The structural design should be congruent with the definition of the concept reflecting the theoretical lens.

The model for the concept—yearning for sleep while enduring distress—was created based on the established core qualities and

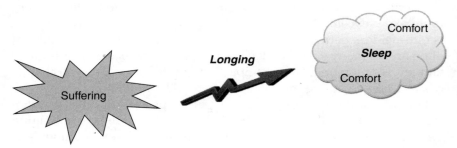

Yearning for sleep while enduring distress is ... *Suffering, yet, longing for comfort*

FIGURE 17.1   Model of New Phenomenon for Research

their relationship to each other. The individual who is yearning for rest is suffering and longing for comfort (in the form of sleep); this is depicted in the model (see Figure 17.1). The shapes represent not only the feelings imposed on the individual by each core quality but also the struggle he or she endures moving from suffering to comfort.

MINI-SYNTHESIS: THE FINAL PHASE

In the systematic process of building structures for research, the final phase involves the writing of a mini-synthesis (Liehr & Smith, 2008). A mini-synthesis is a three-sentence statement that synthesizes the structure-building process (Liehr & Smith, 2008). The first sentence addresses the concept in the context of a population, the second sentence names and defines the concept, and the third sentence suggests implications for future study (Liehr & Smith, 2008).

The mini-synthesis for this concept highlights the impact of sleep disturbances within the population of sleep apnea sufferers. The concept and core qualities are addressed, and the synthesis concludes with a statement regarding the research implications:

Individuals with obstructive sleep apnea endure distress that impacts school, work, family, social life, and health. Yearning for sleep while enduring distress is suffering, yet longing for comfort. A study on early intervention for obstructive sleep apnea may provide evidence on reducing anxiety, improving comfort, and increasing well-being.

CONCLUSION

Developing a unique concept for inquiry is a tedious, iterative process that involves much time, intensive effort, and creativity. The process of building structures for research guides the scholar through the necessary steps to develop an idea from concept to concept that is rich in substance, grounded in theory, and, most importantly, relevant to practice and research. The nursing knowledge explicated during this process promulgates nursing science into deeper realms of caring and healing.

Sleep pattern disturbances and the related symptoms they cause have a direct impact on the human health experience. The concept yearning for sleep while enduring distress adds substance to the existing body of nursing knowledge. The focus on the human health experience reflects the neomodernist practice turn in epistemology that is so critical in conducting meaningful nursing research. This concept will continue to evolve and provide the groundwork for future research.

REFERENCES

Beck, A. T., Epstein, N., Brown, G., & Steer, R. A. (1988). An inventory for measuring clinical anxiety: Psychometric properties. *Journal of Consulting and Clinical Psychology, 56*(6), 893–897.

Brant, J. M., Beck, S., & Miaskowski, C. (2009). Building dynamic models and theories to advance the science of symptom management research. *Journal of Advanced Nursing, 66*(1), 228–240.

Bruce, A., Schreiber, R., Petrovskaya, O., & Boston, P. (2011). Longing for ground in a ground(less) world: A qualitative inquiry of existential suffering. *BMC Nursing, 10*(2), 1–9.

Carnevale, F. A. (2009). A conceptual and moral analysis of suffering. *Nursing Ethics, 16*(2), 173–183.

Cassell, E. J. (1982). The nature of suffering and the goals of medicine. *The New England Journal of Medicine, 306*(11), 639–645.

Costello, R. B. (Ed.). (1991). *Webster's college dictionary*. New York, NY: Random House.

Dodd, M., Janson, S., Facione, N., Faucett, J., Froelicher, E. S., Humphreys, J., & Taylor, D. (2001). Advancing the science of symptom management. *Journal of Advanced Nursing, 33*(5), 668–676.

Edwards, S. D. (2003). Three concepts of suffering. *Medicine, Health Care, and Philosophy, 6*(1), 59–66.

Ferrell, B. R., & Coyle, N. (2008). The nature of suffering and the goals of nursing. *Oncology Nursing Forum, 35*(2), 241–247.

Flemons, W. W., & Reimer, M. A. (1998). Development of a disease-specific health-related quality of life questionnaire for sleep apnea. *American Journal of Respiratory and Critical Care Medicine, 158*(2), 494–503.

Foss, B., & Nåden, D. (2009). Janice Morse' theory of suffering: A discussion in a caring science perspective. *Nordic Journal of Nursing Research & Clinical Studies/Vård i Norden, 29*(1), 14–18.

Fredriksson, L., & Eriksson, K. (2001). The patient's narrative of suffering: A path to health? An interpretative research synthesis on narrative understanding. *Scandinavian Journal of Caring Sciences, 15*(1), 3–11.

Garrard, J. (2011). *Health sciences literature review made easy: The matrix method* (3rd ed.). Sudbury, ON: Jones & Bartlett Learning.

Holm, O. (1999). Analyses of longing: Origins, levels, and dimensions. *Journal of Psychology: Interdisciplinary and Applied, 133*(6), 621–630.

Humphreys, J., Lee, K. A., Carrieri-Kohlman, V., Puntillo, K., Faucett, J., Janson, S., ... the UCSF School of Nursing Symptom Management Faculty Group. (2008). Theory of symptom management. In M. J. Smith & P. R. Liehr (Eds.), *Middle range theory for nursing* (2nd ed., pp. 145–158). New York, NY: Springer.

Liehr, P. R., & Smith, M. J. (2008). Building structures for research. In M. J. Smith & P. R. Liehr (Eds.), *Middle range theory for nursing* (2nd ed., pp. 33–54). New York, NY: Springer.

Malinowski, A., & Stamler, L. L. (2002). Comfort: Exploration of the concept in nursing. *Journal of Advanced Nursing, 39*(6), 599–606.

Mayser, S., Scheibe, S., & Riediger, M. (2008). (Un)reachable? An empirical differentiation of goals and life longings. *European Psychologist, 13*(2), 126–140.

Morse, J. M. (2001). Toward a praxis theory of suffering. *Advances in Nursing Science, 24*(1), 47–59.

Morse, J. M., Bottorff, J. L., & Hutchinson, S. (1994). The phenomenology of comfort. *Journal of Advanced Nursing, 20*(1), 189–195.

Newman, M. A., Sime, A. M., & Corcoran-Perry, S. A. (1991). The focus of the discipline of nursing. *Advances in Nursing Science, 14*(1), 1–6.

Ohman, M., Soderberg, S., & Lundman, B. (2003). Hovering between suffering and enduring: The meaning of living with serious chronic illness. *Qualitative Health Research, 13*(4), 528–542.

Palaian, S. K. (1993). *The experience of longing: A phenomenological investigation* (Doctoral dissertation). Retrieved from http:search.ebscohost.com (Accession number 1995-72770-001)

Paley, J. (1996). How not to clarify concepts in nursing. *Journal of Advanced Nursing, 24*(3), 572–578.

Pink, D. H. (2005). *A whole new mind: Why right-brainers will rule the future* (pp. 119–120). New York, NY: Penguin Group.

Rakel, R. E. (2009). Clinical and societal consequences of obstructive sleep apnea and excessive daytime sleepiness. *Postgraduate Medicine, 121*(1), 86–95.

Reed, P. G. (1995). A treatise on nursing knowledge development for the 21st century: Beyond postmodernism. *Advances in Nursing Science, 17*(3), 70–84.

Reed, P. G. (2006). Scholarly dialogue: The practice turn in nursing epistemology. *Nursing Science Quarterly, 19*(1), 36–38.

Reishtein, J., Pack, A. I., Maislin, G., Dinges, D. F., Bloxham, T., George, C. F. P., ... Weaver, T. E. (2006). Sleepiness and relationships in obstructive sleep apnea. *Issues in Mental Health Nursing, 27*(3), 319–330.

Rhodes, V. A., & Watson, P. M. (1987). Symptom distress—The concept: Past and present. *Seminars in Oncology Nursing, 3*(4), 242–247.

Spielberger, C. D. (1983). *State-Trait anxiety inventory (STAI).* Menlo Park, CA: Mind Garden.

Tutton, E., & Seers, K. (2003). An exploration of the concept of comfort. *Journal of Clinical Nursing, 12*(5), 689–696.

Weaver, T. E., Laizner, A. M., Evans, L. K., Maislin, G., Chugh, D. K., Lyon, K., … Dinges, D. F. (1997). An instrument to measure functional status outcomes for disorders of excessive sleepiness. *Sleep, 20*(10), 835–843.

Wilson, I. B., & Cleary, P. D. (1995). Linking clinical variables with health-related quality of life: A conceptual model of patient outcomes. *Journal of the American Medical Association, 273*(1), 59–65.

Zigmond, A. S., & Snaith, R. P. (1983). The hospital anxiety and depression scale. *Acta Psychiatrica Scandinavica, 67*(6), 361–370.

18

Reconceptualizing Normal

Shelley J. Greif

This chapter describes how the concept building process developed by Liehr and Smith (2008) was used to guide the development of the concept "reconceptualizing normal" after traumatic brain injury (TBI). The structured, 10-phase process was used to identify the idea, beginning with a practice story describing a nursing situation and culminating with a mini-synthesis that merged the knowledge that was gleaned from a theoretical perspective, the literature, and a story from a person who had lived "reconceptualizing normal." In this chapter, a definition of reconceptualizing normal, a model linking core qualities, and a mini-saga that distills the story collected from a person living the phenomenon will be presented.

In my work with children and youth survivors of TBI and their families, I am constantly privileged to enter into a caring relationship with people whose lives have been impacted in ways that they never imagined and for which they are totally unprepared. When children have a moderate to severe TBI, they are treated in a continuum of care that includes triage and emergency care, inpatient hospitalization, inpatient rehabilitation, and outpatient therapy. Emergency medical systems are organized to provide the highest level of intervention necessary to treat the acute injury. These systems include transport to regional trauma centers, transfer to pediatric intensive care as soon as appropriate, and transfer to inpatient rehabilitation as soon as intensive care is no longer necessary. Within this continuum of care, children and their families have support, education, and training from a number of different specialists across multiple disciplines. Physical and cognitive recovery from brain injury can take several years with long periods of time in inpatient settings. Although children and their families are usually eager to return home to familiar activities, there are often significant cognitive, behavioral, and emotional changes that challenge them. Outpatient therapy resources may not be easily accessible geographically or may be limited by caps on insurance. Schools are the primary entity for community reintegration; however, many children with special education needs after TBI are not identified for services, or their learning needs are not associated with the injury (Ylvisaker et al., 2005).

Parents and caregivers are the constants in a child's life when they return home. However, the challenges of recognizing changes in their child's functioning and learning how to effectively support rehabilitation and cognitive development, particularly during the first few critical years postinjury, are often compounded by inconsistent, inadequate, or inaccessible services in the community. This is particularly true in communities that do not have easy access to a large children's hospital with rehabilitation services. In addition, the functional, cognitive, and behavioral changes in the child have an impact on the stress and coping skills of the caregiver (Livingston, Brooks, & Bond, 1985). Children's cognitive recovery will vary, depending on numerous factors that include preinjury conditions and severity of injury. The success of community reintegration depends on the ability of the family to understand and support the child through that process, dealing with and responding effectively to the challenges of behavioral and cognitive changes.

The concept building process, which is the focus of this chapter, begins with a practice story about a nursing situation that is a source of interest. My experience with the families of children who suffered a TBI was the basis for the following practice story about Maria and her family.

PRACTICE STORY

Maria sustained a severe TBI at the age of 16, when she was struck and dragged by a truck while riding a bicycle. She was in intensive care at the local trauma center for 3 weeks, then in inpatient rehabilitation for 1 month. She was discharged after 1 month with follow-up therapies at the local hospital outpatient department. There were no school or day programs available during the summer. In the 2 years prior to her TBI, Maria had two psychiatric hospitalizations for bipolar disorder. Maria's mom is a single working parent and was employed at the time as a manager of a small specialty food shop. She had private insurance. Maria's sister was 1 year older and still living at home, in her senior year of high school.

When she was discharged from inpatient rehabilitation, the critical issues for Maria and her family were her dependence and need for constant supervision. Due to brain injury, her judgment was impaired, she was impulsive, and she was unable to be left by herself. Prior to her injury, she had been an independent teenager, getting around the community on her bicycle, with a great deal of freedom to choose her activities. Now, Maria's independence was curtailed, and her mother had to take an extended leave from her job to provide the daily supervision that Maria needed. One of the things I found significant during this period was Maria's mother's reliance on me, as her nurse, to help her understand her daughter's needs, what was and was not available in the community. We diligently worked at trying to identify and create approaches to meet Maria's pressing need for structure and organization.

Maria wanted to go back to her home school and be with her friends but the school did not have enough specialized services. We identified an alternative school placement for her in a setting that could meet her TBI and mental health needs. Maria enrolled in this special program for students with TBI. One of her emotional issues was an extreme sensitivity to how others felt about her and her perception about how she was being treated. She felt as if people were talking about her and making fun of her at school and refused to go to school after a few weeks. We met with Maria's mother and the school team, but her mom felt that she could not "make her go to school."

Maria spent several months at home with no structure or daily activity. Her mental health deteriorated, and she was admitted to a psychiatric hospital for a suicide attempt. Her mother believed that she needed more services and structure than she was currently able to receive in the community, and we requested special funding for extended inpatient neurorehabilitation. Funding was approved, and Maria had 60 days of inpatient neurorehabilitation services at a facility for individuals with TBI, with a specific program, including school, for teens. By the time she was discharged, she had made progress with respect to attending and participating in classes and improved hygiene and self-care.

However, Maria's mental health continued to deteriorate, and she was eventually admitted to an out-of-state psychiatric facility that serves children and young adults with brain injury and emotional and/or behavioral problems. This hospitalization resulted in considerable improvement in her ability to perform activities of daily living (ADL) and respond appropriately to situations. She still does not initiate activity but responds to cues and direction.

Maria had expressed interest in living independently. Her mother and I worked with adult mental health providers to have her placed in a supported community residential program with daily supervision and coaching. Currently, she is doing well in this environment and has again returned to school. Both she and her mother hope that with these supports she will continue to be able to live in the community, complete school, and participate in a supported work program.

PHENOMENON OF INTEREST

When naming the phenomenon, effort was made to express the experience that I observed in families with children who suffered a TBI in a more general way. This effort to name the phenomenon in the middle of the ladder of abstraction (Smith & Liehr, 2008) was intended to enable use of the ideas in situations other than the one from which the phenomenon arose. Maria's family experience was named "reconceptualizing normal." Both Maria and her mother had to change their daily activities as well as expectations and goals. They have continued to adapt to constantly changing needs. Maria's mother was able to return to work after the first year, however, to a different job. Her new employer is a large company with a strong family support focus, and they have worked with her need for flexibility related to her daughter's needs. She has learned how to be an advocate for her daughter, to make supportive financial and guardianship arrangements, and to constantly explore options and services. Both Maria and her mother have learned how to work with multiple providers and programs to help in her continued recovery, development, and goal of becoming as independent an adult as possible.

THEORETICAL LENS

The first theoretical lens considered for use was the Theory of Family Stress and Adaptation (LoBiondo-Wood, 2008), a middle range theory based on a family crisis model that predicts family adaptation over time. It assumes that families face hardships and changes as a natural part of life; that they develop basic competencies and patterns of functioning, including capabilities to foster growth in family members; that one family competency is the ability to foster recovery following a crisis; that family members draw from and contribute to a network of relationships and resources in the community; and that when faced with crisis, families work to restore order and balance (p. 227). The model called the Double ABCX Model measures the concepts of pile up, existing and new resources, coping, perception of stressor, and adaptation. The model also provides instruments for testing the central concepts. The Theory of Family Stress and Adaptation calls nurses to understand the process and stages of illness and to understand how families adjust and adapt to a crisis situation.

As time went by, and I moved to the literature supporting reconstructing normal, I circled back to consider the theoretical lens for conceptual development and settled on Uncertainty Theory. The Theories of Uncertainty in Illness (Mishel & Clayton, 2008) describe the uncertainty that exists in situations where illness or health impact is unpredictable or ambiguous, or where there is insufficient information to determine the meaning of the event. In discussing one example of the adjustment of families of individuals who have had heart transplants, Mishel and Murdaugh (1987) found that adjustments were continually being made, and belief of return to normal was gradually eroded. They describe the process of adjustment as one which includes an awareness of the need to redefine what is normal. This is similar to what is found in the experience of families following traumatic brain or spinal cord injury. The family in the original practice story described uncertainty as a central essence of their experience, and uncertainty is a pervasive theme throughout the qualitative literature. For parents, there is uncertainty with respect to their child's improvement as well as what to expect from structure providers. Family adaptation strategies reflect how they deal with that uncertainty.

LITERATURE REVIEW

TBI is frequently referred to as the "silent epidemic" because the complications from TBI—such as changes affecting thinking, sensation, language, or emotions—may not be readily apparent. Each year, traumatic brain injuries contribute to a substantial number of deaths and cases of permanent disability. Recent data show that, on average, approximately 1.7 million people sustain a TBI annually (Faul, Xu, Wald, & Coronado, 2010). Children from birth to 4 years of age, teenagers from 15 to 19 years, and adults over the age of 65 are most likely to sustain a TBI, and almost half a million emergency department visits are made annually by children birth to 14 years.

There has been a great deal of interest across multiple disciplines in studying and understanding the impact of TBI and factors that contribute to recovery (Verhaeghe, Defloor, & Grypdonck, 2004). Because TBI affects how someone thinks, feels, and behaves, it has a significant and profound effect on the lives of survivors and their families. Critical in reviewing the impact of TBI is the importance of seeing the person within the numbers, but the quantitative studies often fall short in this regard.

Many social and physical science researchers have examined pre-trauma profile (presence or absence of learning disabilities, parent education, employment, and socioeconomic status) and severity of injury (Glasgow Coma Score [GCS], length of coma, presence of intracranial lesions, and cerebral perfusion pressure) to predict functional and cognitive outcomes of TBI (Catroppa, Anderson, Morse, Haritou, & Rosenfield, 2008; Keenan, Runyan, & Nocera, 2006; Kinsella et al., 1997; Miller & Donders, 2003; Sander et al., 2003; Slomine et al., 2006; Woodward et al., 1999). Injury severity as determined by the GCS is classified as severe if GCS less than 9, moderate if GCS is 9 to 12, and mild if GCS is greater than 12. Children with moderate to severe traumatic brain injuries generally do not perform as well on measures of academic achievement as children with mild brain injury, even several years after the injury. Pretrauma family factors such as education, employment, coping skills, and family dysfunction, as well as pretrauma child factors—particularly the presence of learning disabilities or behavioral problems—are found to be consistent predictors of outcomes 1 to 7 years after injury. Although quantitative studies provide a snapshot of the context generating persistent uncertainty for families whose children have suffered a TBI, qualitative studies most directly address how families get along day by day.

Studies by nurse researchers of families caring for children with TBI are primarily qualitative and focus on what caregivers and survivors experience. Qualitative studies of the lived experience of mothers of children with TBI identify common themes of "learning to parent" and "raising my child all over again" (Wongvatunyu & Porter, 2008a). When young adults return home following a TBI, factors relevant to developmental tasks can resurface, such as functional status, history of mother–child relationship, and community reintegration. Mothers describe the process of getting to know their child again, keeping their child safe, providing support and encouragement, teaching basic functional skills, and responding to and addressing behavioral issues. Wongvatunyu and Porter (2008a) use a descriptive phenomenological method to explore the lifeworld of seven mothers whose young adult children had suffered a moderate or severe TBI. The authors consolidated their findings into five lifeworld features and their component descriptors (p. 1065): (1) having a child who survived a TBI as a young adult: looking for answers that no one has, holding on to the child who has been mine and getting to know my child now: (2) perceiving that life has really changed: living with changes in my own life and in my relationship with my child: (3) having sufficient support/feeling bereft of help: (4) believing that my child is still able: and (5) believing that I can help my child. Mothers saw themselves as first observers: the first to recognize progress in their child and often having to convince health professionals that progress was real.

Kao and Stuifbergen (2004) used a phenomenological approach to explore the meaning of the lived experience of young adult TBI survivors (age 18–25 years) and their maternal caregivers. Participants included nine males and three females who were at least 2 years post-TBI, all of whom were living with their mothers who were the primary caregivers. Additional criteria for inclusion were injury due to motor vehicle accident, posttraumatic amnesia of more than 24 hours, and ability to participate in verbal interview. Colaizzi's phenomenological techniques were used to analyze the data for both the dyads and the individuals. The two broad themes that emerged were sense of abnormality and period of uncertainty. Maternal–child themes included dependence and autonomy, marital menace, and maintaining harmony. Although this study focuses on the mother–child relationship, with mother as the primary caregiver, it does include the impact on family and marital or partner relationship in the inquiry. Survivor reactions of the adult child included subjective response, interfamily response, family isolation from society, and societal response. The researchers recommend that health professionals design more appropriate long-term community interventions to decrease the burden of injury stress, increase self-esteem, and improve quality of life for both survivors and families.

In a phenomenological qualitative study of children's and parents' experiences following children's TBI, Roscigno (2008) described children as struggling to find their place in a social world that is unprepared to handle their differences. The children expressed their idea that going home would get them back to their old life but found that it did not. In addition, they expressed feeling like they would never be the person they were before. Parents' experiences were similar to those found by Wongvatunyu and Porter. They described being grateful to still have their child, yet grieving for the child that they knew. Parents in this study also identified lack of support and insensitivity to their experience as adding considerably to their stress. The sample in this study, which focuses on family and community reintegration after TBI, consisted of 39 children and 42 parents, with families coming from 13 states in the United States. Roscigno suggests that more qualitative inquiry is needed to understand how cultural attitudes and beliefs about the impairments of TBI influence social interactions that occur in child–parent–community everyday engagement.

Duff (2002, 2006) reported using grounded theory method to address family issues when a close relative suffered TBI. This research was conducted in two acute care neurosurgical trauma units in Toronto, Canada, and included 36 participants (11 individuals who were injured and 25 family members). The purpose was to discover the most significant concerns of family members with a close relative who had a TBI and how they dealt with the uncertain trajectory during the initial acute phase of treatment. Data were collected from participants in one to three interviews conducted over a 16-month period. Basic social processes identified were negotiating uncertainty, willing survival, attending to Snow White, reconstructing the person, and making it better. Negotiating uncertainty was the process that occurred between family and members of the health care team as a result of the uncertain trajectory of the impact of the injury, and included negotiating on behalf of the injured person to support and promote recovery. Willing survival is an expression of the faith and beliefs of family members directed toward their injured loved one. Family members described the period of watchful waiting while their loved one was in a coma as attending to Snow White, reflecting the hope expressed in the fairy tale of waking up from an evil spell. As the injured person became better physiologically, family members re-evaluated and reconciled the pre- and postinjury person, reconstructing the person as their way of getting to know them all over again. The final process of making it better occurs when families realize that they cannot return to preinjury abilities and functioning and begin to move forward to help their family member achieve optimal recovery as well as reclaim their own commitments to family and work responsibilities. Duff makes specific recommendations for nursing practice designed to reduce the uncertainty experienced by families and facilitate the way in which families negotiate with members of the health care team. Family survival is dependent on developing survival strategies, and recommendations are made specific to the different stages of the social processes uncovered with the grounded theory method. Duff recognized that one of the limitations of this study was that it was conducted during the acute phase of the recovery trajectory and suggested further research about how families negotiate TBI across the entire trajectory.

Consistent throughout the literature that has been reviewed is the importance of family functioning. Review of qualitative research suggests that what is central to successful adaptation and community reintegration is the family's ability to reconceptualize what is normal, to change expectations about how they and their child will live and experience daily activities (Duff, 2002, 2006; Kao & Stuifbergen, 2004; Mishel & Murdaugh, 1987; Roscigno, 2008; Wongvatunyu & Porter, 2008a, 2008b). Nurse researchers focus much of their attention on the ways in which children and their families respond and adapt to TBI. Middle range theories that emerge from the intersection of practice and research (Smith & Liehr, 2008) are logical guides for nurse researchers interested in studying families of children who have suffered TBI.

GATHER THE STORY

Exploring the idea of reconceptualizing normal came from my nursing practice experience of working with survivors of traumatic brain and spinal cord injuries and their families. The concept initially evolved from my understanding of the theory of family stress and adaptation; however, further thought and discussion led to application of the theory of uncertainty as the overarching structure guiding concept development. The reconstructed story is an expression of the experience of the mother of a 19-year-old survivor of TBI.

Mark was a 16-year-old high school student who had head trauma when he was in a car accident while he was playing with friends and fell off the hood of a car. He was admitted to the trauma center where he was stabilized and diagnosed with skull fractures and TBI. He had surgery to remove part of his skull to alleviate the pressure on his brain. He was in ICU and step down ICU for 3 weeks, then transferred by way of air transport to an out-of-state children's rehabilitation hospital. His rehabilitation included intensive physical, life skills, speech, cognitive, and respiratory therapy. There is tremendous uncertainty in brain injury rehabilitation. Brain healing occurs over a 1- to 2-year period, and the extent of most brain injuries is not completely recognized until 6 months to 1 year after the trauma. In addition, particularly for children and adolescents whose brains are still developing, there are the constant challenges of incorporating new experiences and developmental stages. Mark remained in the out-of-state inpatient and day rehabilitation for 3 months and then returned home to reintegrate into his family, school, and community. Mark returned to his high school parttime within the first year of his accident. However, he began to develop behavioral and emotional problems, including threatening to harm his brother. He once again went out of state for an admission to a TBI rehabilitation center for cognitive therapy. He spent 6 months receiving help relearning how his brain interprets information, how he responds, and how he can manage himself. He returned home again to complete high school and graduate. At the time of his graduation, 3 years had passed since his accident. During the intervening summer, he volunteered at the local YMCA, working with children enrolled in the summer program. He wants to go to college and has just started taking one class at a local college. He is finding it difficult, but his mother has arranged for a vocational evaluation to explore alternatives. His mother, Angela, feels that Mark has shown tremendous resiliency and determination to recover. The entire family has as well.

Angela feels that the major change for their family is recognizing that they are in a constant state of flux and that they can have anything in their lives change in a minute. They have tried as a family to look at change in a positive way and not be threatened because things are not the way they were. She describes the family prior to her son's injury as very structured and predictable in terms of looking at schools and sports, making sure both children had the opportunities available to reach their goals. They still use structure and schedule, but now it is with the understanding of the importance of structure and consistency for someone with a brain injury. Angela also understands that whatever is planned is subject to change. They do not get stressed when plans change and use humor to help cope.

Angela and her husband are very conscientious about how they spend time with each of their children, recognizing that Mark's brain injury has changed his relationship with his brother Robert, the much admired older brother. Angela and her husband have allowed and encouraged Robert to express his feelings and anger as much as possible, recognizing that it is important that he doesn't go to his friends with his anger.

Angela said she expected to go through a severe mourning stage, but it hasn't happened. She is much more sensitive to how parents make a big deal about things that are not so important. Having a child who almost died, she sees parents caught up in the rat race of who they want their child to be and not taking time to know them. She has managed family uncertainty by helping her husband and her son, Robert, to get to know Mark all over again, establishing new patterns and approaches to meet the needs of each member of the family.

Mini-Saga Emerging From the Reconstructed Story

Mark's brain injury changed his family in ways his parents and brother could not anticipate. They are in constant flux, adjusting to ever-changing needs and concerns. His mother manages uncertainty by getting to know Mark all over again, staying open to who he is becoming and always looking forward.

CORE QUALITIES

There is persistent uncertainty associated with how a child will recover from brain injury. Families develop basic competencies and patterns that foster growth, protect their child, and enable recovery. In coping with uncertainty, they demonstrate flexibility and draw on unconditional love that enables them to get to know their child all over again and develop new approaches for everyday living and recovery. Willing openness to know anew (Roscigno, 2008; Wongvatunyu & Porter, 2008b), intentional flexibility (Duff, 2002, 2006; Kao & Stuifbergen, 2004), and unconditional love (Kao & Stuifbergen, 2004; Wongvatunyu & Porter, 2008b) are the core qualities that parents culti-vate as they learn how to manage care for their child and to help their child learn how to manage his or her own care. The support of client and family to re-envision their present and future, to reconceptualize normal, is a continuous process of coordination and communication, focusing on short-term needs and goals within the context of long-term needs and goals. Understanding this phenomenon guides the nurse in providing support and offers opportunities for research intended to help families cope with the trauma of brain injury.

SYNTHESIZED DEFINITION

Reconceptualizing normal is willing openness to know anew through intentional flexibility and unconditional love (Figure 18.1).

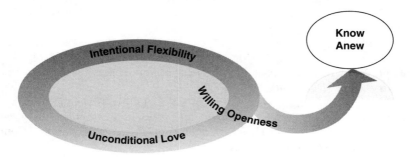

FIGURE 18.1   Model of Reconceptualizing Normal

Mini-Synthesis

When a child survives a traumatic injury, there is a long period of rehabilitation followed by a longer period of community reintegration, requiring new family perspectives. Reconceptualizing normal is willing openness to know anew through intentional flexibility and unconditional love. Understanding what families experience helps guide the nurse's supportive interventions.

CONCLUSION

The approach to developing structures for research using the 10-phase process developed by Smith and Liehr (2008) has been the foundation for development of the concept of reconceptualizing normal. Understanding this phenomenon guides the nurse in providing support and offers opportunities for research with promise for helping families after TBI. However, this understanding extends beyond TBI. Any person who has experienced a life-changing transition will engage in reconceptualizing normal in some way. For instance, the concept may be applied to women who have had mastectomies, children who lose a parent, or people entering a program for substance use recovery. For me, this work has had its roots in decades of working with families whose child has suffered a TBI. I am grateful to the families who have opened their lives to me and allowed me to better understand and help support them in caring for their child after TBI.

REFERENCES

Catroppa, C., Anderson, V. A., Morse, S. A., Haritou, F., & Rosenfield, J. V. (2008). Outcome and predictors of functional recovery 5 years following pediatric traumatic brain injury (TBI). *Journal of Pediatric Psychology, 33*(7), 707–718.

Duff, D. (2002). Family concerns and responses following a severe traumatic brain injury: A grounded theory study. *Axon (Dartmouth, N. S.), 24*(2), 14–22.

Duff, D. (2006). Family impact and influence following severe traumatic brain injury. *Axon, (Dartmouth, N. S.), 27*(2), 9–23.

Faul, M., Xu, L., Wald, M. M., & Coronado, V. G. (2010). *Traumatic brain injury in the United States: Emergency department visits, hospitalizations, and deaths.* Atlanta, GA: Centers for Disease Control and Prevention, National Center for Injury Prevention and Control.

Kao, H.-F. S., & Stuifbergen, A. K. (2004). Love and load–the lived experience of the mother-child relationship among young adult traumatic brain-injured survivors. *The Journal of Neuroscience Nursing, 36*(2), 73–81.

Keenan, H. T., Runyan, D. K., & Nocera, M. (2006). Longitudinal follow-up of families and young children with traumatic brain injury. (Disease/Disorder overview). *Pediatrics, 117*(4), 1291.

Kinsella, G. J., Prior, M., Sawyer, M., Ong, B., Murtach, D., Eisenmajer, R., ... Klug, G. (1997). Predictors and indicators of academic outcome in children 2 years following traumatic brain injury. *Journal of the International Neuropsychological Society, 3,* 608–616.

Liehr, P. R., & Smith, M. J. (2008). Building structures for research. In M. J. Smith & P. R. Liehr (Eds.). *Middle Range Theory for Nursing.* New York, NY: Springer Publishing.

Livingston, M. G., Brooks, D. N., Bond, M. R. (1985). Patient outcome in the year following severe head injury and relatives' psychiatric and social functioning. *Journal of Neurology, Neurosurgery, and Psychiatry, 48*(9), 876–881.

LoBiondo-Wood, G. (2008). Theory of family stress and adaptation. In M. J. Smith & P. R. Liehr (Eds.), *Middle range theory for nursing* (pp. 225–241). New York, NY: Springer.

Miller, L. J., & Donders, J. (2003). Prediction of educational outcome after pediatric traumatic brain injury. *Rehabilitation Psychology, 48*(4), 237–241.

Mishel, M. H., & Clayton, M. F. (2008). Theories of uncertainty in illness. In M. J. Smith & P. R. Liehr (Eds.), *Middle range theory for nursing* (pp. 55–84). New York, NY: Springer.

Mishel, M. H. & Murdaugh, C. L. (1987). Family adjustment to heart transplantation: Redesigning the dream. *Nursing Research, 36*(6), 332–338.

Roscigno, C. (2008). *Children's and parents' experiences following children's moderate to severe traumatic brain injury* (Unpublished doctoral dissertation). University of Washington, Seattle.

Sander, A. M., Sherer, M. S., Malec, J. F., High, W. M., Jr., Thompson, R. N., Moessner, A. M., & Josey, J. (2003). Preinjury emotional and family functioning in caregivers of persons with traumatic brain injury. *Archives of Physical Medicine and Rehabilitation, 84,* 197–203.

Slomine, B. S., McCarthy, M. L., Ding, R., MacKenzie, E. J., Jaffe, K. M., Aitken, M. E., ... Paidas, C. N. (2006). Health care utilization and needs after pediatric traumatic brain injury. *Pediatrics, 117*(4), e663.

Verhaeghe, S., Defloor, T., & Grypdonck, M. (2004). Stress and coping among families of patients with traumatic brain injury: A review of the literature. *Journal of Clinical Nursing, 14,* 1004–1012.

Wongvatunyu, S., & Porter, E. J. (2008a). Helping young adult children with traumatic brain injury: The life-world of mothers. *Qualitative Health Research, 18,* 1062–1074.

Wongvatunyu, S., & Porter, E. J. (2008b). Changes in family life perceived by mothers of young adult TBI survivors. *Journal of Family Nursing, 14*(3), 314–332.

Woodward, H., Winterhalther, K., Donders, J., Hackbarth, R., Kuldanek, A., Sanfilippo, D. (1999). Prediction of neurobehavioral outcome 1–5 years post pediatric traumatic head injury. *Journal of Head Trauma Rehabilitation, 14*(4), 351–359.

Ylvisaker, M., Adelson, P. D., Braga, L. W., Burnett, S. M., Glang, A., Feeney, T., ... Todis, B. (2005). Rehabilitation and ongoing support after pediatric TBI—Twenty years of progress. *Journal of Head Trauma Rehabilitation, 20*(1), 95–109.

19

Yearning to Be Recognized: From Concept Building to Proposal Development to Data Gathering and Analysis

Anthony R. Ramsey

THE FOUNDATION OF CONCEPT BUILDING

Nursing practice in many settings offers the opportunity to care for women experiencing migraine headache. These women utilize health care resources more frequently than women without migraine (Elston-Lafata et al., 2004). Based on the observations in the clinical setting, the headache experience for these women is a powerful force, which invokes physical pain and emotional turmoil. A strong interest in the phenomenon of living with migraine headaches was born in the clinical setting and further developed during a doctoral level nursing theory course. After classes had concluded, I continued to work with my mentor regarding this idea. We concluded that women who experience migraine headache are in fact yearning for the physical and emotional pain to be recognized as real. To better define the concept, I embarked on a journey of exploring the literature and gathering the story of a woman living with migraine headache. In the end, the concept of yearning to be recognized—defined as attending to the voice of suffering that calls for relief—was developed.

Theoretical Lens

The phenomenon of yearning to be recognized is directly linked to story theory (Liehr & Smith, 2008). This theory centers on nurse presence with another to validate suffering through story. In the context of true presence, there is intentional focus on dialogue to summon a story. The migraine experience of pain is the complicating health challenge that initiates the sharing of story. The nurse is charged with remaining free from distraction while embracing the reality of the other through sharing the migraine story. In true presence, the nurse withholds judgment while listening, allowing the identification of story patterns that facilitate understanding of the meaning of suffering with migraine headache to come forth. The human experience of suffering comes in many different forms and is a complicating health challenge. Finally, relief—another attribute of yearning to be recognized—involves the understanding of another. This understanding enables ease that Liehr and Smith describe as an energizing release.

Related Literature

The work of coming to know this idea required a significant literature review to identify essential qualities of the phenomenon. Different search strategies were used including searches on migraine, women, care, validation, pain, and suffering. However, "yearning to be recognized" with these exact words is not found in the nursing or medical literature. Instead, this idea was informed through related concepts in the literature. Suffering, threat to integrity, attentive presence, help seeking, and release of pressure were evidence-based concepts (Fredriksson & Eriksson, 2001; Kahn & Steeves, 1986; Liehr & Smith, 2008; Moloney, Strickland, DeRossett, Melby, & Dietrich, 2006; Norberg, Bergsten, & Lundman, 2001; Sundin, Axelsson, Jansson, & Norberg, 2000) that informed understanding of yearning to be recognized.

Core Qualities/Definition/Model

Webster's Ninth New Collegiate Dictionary defines yearning as "longing persistently, wistfully or sadly." Recognize is defined as "to acknowledge formally; to admit as being one entitled to be heard" (Merriam-Webster, 1988). Based on the supporting literature and the real-world stories of women with migraine headache, the phenomenon of yearning to be recognized was defined as attending to the voice of suffering that calls for relief. The attributes of the phenomenon are attending, voice of suffering, and relief. Attending is defined as being truly present with another story to validate what matters most to the person. The second attribute the voice of suffering is defined as the bodily

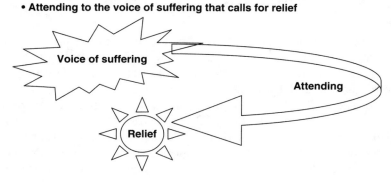

FIGURE 19.1   Yearning to Be Recognized

expression of deep pain. For a person with migraine headache, deep pain is a profound, all-consuming state of unrelenting pressure. Relief is defined as the release of emotional and physical pressure. A model depicting the concept of yearning to be recognized is presented in Figure 19.1.

Relationship of the Model to a Research Proposal

The model of the concept yearning to be recognized served as the foundation for the development of a research proposal. During the proposal planning phases, the model was kept at the forefront as the details of the proposal emerged.

As I planned and developed the research proposal, I wanted to accomplish two goals: (1) to intentionally dialogue with women who are living with migraine headache by following a story path, and (2) to create a structure of meaning for the phenomena of women living with migraine headache based on phenomenological analysis of the stories. Multiple practice conversations prior to and during the development of the research proposal were held to perfect gathering the story of women with migraine headache using a story path (Liehr & Smith, 2008). These conversations included any woman willing to talk about a complicating health challenge that we mutually agreed on. I used participant feedback from the practice conversations to become better prepared. An example of feedback that I continued to utilize was the use of eye contact. Women in the practice conversations stated that they could tell I was deeply connected because of my eye contact and calm demeanor.

EXEMPLAR PROPOSAL

Migraine headache is defined as a headache that lasts up to 72 hours when left untreated. This type of headache is usually limited to one side of the head (unilateral), produces moderate or severe pain, and may be aggravated by physical activity. Lipton, Stewart, Diamond, Diamond, and Reed (2001) examined the prevalence and burden of migraine in the United States—29,727 individuals from across the country responded to a mailed survey. It was determined that 16.6% of women living in the mid-Atlantic region experience migraine. Ninety-one percent of these women reported some form of functional impairment with migraine and 31% missed at least 1 day of work in the 3 months before the survey. In this landmark study, Lipton et al. found that women were three times more likely to experience migraine headache than men. When women experience migraine headache, they feel intense physical pain (Lipton et al., 2001) that is often accompanied by nausea and vomiting, blurred vision, and feelings of complete disability (Kolotylo & Broome, 2000a).

Migraine headache is a chronic illness with significant comorbidities. The headaches and comorbidities produce increased societal costs. A study revealed that nurses with migraine headache experienced a lower quality of life because of the headache (Durham et al., 1998). Migraine patients use the emergency department for care more than nonmigraine patients and incur more medical care costs than those who do not experience migraine (Elston-Lafata et al., 2004). Researchers have identified other conditions that coexist with migraine headache. One such condition is depression, which frequently accompanies migraine and may be compounded when health care providers fail to acknowledge migraine headache (Kolotylo & Broome, 2000b; Wikberg, Jansson, & Lithner, 2000). Because migraine headache is a significant problem with possible comorbidities for individuals who experience this chronic condition, and because migraine headache is related to increased societal costs, it is essential for nurses to better understand the overall experience of these patients.

The prevalence, symptoms, and effects of migraine headache have been studied extensively. However, there is little research designed to explore the meaning of living with migraine headache for women who experience this complicating health challenge. Phenomenological research may provide a better understanding of the migraine headache experience, which, in turn, will lead to improved nursing care.

Purpose

The purpose of this study is to better understand the experience of women living with migraine headache through exploring the question, "What is the structure of meaning for women living with migraine headache?" A structure of meaning emerges when a story of the lived experience is dwelled with and reflected on, leading to the interpretation of qualities that go together to create a structure that captures the meaning of the lived experience. Understanding the experience of women with migraine headache through the development of a structure of meaning will enable nurses to become better informed about various factors related to living with this often debilitating condition. Nurses who have enhanced appreciation of the phenomenon are better prepared to provide optimal care for those who suffer migraine headache and ultimately to help to improve the quality of their lives. Finally, this qualitative study may serve as a stimulus for future nursing research related to migraine headache.

Theoretical Perspective

Theoretical guidance for this proposal includes hermeneutic phenomenology (van Manen, 1997) and story theory (Liehr & Smith, 2008). Van Manen (1997) postulates that phenomenology is an act of caring, because to understand another's world is to care for that person. Furthermore, phenomenology involves the understanding of what is unique to a person (van Manen, 1997). The aim of phenomenology is to better understand the essential nature of everyday experiences, achieved as a person consciously reflects on life experience and interprets the associated feelings and thoughts in dialogue with another person. From this reflection, embedded meaning surfaces for both the study participant and the researcher. As the researcher reflects on the participant's story, a deeper understanding of meaning emerges (van Manen, 1997). The philosophical underpinnings of hermeneutic phenomenology maintain that reflecting on a lived experience provides a rich understanding of meaning. The search for individual meaning in relation to living with migraine headache provides a natural fit with the interpretive phenomenology method described by van Manen.

To further guide understanding of the human health experience of migraine headache, story theory, a middle range nursing theory, served as the additional framework for inquiry. The purpose of this theory is to "describe and explain story as the context for a nurse–person health promotion process" (Liehr & Smith, 2008, p. 205). Three interrelated concepts compose the basis of story theory. The first, intentional dialogue, is the "purposeful engagement with another to summon the story of a complicating health challenge" (Liehr & Smith, 2008, p. 209). The second concept is connecting with self-in-relation, which is "the active process of recognizing self as related with others in a story-plot" (p. 210). The final concept, creating ease, "is an energizing release experienced as the story comes together in movement toward resolving" (p. 212).

When applied to nursing research, story theory places the participant at the center of attention while the nurse researcher serves as an engaged guide. When conducting research involving women with migraine headache, the researcher asks the participant, "What is it like to live with migraine headaches?" (Liehr & Smith, 2008). As the story unfolds, the nurse researcher is charged with aiding the participant to clarify and connect the everyday thoughts and feelings of living with the health challenge of migraine headaches. This connection leads to the realization of control over the situation and the researcher gains a thorough understanding of the participant's experiences. Once the participant has verbalized this experience, a sense of freedom and ease may result, leading to the formation of a new pattern of thought. Ultimately, the person has, through story, attained a contextual realization.

The human health experience of migraine headache is a significant health issue for women (Lipton et al., 2001). These headaches produce intense localized pain, often accompanied by nausea, vomiting, and/or blurred vision (Lipton et al., 2001). Women with migraine may experience anxiety, depression, and/or feelings of isolation in addition to the pain of the migraine (Mongini et al., 2005). Furthermore, women report that migraine contributes to missed work and time with family (Lipton et al., 2001), possibly creating increased feelings of anxiety and/or depression. The increase in anxiety and/or depression is associated with increased occurrence of migraine headache. The suffering embedded in this lived experience calls for the study of the migraine headache experience to provide a foundation for caring/healing practices and enhanced quality of life. It is expected that the findings of this study will contribute to the body of knowledge on the human health experience of migraine headache.

Relevant Literature

It is evident from a historical perspective that migraine headache has been described by scientists, physicians, and other writers for thousands of years. Early descriptions appeared as poems or through other written expressions. The earliest documentation of migraine headache noted in the literature was 9,000 years ago (Magiorkinis, Diamantis, Mitsikostas, & Androutsos, 2009). Authors believe that early writings and descriptions resulted, in part, from personal experiences with headache (Silberstein, Lipton, & Dodick, 2008). Through observation and research, an understanding of the pathophysiology, triggers, and treatment of migraine headache has emerged. This understanding has contributed to advances that provide relief for many people who suffer with migraine headache. Although diagnosis and treatment of migraine headache has been discussed from a variety of perspectives, historically there has been little to no research that focuses on understanding the nature of what it is like for people to live with migraine headache.

The migraine headache work reported by Birtch in 1910 was the beginning of migraine literature, describing experimental processes frequently utilized during this period. Moffitt (1911) reported that his observations indicated that migraine is a disease of the brain, inherited from family members. Later, in the 1930s and 1940s, vasodilatation of cephalic arteries was reported to be the primary cause of migraine headache, a theory that has stood the test of time. Drugs such as ergotamine and caffeine were employed to induce vasoconstriction and relieve migraine pain (Silberstein et al., 2008).

Vujevich (2007) reported that hormones make migraines different for women than for men. Brandes (2006) concluded that migraine headaches related to menstruation are more difficult to treat and that this may be true, in part, because estrogen withdrawal stimulates migraine. With the exception of dysmenorrhea, menstrual migraine is the most frequently reported menses-related symptom (Mannix, 2008). However, menstrual-related migraine is, for the most part, treated in the same fashion as nonmenstrual migraine. The prophylactic drugs—such as low-dose estrogen, beta-blockers, propranolol, and amitriptyline—are all reported as frequently prescribed drugs intended to decrease the occurrence of migraine. To abort migraine, ergotamine, the triptans, and nonsteroidal anti-inflammatory drugs are employed. Frequently used nonpharmacological treatments include ice to the head, avoidance of triggers, and stress reduction (Weitzel, Strickland, Smith, & Goode, 2001).

Researchers have linked personality characteristics to migraine headache. A study examined the personality of 70 women with migraine headache through the use of the Myers-Briggs Trait Indicator (Gallagher, Mueller, Steer, & Ciervo, 1998). The authors found that women who suffered migraines were characterized by an overreaction to stressful situations, unrealistically high expectations, and the avoidance of controversy. The Temperament and Character Inventory, another well-validated tool, was used to assess 49 women with migraine headache (Mongini et al., 2005). The women with migraine scored significantly higher in the areas of harm avoidance, persistence, and level of anxiety (Mongini et al., 2005).

Instruments reported in the literature to assess migraine headache pain are the Diagnostic Diary (Nappi et al., 2006), the Migraine Assessment Tool (Marcus, Kapelewski, Jacob, Rudy, & Furman, 2004), and the Migraine-Specific Quality of Life Questionnaire Version 2.1 (Martin et al., 2000). The predominantly used instrument is the Migraine Disability Assessment Questionnaire (Stewart, Lipton, Dowson, & Sawyer, 2001).

A review of the qualitative literature revealed seven pertinent articles that addressed some aspect of living with migraine headache. These studies used a variety of methodologies, including grounded theory, focus groups, content analysis, and concept development. The findings of the studies indicated that participants had difficulty communicating headache pain; they had an intense desire for relief from the pain; and the impact of migraine headache pain strongly affected their daily life. Using a semistructured interview with 13 participants, Peters, Abu-Saad, Vydelingum, Dowson, and Murphy (2004, 2005) arrived at three themes describing the migraine headache: headache as severe pain, headache as a health issue, and the impact of headache on performance of everyday tasks.

In a grounded theory study, Peters et al. (2004) found that participants had low expectations regarding care from the general practitioners they saw for their migraine headache and that little attention was given to uncovering the cause of their headache. Belam et al., using a grounded theory method, found that "Handling the Beast" was the metaphor that emerged as an overarching theme (Belam et al., 2005, p. 89). The "Beast" was handled through making sense of the problem, putting up with it, and doing something about it.

Using a focus group approach, Ruiz de Velasco, Gonzalez, Etxeberria, and Garcia-Monco (2003) found that migraine headache diminished quality of life for patients, especially in the areas of work, personal relationships, and recreation. Meyer (2002) described how women may constantly be on guard for a potential migraine. Women with a history of migraine routinely ask themselves, "Could this bring on a headache?" (Meyer, 2002, p. 1226).

Moloney et al. (2006) assessed the experiences of middle-age women with migraine headache with story, focus groups, and questionnaires. Three patterns identified in the findings were the changing nature of headache over time, migraine triggers and control over headache, and the influence of migraine headache on relationships and daily life.

The literature presented in this section examined migraine headache through various qualitative research methods. Lack of attention from health care providers, social stigma with migraine, and statements of dependence on self are themes located in this literature review. Each of these themes generally addresses extrinsic factors/strategies associated with suffering migraine headache. However, the meaning of living with migraine headache has never been investigated using a phenomenological approach, which promises to capture the intrinsic nature of suffering migraine headaches. The themes from the studies and the identified gap in the literature provide substantive support for phenomenological research asking the question, "What is the structure of meaning for women living with migraine headache?"

Preliminary Work

Because this study was phenomenological in nature, I believed that it was important for me to critically review my thoughts and feelings regarding migraine headache. This reflection created an avenue for "examining personal commitments and prejudices prior to beginning data collection" (Cohen, 2000a, p. 38). I have never had a migraine headache and rarely experience any type of headache. My interest in migraines began while I was working as an emergency department nurse. In this setting, I would often encounter women with severe headaches. Some of these women shared with me that they often felt as if they would never live a migraine-free life. Some held hope that relief would one day be found.

As I began doctoral studies, my research interest returned to these women. I developed a migraine clinic at a local health care facility for uninsured patients and hold this migraine clinic once each month. This clinic has allowed me to experience the happiness of reducing a woman's migraine headache occurrence from ten headaches per month to two headaches per month. Conversely, I have experienced the frustration of working with a woman for over 1 year with no significant reduction in headache occurrence. The fact that I can provide the same level of care and have two opposite patient outcomes led me to wonder why some women respond to treatment plans and others do not. This thinking— combined with a significant gap in the literature related to the meaning of living with migraine for women and my personal inexperience with headache—reaffirmed my commitment to the question, "What is the structure of meaning for women living with migraine headache?"

An e-mail query seeking interested participants was sent to women who held an account at a mid-Atlantic university. By the end of the day that the query was distributed, 59 people had responded saying they would like to volunteer for this study of migraine headache. Within 1 week of the advertisement distribution, a total of 93 people responded stating their interest in study participation. For me, this response affirmed the importance of the concept that was the foundation for this work; these women were yearning to be recognized.

Design

This was a phenomenological study that addressed the research question: "What is the structure of meaning for women living with migraine headache?" Because phenomenology focuses on how people make meaning of experiences, it was identified as the appropriate approach for this study (Cohen, 2000b).

Protection of Human Subjects

Institutional review board approval was obtained. It specified that recruitment of participants was to be achieved by sending an e-mail with a study advertisement to everyone who held an account at a local university and by placing advertisement flyers in various buildings located on the university campus. This advertisement included a description of the study and contact information for anyone wishing to participate in the research. Those volunteering to participate would be given a letter describing the study, informing them of their right to refuse to participate in all or any part of the study, methods to protect privacy, such as separating identifying information from data, and a statement that any publications or public presentations of findings would not include their names or any identifying information. All participants were required to sign a consent form before the conversation. Each participant was told that she could refuse to provide demographic data and/or stop the conversation at any point. The investigator provided emergency telephone numbers of health professionals including mental health professionals in case the participant experienced distress during the conversation. Participant confidentiality was assured. The transcriptionist had no access to participant information, and recordings were to be erased after data analysis was complete. The demographic data and transcribed conversations were to be secured in a locked file cabinet within a locked office, remaining there for 7 years before being destroyed.

Data Collection

Exclusion criteria included women who were younger than 18 years, those reporting headache other than migraine, and those who did not speak English. Volunteers were called to set a place for gathering the story. All of the conversations were conducted in a room where privacy could be held in high regard to protect the confidential content of the conversation.

The researcher began the meeting with each participant in the same way, by providing the background of the study and the study's intent. Each participant was given a detailed oral description of the conversation process, as well as the transcription and analysis processes. Participants then read the consent form and the health insurance portability and accountability forms. All participant questions were answered before obtaining signatures. Demographic data, including participant age, age at migraine diagnosis, intimate relationship status, pregnancy history, educational level, profession, health insurance status, and place of professional migraine care, were collected. Each participant received copies of all forms used to conduct this study.

After consents were signed, the investigator began the conversation by first writing on a blank piece of paper, "the story of living with migraine headache" (Liehr & Smith, 2008, p. 217). Audio recording began with the researcher asking the participant, "What is it like to live with migraine headache?" The conversation starts with living with migraine in the present. Liehr and Smith (2008) suggest that the researcher begin with the present, then focus on the past, and then the future. The researcher maintained this present–past–future path of inquiry while attending to van Manen's (1997) suggestion that the researcher stay with the original question throughout the conversation. Van Manen further stated that with patience and silence, the participant can stay with the original question. If the participant became idle, repeating the last sentence stimulated thought for her to proceed. The recordings were sent to the transcriptionist, who returned each recording and transcript within 3 days of the conversation. The researcher then listened to the recordings to verify the transcriptions.

Data Analysis

Various methods of interpreting phenomenological data exist in the nursing literature. For the purposes of analyzing the conversations of women in this study, van Manen's method was utilized. According to van Manen, theme is a simplified formulation of the focus or point of an experience. To capture theme, van Manen (1997) suggested that the researcher first look at the text as a whole, asking the question "What does this mean?" and writing a phrase that captures that meaning. Next, he suggested that after several readings, the researcher circle essential descriptions of the phenomenon of interest. Finally, each essential description is examined with the question "What does this reveal about the experience?" (van Manen, 1997, p. 93) The task is then to determine commonalities (themes) and capture them with words. Finally, the researcher should ask if the phenomenon would lose its meaning without the theme. Identifying themes from the conversation allows the researcher to grasp the essence of the phenomena, or "touch the core of the notion we are trying to understand" (van Manen, 1990, p. 88).

Van Manen (1997) asserts that although gathering stories and analyzing themes are two different processes, the processes are related. Analysis is always in the background when gathering the story and then becomes foreground in the analysis of themes. After gathering the stories about living with migraine headache, the transcribed stories were read and reread to uncover the structure of the story, which was how the experience began, how it is in the present, and thoughts about the future. A reconstructed story for each participant was written in the participant's words. The reconstructed story was composed with a beginning, middle, and end (Liehr & Smith, 2008). The next phase of the analysis was selective highlighting of statements indicating a quality of the lived experience recorded in the reconstructed stories. The qualities were listed for all participants and then lifted in abstraction to interpret the themes of the structure of meaning. Each of these themes is a synthesis that taps essential meaning encompassed in the stories. The themes were then incorporated into a structure of meaning for the experience of living with migraine headache. This structure of meaning comprises the findings of the study.

Rigor

The rigor of qualitative research is upheld through the establishment of credibility, auditability, confirmability, and fittingness (Sandelowski, 1986). Credibility increases the confidence in the truthfulness of the data. To establish credibility, the investigator engages in prolonged engagement, meaning that the researcher invests a sufficient amount of time to develop a true understanding of what it is like to live with migraine headache. The researcher thoroughly engages with the data during the conversation process, again while listening to recordings and reviewing transcripts, during conferences reflecting on the data with various committee members, and during the process of building a structure of meaning.

The investigator also embraces triangulation to establish credibility. This was to be achieved by gaining data from three sources: the conversation, observation of the participants, and the transcript and field notes related to the recorded conversation. To further establish credibility, the researcher identifies a nurse scholar with experience in qualitative analysis to serve as an external check confirming or refuting data analysis processes by following the transcriptions as well as the notes and analytic interpretations generated by the researcher. Several conferences with the nurse scholar are required to assure credibility.

Auditability involves the establishment of a data trail. This trail is located in journal documents that the investigator keeps throughout the research process. The journal includes the notes the investigator maintained from the conversation phase throughout the analysis phase and the conversation transcripts that include each stage of the analysis notes.

Confirmability "refers to the objectivity or neutrality of the data" (Polit & Hungler, 1997, p. 307). This implies that two or more people will review the data and agree to the meaning conveyed, thereby minimizing researcher bias. Confirmability is established through member checks, external checks, and a well-developed audit trail (Polit & Hungler, 1997). Fittingness or applicability—defined as the data fitting circumstances beyond the study—comes to light by verifying that credibility, auditability, and confirmability have been given necessary attention (Sandelowski, 1986).

EVALUATION OF THE STRUCTURE BUILDING PROCESS

The concept of yearning to be recognized was held tacitly before entering doctoral studies. What I knew to be true was that women with migraine who visited the emergency department or even the primary care setting were often labeled as "drug seekers," "frequent flyers," or "the headache in room 2." As I reflected on these women during a nursing theory course for doctoral studies, I knew there was a name for what I was seeing and hearing. Furthermore, I knew these women had unique stories that must be captured so that nursing can best understand what it is like to live with migraine headache.

It was through the assistance of a most knowledgeable professor and my fellow classmates that the concept started to emerge in our summer course. However, concept building is not a process that can be completed in just a few weeks. The work of building the concept of yearning to be recognized continued into the following years up to the point of finalization of the research proposal presented in this chapter.

Liehr and Smith (2008) identified 10 steps in building a structure for research. The first step is to capture phenomena in a clinical setting. This was achieved by reflecting on my experiences with women who presented with migraine headache in outpatient and inpatient settings. The second step in the approach is to name the phenomena. Working with my professor, we struggled to find the right name. We first used "making valid," but as we continued to think and talk, yearning to be recognized surfaced. Following Liehr and Smith's (2008) systematic approach, I then identified a philosophical perspective and middle range theory that fit the phenomena and allowed me to work up and down the ladder of abstraction. As previously mentioned, I extensively explored the literature, the fourth step. The fifth step was to gather the story of someone who lived with migraine headache. This step calls for writing a reconstructed story that captures the core qualities of the phenomena. This reconstructed story allowed me to edge closer to realizing a concept that could guide my research.

The remaining steps of Liehr and Smith's approach include the creation of a mini-saga, identification of the core qualities of the phenomena within a synthesized definition of the phenomena, a model, and a mini-synthesis (Liehr & Smith, 2008). The mini-saga, a short version of the reconstructed story, must be 50 words exactly. Although difficult and time consuming, creating the mini-saga allowed me to acknowledge the essence of the story of living with migraine headache. I went on to utilize the mini-saga on numerous occasions as I considered the essence of the stories I gathered in preparation for and during dissertation research.

As noted early in this chapter, the definition of yearning to be recognized is attending to the voice of suffering that calls for relief. Arranging the words in this manner allowed the core qualities and how they relate to each other to be presented in a concise manner. Creating this definition was critical for the concept building that led to a proposal for research. The definition was expressed in a model. The model for yearning to be recognized allows for visualization of the concept, enabling a next step where logical thinking about what has been learned comes into the forefront. The mini-synthesis requires one sentence that suggests a direction for research, thereby planting the seeds for research ideas and providing the grounding necessary for proposal development.

Data collected during dissertation research will serve to reconsider the model developed during the concept building process. It is possible that changes will be made guided by study findings. The expectation is that over time, the model of yearning to be recognized will be refined as it is used to study not only women with migraine, but also other populations who face this human health experience.

REFERENCES

Belam, J., Harris, G., Kernick, D., Kline, F., Lindley, K., McWatt, J., ... Reinhold, D. (2005). A qualitative study of migraine involving patient researchers. *British Journal of General Practice, 55*(511), 87–93.

Birtch, F. W. (1910, August). Report of a case of sick-headache. *California State Journal of Medicine, VIII*(8), 281–282.

Brandes, J. L. (2006, April 19). The influence of estrogen on migraine: A systematic review. *Journal of the American Medical Association, 295*(15), 1824–1830.

Cohen, M. Z. (2000a). Ethical issues and ethical approval. In M. Z. Cohen, D. L. Cohen, & R. H. Steves, *Hermenuetic phenomenological research: A practical guide for nurse researchers* (pp. 37–44). Thousand Oaks, CA: Sage.

Cohen, M. Z. (2000b). Introduction. In *Hermenutic phenomenological research: A practical guide for nurse researchers* (pp. 1–12). Thousand Oaks, CA: Sage.

Durham, C. F., Alden, K. R., Dalton, J., Carlson, J., Miller, D. W., Englebardt, S. P., & Neelon, V. J. (1998). Quality of life and productivity in nurses reporting migraine. *Headache, 38,* 427–435.

Elston-Lafata, J., Moon, C., Leotta, C., Kolodner, K., Poisson, L., & Lipton, R. B. (2004). The medical care utilization and costs associated with migraine headache. *Journal of General Internal Medicine, 19*(10), 1005–1012.

Frederiksson, L., & Eriksson, K. (2001). The patient's narrative of suffering: A path to health? An interpretive research synthesis on narrative understanding. *Scandinavian Journal of Caring Sciences, 15,* 3–11.

Gallagher, R. M., Mueller, L., Steer, R., & Ciervo, C. A. (1998). Myers-Briggs personality type classification of migrainous women. *Headache Quarterly, Current Treatment and Research, 9*(2), 149–152.

Kahn, D. L., & Steeves, R. H. (1986). The experience of suffering: Conceptual clarification and theoretical definition. *Journal of Advanced Nursing, 11*(6), 623–631.

Kolotylo, C. J., & Broome, M. E. (2000a). Predicting disability and quality of life in a community-based sample of women with migraine headache. *Pain Management Nursing, 1*(4), 139–151.

Kolotylo, C. J., & Broome, M. E. (2000b). Exploration of migraine pain, disability, depressive symptomatology, and coping: A pilot study. *Health Care for Women International, 21*(3), 203–218.

Liehr, P. R., & Smith, M. J. (2008). Story theory. In M. J. Smith & P. R. Liehr (Eds.), *Middle range theory for nursing* (2nd ed., pp. 205–224). New York, NY: Springer Publishing.

Lipton, R. B., Stewart, W. F., Diamond, S., Reed, M. L., & Reed, M. (2001). Prevalence and burden of migraine in the United States: Data from the American Migraine Study II. *Headache, 41*(7), 646–657.

Magiorkinis, E., Diamantis, A., Mitsikostas, D., & Androutsos, G. (2009). Headaches in antiquity and during the early scientific era. *Journal of Neurology, 256*(8), 1215–1220.

Mannix, L. K. (2008). Menstrual-related pain conditions: Dysmenorrhea and migraine. *Journal of Women's Health, 17*(5), 879–891.

Marcus, D. A., Kapelewski, C., Jacob, R. G., Rudy, T. E., & Furman, J. M. (2004). Validation of a brief nurse-administered migraine assessment tool. *Headache, 44*(4), 328–332.

Martin, B. C., Pathak, D. S., Sharfman, M. I., Adelman, J. U., Taylor, F., & Kwong, W. J. (2000). Validity and reliability of the Migraine-Specific Quality of Life Questionnaire (MSQ version 2.1). *Headache, 40*(3), 204–215.

Merriam-Webster. (1988). *Webster's ninth new collegiate dictionary* (9th ed.). Springfield, MA: Author.

Meyer, G. A. (2002). The art of watching out: Vigilance in women who have migraine headache. *Qualitative Health Research, 12*(9), 1220–1234.

Moffitt, H. C. (1911). Clinical observations on migraine. *California State Journal of Medicine, 9*(9), 358–361.

Moloney, M. F., Strickland, O. L., DeRossett, S. E., Melby, M. K., & Dietrich, A. S. (2006). The experiences of midlife women with migraines. *Journal of Nursing Scholarship, 38*(3), 278–285.

Mongini, F., Fassino, S., Rota, E., Deregibus, A., Levi, M., Monticone, D., & Abbate-Daga, G. (2005). The temperament and character inventory in women with migraine. *Journal of Headache and Pain, 6*(4), 247–249.

Nappi, G., Jensen, R., Nappi, R. E., Sances, G., Torelli, P., & Olesen, J. (2006). Diaries and calendars for migraine: A review. *Cephalalgia, 26*(8), 905–916.

Norberg, A., Bergsten, M., & Lundman, B. (2001). A model of consolidation. *Nursing Ethics, 8*(6), 544–553.

Peters, M., Abu-Saad, H. H., Vydelingum, V., Dowson, A., & Murphy, M. (2004). Migraine and chronic daily headache management: A qualitative study of patients' perceptions. *Scandinavian Journal of Caring Sciences, 18*(3), 294–303.

Peters, M., Abu-Saad, H. H., Vydelingum, V., Dowson, A., & Murphy, M. (2005). The patients' perceptions of migraine and chronic daily headache: A qualitative study. *The Journal of Headache and Pain, 6*(1), 40–47.

Polit, D. F., & Hungler, B. P. (1997). *Essentials of nursing research: Methods, appraisal, and utilization* (4th ed.). Philadelphia, PA: Lippincott.

Ruiz de Velasco, I., Gonzalez, N., Etxeberria, Y., & Garcia-Monco, J. C. (2003). Quality of life in migraine patients: A qualitative study. *Cephalalgia, 23,* 892–900.

Sandelowski, M. (1986). The problem of rigor in qualitative research. *Advances in Nursing Science, 8*(3), 27–37.

Silberstein, S. D., Lipton, R. B., & Dodick, D. W. (Eds.). (2008). *Wolff's headache and other head pain* (8th ed.). Oxford, NY: Oxford University Press.

Smith, T., Blumenthal, H., Diamond, M., Mauskop, A., Ames, M., McDonald, S., … Burch, S. (2007). Sumatriptan/naproxen sodium for migraine: Efficacy, health related quality of life, and satisfaction outcomes. *Headache, 47*(5), 683–692.

Stewart, W. F., Lipton, R. B., Dowson, A. J., & Sawyer, J. (2001). Development and testing of the Migraine Disability Assessment (MIDAS) Questionnaire to assess headache-related disability. *Neurology, 53*(5), 988–994.

Sundin, K., Axelsson, K., Jansson, L., & Norberg, A. (2000). Suffering from care as expressed in the narratives of former patients in somatic wards. *Scandinavian Journal of Caring Sciences, 14*(1), 16–22.

Van Manen, M. (1990). *Researching lived experience: Human science for an action sensitive pedagogy* (1st ed.). New York, NY: State University of New York Press.

Van Manen, M. (1997). *Researching lived experience: Human science for an action sensitive pedagogy* (2nd ed.). Ontario, Canada: The Althouse Press.

Vujevich, K. (2007). What makes women's migraines different. *The Clinical Advisor*, 33–38.

Weitzel, K. W., Strickland, J. M., Smith, K. M., & Goode, J. R. (2001). Gender-specific issues in the treatment of migraine. *Journal of Gender-Specific Medicine, 4*(1), 64–74.

Wikberg, A., Jansson, L., & Lithner, F. (2000). Women's experience of suffering repeated severe attacks of acute intermittant porphyria. *Journal of Advanced Nursing, 32*(6), 1348–1355.

20

Catastrophic Cultural Immersion: From Concept Building to Proposal Development to Data Gathering and Analysis

Lisa Marie Wands

THE FOUNDATION OF CONCEPT BUILDING

Building a concept for research using my own experience as a starting point was immensely useful, specifically my values as a person, nurse, and future researcher were honored and my intimate knowledge of a phenomenon initiated the process. Observing firsthand the fortitude and purpose with which post-Hurricane Katrina flood survivors faced the task of cleaning up and moving on with their lives inspired me to think about how people pick themselves up after a catastrophe and forge ahead into the unknown future. I thought about how they lived their lives prior to Katrina compared to after the storm. Many were living simple, normal lives: going to work, coming home, making dinner for their families, planning for the future. Suddenly, all of their material possessions were gone with the storm surge; there was no workplace to go to, no house to come home to, no kitchen to make dinner in. With all of those things gone, planning for the future meant thinking about how to get through the next day. Their new lives as hurricane survivors required redefining what it meant to live a normal life, to be normal.

Working with a broad definition of culture as a system made up of a group of people who shared their experience, survivors of catastrophes can be viewed as being members of a unique culture. When people experience a catastrophic event, such as a hurricane, they find themselves immersed in a culture of which they may have had no knowledge prior to the event. In considering how this phenomenon of interest could be articulated as a potential concept for research required thinking about the concept at a higher level of abstraction and separating the concept from the specific population of post-Hurricane Katrina flood survivors. Labeling the concept Catastrophic Cultural Immersion was meant to capture an experience that is prompted by upheaval and results in being submerged in a new contextual environment.

Definition

Catastrophic cultural immersion is the abrupt displacement of persons who then struggle to transcend the sudden unfamiliarity of a new culture in which they find themselves immersed.

Evolution of the Model

Most of the dialogue I have shared with others about this model has provided affirmation that the concepts are relevant and easily understandable. I have received comments that the arrow noting Struggle to Transcend should be wavy instead of straight to better imply that the journey of transcending unfamiliarity is not easy. I think this suggestion has merit, but I also feel that the stutter of bars at the beginning of the arrow represent the struggle. A most poignant question was asked by my former dean, Ann Boykin, when she asked where nursing was located within the model. Because this model was meant to guide *nursing* research, this was an important question; answering it helped me to hone in on the practicality and applicability of the model. The answer is that nursing has the ability to assist with the struggle to transcend times when people find themselves abruptly immersed in unfamiliarity; therefore, nursing is located in that stutter of bars at the beginning of the struggle. As illustrated in Figure 20.1, nursing was added as a component to the model to show this.

Using the Model to Design Research

The idea of catastrophic cultural immersion began in the context of natural disaster, but during my doctoral studies my interest grew for populations of war survivors. Engaged in cross-cultural work that focused on the long-term experience of surviving the World War II attacks on Pearl Harbor or Hiroshima prompted thinking about how

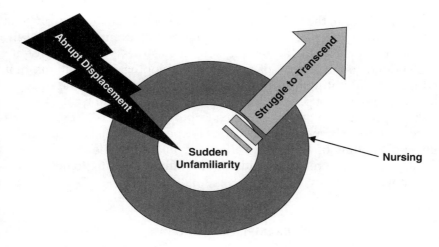

FIGURE 20.1   Catastrophic Cultural Immersion

living through war impacts people's lives on many levels. Coupled with the military campaigns the United States continues to engage in overseas and the daily reports on social media platforms about the difficulties veterans face when working to reintegrate into life at home after military service, I envisioned how their experience of coming home was a relevant example of catastrophic cultural immersion.

Concepts of the model are present in the veteran's health experience of returning home from war to a place that was once familiar but which has been altered by time and absence, requiring the veteran to negotiate everyday living in the culture of this unexpectedly new environment while resolving conflicts between military and civilian sense of self. For veterans who return home from war, a reevaluation of self needs to take into account changes that have occurred in the home environment while they were away, such as children passing developmental milestones, and changes that have occurred within themselves as a result of their war experience. Returning veterans may struggle with disconnecting from military-driven thinking to reconnect with home life and loved ones. Personality traits, such as aggressiveness, venerated by the military may not be conducive to reintegration into relationships.

Viewing the challenge of coming home from war through the lens of catastrophic cultural immersion allows for a new perspective not found in extant literature on the veteran population. While specific problems, such as post-traumatic stress disorder (PTSD), have been studied at length, the individual experience of coming home from war has not been viewed or studied as a catastrophic event in and of itself. Nurses can play a role in helping veterans as they work to negotiate the sudden unfamiliarity of home by developing interventions that address complicating health issues that arise in relation to the struggle to transcend abrupt postdeployment displacement. Using catastrophic cultural immersion as a guiding concept honors the veteran's experience of coming home as an immersive experience that can potentially affect all realms of health and life. Understanding the challenges of reintegration can create a foundation for nurses desiring to help veterans move on with living.

EXEMPLAR PROPOSAL

Approximately 2.4 million men and women served in the military campaigns Operation Enduring Freedom (OEF) and Operation Iraqi Freedom (OIF) in Middle Eastern countries since September 11, 2001 (Spelman, Hunt, Seal, & Burgo-Black, 2012). The United States maintains an all-volunteer military, meaning that these individuals signed up for military duty by choice, leaving their homes and families to protect and defend the nation. After fulfilling contractual obligations, veterans return home to resume normal lives and reoccupy previously held social roles, such as spouse. Very often, the process of reintegrating into civilian life is challenging as changes have occurred at home while the serviceman or woman was deployed (Doyle & Peterson, 2005). Physical injury or psychological trauma may make reintegration more difficult for some. While the health care community has concentrated on developing ways to address the needs of veterans suffering from certain service-related afflictions, such as traumatic brain injury (TBI) and PTSD, it is equally important to understand and support the all-encompassing experience of reintegrating into life at home for any veteran, as difficulties with the transition can have a direct impact on veteran health. The transition from living in a chaotic war zone to resuming a fulfilling life at home is deeply embedded in the context of relationships to self and to others. As such, nursing focused on supporting all realms of life and health can provide support to individuals who struggle through the transition.

The purpose of this mixed methods study was to explore the experience of coming home from war for veterans of the current military conflicts in the Middle East. The specific aims of this study integrate qualitative (specific aims 1 and 2) and quantitative (specific aim 3) approaches to:

1. Describe complicating health issues for veterans of the current war in the Middle East in the context of the challenge of coming home from war;
2. Describe how veterans of the current war in the Middle East move to resolve complicating health issues that emerge within the context of the challenge of coming home from war;
3. Identify dimensions of health for veterans coming home from the current war in the Middle East through self-reported health status (SF-36v2); and
4. Explore similarities and distinctions among complicating health issues, movement toward resolving, and dimensions of health identified through qualitative and quantitative analyses.

Background and Significance

While deployed to combat zones in the Middle East, military personnel must learn to survive in an environment when threat to life can come from anywhere at any time. Data collected during 2003 revealed that 93% of Army personnel deployed to Iraq had been under fire, and 95% had seen the bodies of people killed as a result of combat (Hoge et al., 2004). Harsh foreign physical surroundings, strenuous demands of a rigorous military schedule, and constant vigilance were required to ensure the safety of self and fellow soldiers to create an environment far removed from life within the protected boundaries of country and home. Out of necessity, traits of survivor and warrior, such as secrecy and domination, govern the psyche of the soldier (National Center for PTSD, 2006), and strong bonds are forged with fellow soldiers allowing for feelings of safety and security in an otherwise threatening environment (Flinn, 2007).

Once back at home, veterans may simultaneously struggle with disconnecting from their military identity and soldier comrades while defining new connections with friends, family, and society (Flinn, 2007). Veterans may be reluctant to communicate with family and friends, not only because loved ones cannot place the veteran's experiences of war in an accurate context but also out of fear of judgment for actions necessitated by combat duty (Committee on Veterans Affairs, 2005; Hutchinson & Banks-Williams, 2006). Changes in home environment and organization may leave the veteran questioning his or her ability to contribute to the family (Faber, Willerton, Clymer, MacDermid, & Weiss, 2008), while abrupt resumption of previously held responsibilities may leave family members feeling usurped, underappreciated, or undermined (Doyle & Peterson, 2005). Societal opinion against the war may lead a veteran to feel a sense of public rejection (Hutchinson & Banks-Williams, 2006). These factors can leave the veteran feeling confused, frustrated, or unsupported, which may consequently lead to adverse health outcomes.

In extant literature, the health of veterans is most often discussed in a fragmented manner. The most prevalent discussions center on veteran physical and mental health. Irrefutably, these realms warrant attention as significant numbers of veterans suffer with issues related to these domains. About 49,000 service members have been physically wounded in action since 2001 in the OEF/OIF military campaigns as of August 2012 (Department of Defense 2012). Advances in warfare technology resulted in both more powerful weapons and improved body armor protection, resulting in a larger proportion of combatants surviving injuries (Gawande, 2004); however, the severity of injuries can often be great. Almost 1,500 amputations have been performed in-field, and more than 40,000 service personnel suffered a TBI as of June 2012 (Department of Defense 2009). Unfortunately, the actual incidence of TBI is likely greater according to Tanelian and Jaycox (2008) who cited poor documentation of blast exposure and failure to identify potential cases as causes of under-counting TBI rates.

In 2004, Hoge et al. reported results of an important study of the prevalence of mental health issues among 6,201 Army and Marine personnel either before deployment to Iraq or after deployment to Iraq or Afghanistan. The participant population was mostly Army personnel ($n = 5,386$), and most of the testing was done postdeployment ($n = 3,671$). Postdeployment surveys were given 3 to 4 months after Army soldiers ($n = 1,962$) who had been stationed in Afghanistan and Army soldiers and Marines ($n = 1,709$) who had been stationed in Iraq returned stateside. Findings of the study revealed that major depression, PTSD, or alcohol abuse "was significantly higher among soldiers after deployment than before deployment particularly with regard to PTSD" (p. 17). Participants surveyed postdeployment met criteria for depression at rates ranging 6.9% to 7.9%; anxiety at rates ranging 6.6% to 7.9%; and PTSD at rates ranging 6.2% to 12.9%. Limitations of this study led the authors to assert that these findings are conservative.

Although not extensive, some work has been done to investigate other realms of OEF/OIF veteran health in addition to physical and mental domains. Faber et al. (2008) studied issues of loss and separation in a small sample of families in which at least one member was an Army Reservist who served in Iraq; during deployment, families reported stress in relation to not knowing what was happening with their Reservist, not having control over the situation, and redistribution of family roles and responsibilities. In addition, uncertainty was a prevailing theme after the Reservist returned home. Barker and Berry (2009) studied the impact of parent deployment on young children in 57 families with one parent serving active duty; results of the study showed an increase in child behavior problems and attachment behavior problems among children whose parent served a tour of duty. Greater length of deployment and multiple deployments had an increased effect on child behavior, and parents reported feelings of depression and stress in relation to the experience of deployment.

Physical and mental health of personnel serving in all branches of U.S. military are assessed prior to deployment, immediately postdeployment, and again 3 to 6 months after arriving home (Armed Forces Health Surveillance Center, 2012). Service members generally rate their overall health as worse immediately postdeployment compared to predeployment and worse yet again at a third evaluation 3 to 6 months after arriving home. In this ongoing surveillance of health, veterans self-report health status on a 5-item Likert-type scale ranging from poor to excellent. For the period from June 2011 to May 2012, active-duty personnel responded that their health was fair or poor at a rate of about 2% prior to deployment, 8% to 10% at postdeployment, and 10% to 13% 3 to 6 months postdeployment. These postdeployment screenings are important for the identification of health needs and the arrangement of care to address needs (Doyle & Peterson, 2005); anecdotal evidence, however, reveals that some military personnel are not completely truthful when answering questions on immediate postdeployment health surveys because they fear a delay in release from the military and their greatly anticipated reunion with loved ones (Committee on Veterans Affairs, 2005; Davis et al., 2007; Gaylord, 2006). It is possible that more truthful self-assessment of health occurs at the 3-to-6-month mark postdeployment; however, adverse psychological impact of military experiences may manifest over the span of months following the veteran's return home, thereby resulting in declining reports of health over time (Armed Forces Health Surveillance Center, 2008).

As presented, health of veterans is most often reported in literature in a fragmented manner; dimensions of health are discussed in isolation. The reality, however, is that no dimension of health exists in solitude. When one dimension is affected, other realms are often affected. Several nursing theorists, including Boykin and Schoenhofer

(2001), submit that breaking down an individual into parts negates the ability to come to know the person and to acknowledge the person as a whole being. For example, the essence of a person experiencing PTSD is not fully captured by the diagnosed mental disorder; rather, he or she lives a life that includes flashbacks and intrusive thoughts. Assessing the prevalence of PTSD among veterans relying on the number of times certain symptoms arise does not inform nursing practice of what it means to live with flashbacks or how individuals overcome intrusive thoughts. To truly inform nursing practice, nursing research must be undertaken using a lens of wholeness and a "perspective of what it means to be human" (Boykin & Schoenhofer, 2001, p. 5); this guiding principle provides philosophical direction for designing this study and viewing the experience of coming home from war as an all-encompassing event of catastrophic cultural immersion. In order to capture the all-encompassing human experience of coming home from war through the conceptual lens of catastrophic cultural immersion, a decision was made to gather stories using story inquiry methodology.

From the perspective of the ladder of abstraction (Smith & Liehr, 2008), Boykin and Schoenhofer's work is at the highest level of abstraction while catastrophic cultural immersion is at a lower conceptual level. Story inquiry method, while consistent with the guiding structures, provided distinct empirical direction for story gathering and story analysis.

Preliminary Studies Preparing Research for Proposed Work

I gained experience using story inquiry methodology with two other research projects. In one study, data analysis was guided by story inquiry method (Liehr & Smith, 2007) to explore the challenges that older adults encounter as they negotiate lifestyle changes dictated by their dependence upon hemodialysis for survival (Hain, Wands, & Liehr, 2011). Data collection for this study was conducted using the story path approach. Data from 56 participants receiving outpatient hemodialysis were analyzed by a team of three: Principal Investigator (PI) Debra Hain, DNS, ARNP-BC; Patricia Liehr, PhD, RN (PL); and me (LMW). Two of the team members (PI and LMW) independently read and reread 10 participant stories at a time to discover what "mattered most" to the storyteller in each story. The two researchers met to discuss findings from each 10-story group and reach agreement regarding the central ideas found in the stories. Infrequent disagreement regarding identification of the key element of a story was resolved through discussion. The third team member (PL) reviewed 20% of the stories to verify findings. Stories that were found to have similar character were grouped together into three units, which were each named with a theme identifying the overriding health challenge of the group. The three themes were: living a restriction-driven existence, balancing independence/dependence, and struggling with those providing care. The next analytic process was to identify movement toward resolving health challenges. Keeping the stories divided into theme-associated units, the team followed the same inductive approach to identify movement toward resolving, which are practical approaches participants used to overcome their health challenge. Approaches used to resolve the health challenge of living a restriction-driven existence included: looking forward; keeping it all in perspective; existing, not living; acknowledging but resisting limitations; and keep fighting. Approaches used to resolve the health challenge of balancing independence/dependence included: struggling to keep control; seeking self-perspective through connections; and choosing a positive outlook. Approaches used to resolve the health challenge of struggling with those providing care included: recognizing feelings of discontent; choosing a positive outlook; and taking a stand. Each of the health challenge-themed groups also contained an approach called just do it; however, the meaning for this approach was group-specific, highlighting the contextual nature of approaches used to resolve the health challenge (Hain et al., 2011).

The other study through which I gained experience with story inquiry methodology was an exploration of how the experience of living through the attacks on Pearl Harbor, Hawaii, in 1941 or the atomic bombing of Hiroshima, Japan, in 1945 affected health over time (Liehr, Nishimura, Ito, Wands, & Takahashi, 2011; Takahashi, Nishimura, Ito, Wands, & Liehr, 2009). Data collection for this study was conducted using the story path approach. Data from 51 participants, 28 Hiroshima survivors in Japan and 23 Pearl Harbor survivors in the United States, were analyzed by an international team of five: Co-Principal Investigators Patricia Liehr, PhD, RN (PL) and Ryutaro Takahashi (RT); Mio Ito, PhD, RN (MI); Chie Nishimura, BSN, RN (CN); and me (LMW). Data analysis was guided by story inquiry method (Liehr & Smith, 2011) and was conducted in three phases; communication was accomplished through electronic means, including e-mail and Skype™, and occasional face-to-face meetings. The first phase used an inductive approach to identify turning points and turning point-related descriptive expressions for 10 representative participants, 5 from Hiroshima and 5 from Pearl Harbor) (Takahashi et al., 2009). The second phase used a deductive approach to identify content from the remaining 41 participants that fit with existing turning points and descriptive expressions named in preliminary analysis (Liehr et al., 2011). In the third phase, the research team employed an inductive approach to consider content that did not fit into existing turning points and descriptive expressions identified during the second phase. Finally, descriptive expressions associated with each turning point were synthesized into themes that reflected the complexity of the broader range of content. Three turning points were identified for each participant group, and two to four themes were identified for each turning point. The turning points for Hiroshima survivors are: facing the disorienting aftermath of people and places with fall of the A-bomb; becoming Hibakusha (Japanese term for officially certified atomic bomb survivors); and reaching out to create meaning/purpose that is consistent with cherished peace. The turning points for Pearl Harbor survivors are: coming to grips with the reality of a Japanese attack and scrambling to respond; honoring the memory of their war experience and trying to set it aside to get on with usual valued activities; and embracing connection as a source of comfort and understanding. Turning point-associated themes are reported in the Liehr, Nishimura, Ito, Wands, and Takahashi 2011 published manuscript.

Methods

Design

This mixed methods study design integrated both qualitative and quantitative approaches to gain understanding of the issues that complicate health for veterans and approaches veterans used to resolve complicating health issues associated with the challenge of coming home from war. The qualitative approach was guided by story inquiry method, which is derived from story theory. Story inquiry method is a structured approach for gathering and analyzing stories about a health challenge from a group of individuals who share a particular experience (Liehr & Smith, 2007, 2011); for this study, the shared experience of coming home from war provided the context for discovery of issues that complicate health. Story inquiry method guided data collection through intentional dialogue between nurse researcher and the person sharing the story. Through this approach, the researcher engages the research participant to share what "matters most" about the health challenge. As the health challenge story unfolds, connections between self and others and self and critical moments in time are brought to light for both story sharer (research participant) and intentioned listener (nurse researcher). While sharing the story of the health challenge, the participant may discover meaning, may experience a sense of ease, and may become aware of moving toward resolving the complicating health challenge, in this case, the challenge of coming home from war.

Story inquiry method also guided qualitative data analysis by directing identification of complicating health issues for veterans returning home from war and descriptions of movement toward resolving complicating health issues. Intentional dialogue about a health challenge ensues in the sharing of one's story, encompassing high points, low points, turning points, and insights about movement toward resolving (Liehr & Smith, 2008). For the purposes of this study, the focus was directed to identifying complicating health issues and movement toward resolving health issues, which would indicate progress in living with the challenge of coming home from war.

Quantitative data about participants' health was gathered using the 36-item Short-Form Health Survey, Version 2 (SF-36v2), which participants completed independently as the final segment of data collection. This instrument is used to assess overall physical and mental health status on two summary scales aggregated from eight subscales measuring key operational indicators of health (Ware, 2004); the eight subscales of the SF-36v2 are physical functioning (PF); performance in physical role (RP); performance in emotional role (RE); vitality (V); social functioning (SF); bodily pain (BP); general health perceptions (GHP); and mental health (MH) (Ware et al., 2007). The SF-36v2 also contains a one-item query to measure Reported Health Transition (HT), which asks respondents how current health compares to health one year previous. Wetzler, Lum, and Bush (2000) encourage the use of the SF-36 in clinical practice to measure overall health while emphasizing concern for the whole person.

Version 2 of the SF-36 was released as an improved edition in 2007; internal consistency reliabilities for the eight subscales range from 0.83 for the GHP subscale to 0.95 for the RP subscale (Ware et al., 2007). The SF-36v2 was affirmed as an appropriate tool for use with a veteran population in the Millennium Cohort Study in which the instrument was administered to 77,000 veterans; internal consistency reliabilities for the eight subscales ranged from 0.80 on the MH subscale to 0.92 on the PF subscale (Smith, Smith, Jacobson, Corbeil, & Ryan, 2007).

Creswell's (2003) four criteria for choosing a mixed methods strategy of inquiry were considered for study design; these four tenets are implementation, priority, integration, and theoretical perspective. The first criterion, implementation, refers to data collection. For this study, qualitative and quantitative data were collected concurrently during one session. The second criterion, priority, refers to the weight that data are assigned. This study was meant to explore and describe the experience of coming home for veterans and was intended to have detailed description from a small sample; therefore, qualitative data were given more weight. The third criterion, integration, refers to how and when the data are combined. For this study, qualitative data were analyzed first to discover complicating health issues and then to identify strategies employed to overcome complicating health issues. The SF-36v2 was then analyzed to reveal dimensions of health. Finally, qualitative findings were considered through each of the dimensions assessed with the quantitative tool. The fourth criterion is the consideration of whether a theoretical perspective will guide the work. For this study, story theory (Liehr & Smith, 2008) was used to guide qualitative data collection and analysis through story inquiry method (Liehr & Smith, 2011).

Population/Recruitment/Setting

Participants were recruited for this study at Florida Atlantic University (FAU) through the use of a recruitment flyer and electronic announcements. Although accurate enrollment numbers of student veterans were not available at the time, recruitment of a sufficient number of participants was expected in part due to the implementation of the Post-9/11 GI Bill, which expanded education benefits for veterans in 2009 (Department of Veterans Affairs, 2009). Under this bill, individuals who served in the military on or after September 10, 2001 are provided financial support to further their education. Permission was given by the Institutional Review Board (IRB) to distribute recruitment flyers through the Financial Aid office, specifically through the person who acted as liaison for student veteran benefits between FAU and Veterans Affairs, as well as through the university's three student health clinics and on campus bulletin boards. Recruitment announcements were also distributed in university-wide electronic announcement deliveries.

The following inclusion criteria guided purposive selection of study participants:

- Participants had served in the U.S. Armed Forces, any branch, part or full time.
- Participants may have been actively serving or retired from the military at the time of interview.

- Participants had been deployed to and returned home from at least one tour of duty in Iraq or Afghanistan since September 2001.
- Participants were 21 years of age or older.
- Participants were students at FAU.
- Participants were able to speak and read English.
- Participants gave consent to participate.

Participation in this study was completely voluntary; persons desiring to participate contacted me independently by means of contact information included on flyers and in announcements. Twenty-five participants were sought for inclusion in the study. All respondents meeting the study's inclusion criteria were accepted as participants. Participation was encouraged through the offer of a $5 gift card to either Starbucks or McDonald's; participants were given choice of vendor once all data were collected. Participants met with me and all data were collected in one session per participant in one of FAU's student health clinics during normal operating hours.

Procedure

Conference rooms in the FAU student health clinics were provided, which allowed for uninterrupted privacy for one-on-one interviews as well as a quiet environment in which to audiotape the interviews without interference. The researcher thoroughly explained the study to the participant and answered any questions the participant had prior to providing written consent or engaging in data collection.

Audiotaping began once consent was obtained and continued throughout the researcher–participant dialogue. Sociodemographic data were collected at the beginning of the interview and included age, gender, marital status, number of children and their ages, years of military service, and level of education. Participants were asked about past deployments to Iraq or Afghanistan, including how many times they had deployed, how long the deployments lasted, and the date of their most recent return home. In addition, participants were asked if they had knowledge that they would be returning to Iraq or Afghanistan in the future.

Qualitative data collection began by introducing the participant to a story line (Liehr & Smith, 2000, 2008). Each participant was offered a piece of paper upon which a horizontal line, symbolizing the person's story of the challenge of coming home, had been drawn. A mark was made close to the beginning of the line at the left side of the paper; this mark was labeled with the date of the participant's most recent return home. Participants were asked to make a second mark on the line that represented their current standing in their story of the challenge of coming home. Use of the story line is intended to anchor the participant in the present moment and act as a starting point for a discussion of health in the present (Liehr & Smith, 2000, 2008). Noting a returned home date on the story line at the beginning of the dialogue was intended to direct participants' stories to the experience of coming home from war as opposed to going to or being at war.

Participants were first asked to define health, and dialogue ensued about health in the present moment focusing on the issues they were facing. Once present health had been fully explored, participants were asked to recall the experience of coming home from war. During discourse about health issues experienced in the past, some participants talked about experiences they had while actively serving in the Middle East. The researcher followed through with these discussions, allowing participants to share as much as they felt comfortable sharing. When appropriate, the researcher redirected participants to focus on their coming home experience. Participants were asked to reflect on how their experiences since coming home have contributed to their current health, thereby making the link between past and present. The final segment of the story path interview entailed asking participants about their hopes and dreams for the future and how those aspirations might have been impacted, if at all, by the experience of coming home from war. Length of interview ranged from 20 to 54 minutes; average interview time was 35 minutes. No participants reported or exhibited any outward signs of emotional distress during this qualitative component of the study.

Once the dialogic portion of the interview was finished, audio recording was discontinued and the participant was asked to complete the SF-36v2; this took approximately 5 to 10 minutes. Participants completed the instrument independently, although the researcher stayed in the interview room with them.

Analysis Plan

Descriptive statistics were used to summarize sociodemographic information about the study population; this information provides important contextual data about the study sample, which may inform understanding about study participants but cannot be generalized to a larger population.

Qualitative Analysis

Qualitative data analysis was guided by story inquiry method (Liehr & Smith, 2007, 2008, 2011) to address the first two specific aims of this study: (1) describe complicating health issues for veterans of the current war in the Middle East in the context of the challenge of coming home from war; and (2) describe how veterans of the current war in the Middle East move to resolve complicating health issues. The researcher transcribed audiotaped interviews and then listened to the tapes in their entirety while checking story transcriptions for errors. An inductive approach to qualitative data analysis was followed, which moved from the words of the participants to themes that describe complicating health issues. In this phase, passages in which the storyteller described a complicating health issue were highlighted. Like passages were grouped together, and redundancies and distinctions were noted. Where redundancies occurred, descriptive passages were synthesized to capture the essence of the participants' words. Finally, a health issue theme was identified for each group of passages. This process was repeated for identification of themes describing movement toward resolving complicating health issues.

Trustworthiness of Qualitative Analysis

Qualitative data are very rich when collected from participants. People express themselves in a myriad of ways, and it is imperative that the research stay true to the participants' intended ideas and meaning. In qualitative research, trustworthiness of data analysis occurs when the researcher makes certain that identified themes do not depart from the idea path intended by participants. According to Creswell (2007), there are several strategies that qualitative researchers can employ to validate study findings. One strategy is to check with participants to be sure that the researcher is not misconstruing meanings conveyed during the interview. The researcher can summarize the participant's ideas and offer them back to the participant requesting validation or correction of the researcher's rendering of the participant's story with such phrases as, "What I am hearing you say is X. Is that right?" Another validation strategy is through peer review of reported findings, which, for this study, occurred through the experienced perspectives of the researcher's dissertation committee members. At least 20% of the data were independently reviewed by the researcher's dissertation committee chairperson, and findings were compared to ensure that the researcher stayed focused on and consistent with data interpretation. According to Creswell (2007), qualitative researchers should employ at least two validation strategies to adequately ensure that reported findings are truly reflective of participants' experiences.

Quantitative Analysis

Use of the SF-36v2 was employed in order to address the third specific aim: (3) identify dimensions of health for veterans coming home from the current war in the Middle East through self-reported health status. All participants completed all items of the instrument. Participants' responses were entered into the QualityMetric Health Outcomes™ Scoring Software, Version 4.0. Internal consistency was assessed for each of the eight subscales, and comparisons of participants' scores to general population norms were made. The scoring software also estimated a percentage of the sample that is at risk for depression.

Mixing Methods

Qualitative findings and quantitative results were combined to address the fourth specific aim of the study: (4) explore similarities and distinctions among complicating health issues, movement toward resolving, and dimensions of health identified through qualitative and quantitative analysis. Issues that complicate health for veterans experiencing the challenge of coming home from war and approaches to resolve health issues as discovered through qualitative data analysis were compared to health dimensions, as represented by the eight subscales of the SF-36v2, to discover similarities and distinctions.

EVALUATION OF STRUCTURE BUILDING PROCESS

This study was designed to explore the all-encompassing health experience of coming home from war for veterans of the current military conflicts in the Middle East. The conceptual foundation for the study framed a perspective that coming home from war can be viewed as a catastrophic event. Catastrophic cultural immersion is defined as the abrupt displacement of persons into sudden unfamiliarity from which they struggle to transcend (Wands, 2008). During times of war, military culture is centered on survival; service members are taught skills "to survive and succeed in war" (National Center for PTSD, 2006, p. 2).

These skills often impair communication in non military environments, which can create difficulties as veterans begin reintegrating into civilian life. Viewing culture simply as stemming from a shared experience, Hobbs (2008) stated that veterans are "no longer true civilians [but rather] ex-soldiers that enter the culture of veterans" (p. 337). The catastrophic cultural immersion model depicts the conceptual lens that will be used to consider study findings describing the transition from military culture to veteran culture.

Utilizing the catastrophic cultural immersion model to design a research study provided me with a particular perspective with which to view a phenomenon in which I had interest. The experience of coming home from war has the potential to impact every facet of life for veterans, and this experience can be and has been viewed in a myriad of ways in the development of research studies. Some researchers have focused on factors that influence physical health, while others concentrated on veterans' mental health and on specific diagnoses, such as PTSD, prevalent among this population. In creating my own concept for research, I was able to embed my core disciplinary value that persons are complex whole beings whose parts do not function in isolation. This principal concept is unlikely to change as I move forward with my career as a nurse researcher, and I believe that I will be able to utilize this model for future work with additional groups of veterans as well as with other populations. I look forward to the continued evolution of the model as I complete work and continue thinking about the concept of catastrophic cultural immersion.

REFERENCES

Armed Forces Health Surveillance Center. (2008, July). Update: Deployment health assessments, U.S. Armed Forces. *Medical Surveillance Monthly Report, 15*(6), 20–25.

Armed Forces Health Surveillance Center. (2012, June). Deployment health assessments. U.S. Armed Forces. *Medical Surveillance Monthly Report, 19*(6), 24–27.

Barker, L. H., & Berry, K. D. (2009). Developmental issues impacting military families with young children during single and multiple deployments. *Military Medicine, 174*(10), 1033–1040.

Boykin, A., & Schoenhofer, S. O. (2001). *Nursing as caring: A model for transforming practice.* Sudbury, MA: Jones and Bartlett.

Committee on Veterans Affairs. (2005, August 3). *Seattle field hearing: Coming home from combat—are veterans getting the help they need?* (Senate Hearing 109–328). Washington, DC: U.S. Government Printing Office.

Creswell, J. W. (2003). *Research design: Qualitative, quantitative, and mixed methods approaches* (2nd ed.). Thousand Oaks, CA: Sage.

Creswell, J. W. (2007). *Qualitative inquiry & research design: Choosing among five approaches* (2nd ed.). Thousand Oaks, CA: Sage.

Davis, J. D., Engel, C. C., Mishkind, M., Jaffer, A., Sjoberg, T., Tinker, T., ... O'Leary, T. (2007). Provider and patient perspectives regarding health care for war-related health concerns. *Patient Education and Counseling, 68*(1), 52–60.

Department of Defense. (2012). *Operation Iraqi Freedom (OIF) U.S. casualty status fatalities.* Retrieved from http://www.defenselink.mil/news/casualty.pdf

Department of Veterans Affairs. (2009). *Federal benefits for veterans.* Washington, DC: Author.

Doyle, M. E., & Peterson, K. A. (2005). Re-entry and reintegration: Returning home after combat. *Psychiatry Quarterly, 76*(4), 361–370.

Faber, A. J., Willerton, E., Clymer, S. R., MacDermid, S. M., & Weiss, H. M. (2008). Ambiguous absence, ambiguous presence: A qualitative study of military reserve families in wartime. *Journal of Family Psychology, 22*(2), 222–230.

Flinn, E. S. (2007). Living nursing presence with soldiers returning from Iraq and Afghanistan: Quality of life issues for returning soldiers. *Nursing Science Quarterly, 20*(3), 218–219.

Gawande, A. (2004). Casualties of war – Military care for the wounded from Iraq and Afghanistan. *New England Journal of Medicine, 351*(24), 2471–2475.

Gaylord, K. M. (2006). The psychosocial effects of combat: The frequently unseen injury. *Critical Care Nursing Clinics of North America, 18*, 349–357.

Hain, D. J., Wands, L. M., & Liehr, P. (2011). Approaches to resolve health challenges in a population of older adults undergoing hemodialysis. *Research in Gerontological Nursing, 4*(1), 53–62.

Hobbs, K. (2008). Reflections on the culture of veterans. *AAOHN Journal, 56*(8), 337–341.

Hoge, C. W., Castro, C. A., Messer, S. C., McGurk, D., Cotting, D. I., & Koffman, R. L. (2004). Combat duty in Iraq and Afghanistan, mental health problems, and barriers to care. *The New England Journal of Medicine, 351*(1), 13–22.

Hutchinson, J., & Banks-Williams, L. (2006). Clinical issues and treatment considerations for new veterans: Soldiers of the wars in Iraq and Afghanistan. *Primary Psychiatry, 13*(3), 66–71.

Liehr, P., Nishimura, C., Ito, M., Wands, L. M., & Takahashi, R. (2011). A lifelong journey of moving beyond wartime trauma for survivors from Hiroshima and Pearl Harbor. *Advances in Nursing Science, 34*(3), 215–228.

Liehr, P., & Smith, M. J. (2000). Using story theory to guide nursing practice. *International Journal for Human Caring, 4*, 13–18.

Liehr, P., & Smith, M. J. (2007). Story inquiry: A method for research. *Archives of Psychiatric Nursing, 21*(2), 120–121.

Liehr, P., & Smith, M. J. (2008). Story theory. In M. J. Smith & P. R. Liehr (Eds.), *Middle range theory for nursing* (2nd ed., pp. 205–224). New York, NY: Springer.

Liehr, P., & Smith, M. J. (2011). Refining story inquiry as a method for research. *Archives of Psychiatric Nursing, 25*(1), 74–75.

National Center for PTSD. (2006). *Returning from the war zone.* Washington, DC: Department of Veterans Affairs.

Smith, M. J., & Liehr, P. (2008). Theory-guided translation: Emphasizing human connection. *Archives of Psychiatric Nursing, 22*(3), 175–176.

Smith, T. C., Smith, B., Jacobson, I. G., Corbeil, T. E., & Ryan, M. K. (2007). Reliability of standard health assessment instruments in a large, population-based cohort study. *Annals of Epidemiology, 17,* 525–532. doi:10.1016/j.annepidem.2006.12.002.

Spelman, J. F., Hunt, S. C., Seal, K. H., & Burgo-Black, A. L. (2012). Post deployment care for returning combat veterans. *Journal of General Internal Medicine, 27*(9), 1200–1209.

Takahashi, R., Nishimura, C., Ito, M., Wands, L. M., & Liehr, P. (2009). Health stories of Hiroshima and Pearl Harbor survivors. *Journal of Aging, Humanities, and the Arts, 3*(3), 160–174.

Tanelian, T., & Jaycox, L. H. (Eds.). (2008). *Invisible wounds of care: Psychological and cognitive injuries, their consequences, and services to assist recovery.* Santa Monica, CA: RAND Corporation. Retrieved from http://www.rand.org/pubs/monographs/2008/RAND-MG720.pdf

Wands, L. M. (2008). Exemplar #2: Catastrophic cultural immersion. In M. J. Smith & P. R. Liehr (Eds.), *Middle range theory for nursing* (2nd ed., pp. 46–54). New York, NY: Springer.

Ware, J. E. (2004). SF-36 health survey update. In M. E. Maruish (Ed.), *The use of psychological for treatment planning and outcomes assessment: Instruments for adults* (3rd ed., Vol. 3, pp. 693–718). Mahwah, NJ: Erlbaum.

Ware, J. E., Kosinski, M., Bjorner, J. B., Turner-Bowker, D. M., Gandek, B., & Maruish, M. E. (2007). *User's manual for the SF-36v2 Health Survey* (2nd ed.). Lincoln, RI: QualityMetric.

Wetzler, H. P., Lum, D. L., & Bush, D. M. (2000). Using the SF-36 health survey in primary care. In M. E. Maruish (Ed.), *Handbook of psychological assessment in primary care settings* (pp. 583–621). Mahwah, NJ: Erlbaum.

Appendix

Middle Range Theories: 1988–2012

TABLE A.1

Year	Full citation (APA)	Name of theory
1988	Mishel, M. H. (1988). Uncertainty in illness. *Image: Journal of Nursing Scholarship, 20*(4), 225–231.	Uncertainty in illness
1990	Mishel, M. H. (1990). Reconceptualization of the uncertainty in illness theory. *Image: Journal of Nursing Scholarship, 22*(4), 256–262.	
1989	Thompson, J. E., Oakley, D., Burke, M., Jay, S., & Conklin, M. (1989). Theory building in nurse-midwifery: The care process. *Journal of Nurse-Midwifery, 34*(3), 120–130.	Nurse midwifery care
1990	Kinney, C. K. (1990). Facilitating growth and development: A paradigm case for modeling and role-modeling. *Issues in Mental Health Nursing, 11*, 375–395.	Facilitating growth and development
1991	Reed, P. G. (1991). Toward a nursing theory of self-transcendence: Deductive reformulation using developmental theories. *Advances in Nursing Science, 13*(4), 64–77.	Self-transcendence
1991	Burke, S. O., Kauffmann, E., Costello, E. A., & Dillon, M. C. (1991). Hazardous secrets and reluctantly taking charge: Parenting a child with repeated hospitalizations. *Image: Journal of Nursing Scholarship, 23*(1), 39–45.	Hazardous secrets and reluctantly taking charge
1991	Thomas, S. P. (1991). Toward a new conceptualization of women's anger. *Issues in Mental Health Nursing, 12*, 31–49.	Women's anger

(Continued)

TABLE A.1   (Continued)

Year	Full citation (APA)	Name of theory
1991	Swanson, K. M. (1991). Empirical development of a middle range theory of caring. *Nursing Research, 40*(3), 161–166.	Caring
1994	Powell-Cope, G. M. (1994). Family caregivers of people with AIDS: Negotiating partnerships with professional health care providers. *Nursing Research, 43*(6), 324–330.	Negotiating partnership
1995	Lenz, E. R., Suppe, F., Gift, A. G., Pugh, L. C., & Milligan, R. A. (1995). Collaborative development of middle-range nursing theories: Toward a theory of unpleasant symptoms. *Advances in Nursing Science, 17*(3), 1–13.	Unpleasant symptoms
1997	Lenz, E. R., Pugh, L. C., Milligan, R. A., Gift, A., & Suppe, F. (1997). The middle-range theory of unpleasant symptoms: An update. *Advances in Nursing Science, 19*(3), 14–27.	Unpleasant symptoms
1995	Jezewski, M. A. (1995). Evolution of a grounded theory: Conflict resolution through culture brokering. *Advances in Nursing Science, 17*(3), 14–30.	Cultural brokering
1995	Tollett, J. H., & Thomas, S. P. (1995). A theory-based nursing intervention to instill hope in homeless veterans. *Advances in Nursing Science, 18*(2), 76–90.	Homelessness– hopelessness
1996	Good, M., & Moore, S. M. (1996). Clinical practice guidelines as a new source of middle-range theory: Focus on acute pain. *Nursing Outlook, 44*(2), 74–79.	Balance between analgesia and side effects
1998	Good, M. (1998). A middle-range theory of acute pain management: Use in research. *Nursing Outlook, 46*(3), 120–124.	Acute pain management
1997	Auvil-Novak, S. E. (1997). A middle-range theory of chronotherapeutic intervention for postsurgical pain. *Nursing Research, 46*(2), 66–70.	Chronotherapeutic intervention for postsurgical pain
1997	Olson, J., & Hanchett, E. (1997). Nurse-expressed empathy, patient outcomes, and development of a middle-range theory. *Image: Journal of Nursing Scholarship, 29*(1), 71–76.	Nurse-expressed empathy and patient distress

Year	Full citation (APA)	Name of theory
1997	Brooks, E. M., & Thomas, S. (1997). The perception and judgment of senior baccalaureate student nurses in clinical decision making. *Advances in Nursing Science, 19*(3), 50–69.	Intrapersonal perceptual awareness
1997	Polk, L. V. (1997). Toward a middle-range theory of resilience. *Advances in Nursing Science, 19*(3), 1–13.	Resilience
1997	Gerdner, L. (1997). An individualized music intervention for agitation. *Journal of the American Psychiatric Nurses Association, 3*(6), 177–184.	Individualized music intervention for agitation
1997	Acton, G. J. (1997). Affiliated-individuation as a mediator of stress and burden in caregivers of adults with dementia. *Journal of Holistic Nursing, 15*(4), 336–357.	Affiliated individuation as mediator of stress
1998	Eakes, G. G., Burke, M. L., & Hainsworth, M. A. (1998). Middle-range theory of chronic sorrow. *Image: Journal of Nursing Scholarship, 30*(2), 179–184.	Chronic sorrow
1998	Huth, M. M., & Moore, S. M. (1998). Prescriptive theory of acute pain management in infants and children. *Journal of the Society of Pediatric Nurses, 3*(1), 23–32.	Acute pain management in infants and children
1998	Levesque, L., Ricard, N., Ducharme, F., Duquette, A., & Bonin, J. (1998). Empirical verification of a theoretical model derived from the Roy Adaptation Model: Findings from five studies. *Nursing Science Quarterly, 11*(1), 31–39.	Psychological adaptation
1998	Ruland, C. M., & Moore, S. M. (1998). Theory construction based on standards of care: A proposed theory of the peaceful end of life. *Nursing Outlook, 46*(4), 169–175.	Peaceful end of life
1998	Kearney, M. H. (1998). Truthful self-nurturing: A grounded formal theory of women's addiction recovery. *Qualitative Health Research, 8*(4), 495–512.	Truthful self-nurturing
1998	Burns, C. M. (1998). A retroductive theoretical model of the pathway to chemical dependency in nurses. *Archives of Psychiatric Nursing, 21*(1), 59–65.	Pathway to chemical dependency in nurses

(Continued)

TABLE A.1   *(Continued)*

Year	Full citation (APA)	Name of theory
1999	Jirovec, M. M., Jenkins, J., Isenberg, M., & Baiardi, J. (1999). Urine control theory derived from Roy's conceptual framework. *Nursing Science Quarterly, 12*(3), 251–255.	Urine control theory
1999	Smith, A. A., & Friedemann, M. (1999). Perceived family dynamics of persons with chronic pain. *Journal of Advanced Nursing, 30*(3), 543–551.	Family dynamics of persons with chronic pain
1999	Smith, M. J., & Liehr, P. (1999). Attentively embracing story: A middle-range theory with practice and research implications. *Scholarly Inquiry for Nursing Practice: An International Journal, 13*(3), 187–204.	Attentively embracing story
2000	Doornbos, M. M. (2000). King's systems frameworks and family health: The derivation and testing of a theory. *The Journal of Theory Construction & Testing, 4*(1), 20–26.	Family health
2000	Meleis, A. I., Sawyer, L. M., Im, E., Messias, D. K. H., & Schumacher, K. (2000). Experiencing transitions: An emerging middle-range theory. *Advances in Nursing Science, 23*(1), 12–28.	Experiencing transitions
2000	August-Brady, M. (2000). Prevention as intervention. *Journal of Advanced Nursing, 31*(6), 1304–1308.	Prevention as intervention
2000	Leenerts, M. H., & Magilvy, J. (2000). Investing in self-care: A midrange theory of self-care grounded in the lived experience of low-income HIV-positive white women. *Advances in Nursing Science, 22*(3), 58–75.	Self-care
2000	Sanford, R. C. (2000). Caring through relation and dialogue: A nursing perspective for patient education. *Advances in Nursing Science, 22*(3), 1–15.	Caring through relation and dialogue for patient education
2001	Wuest, J. (2001). Precarious ordering: Toward a formal theory of women's caring. *Health Care for Women International, 22*, 167–193.	Precarious ordering: Theory of women's caring
2001	Kolcaba, K. (2001). Evolution of the mid range theory of comfort for outcomes research. *Nursing Outlook, 49*(2), 86–92.	Comfort
2001	Hills, R. G. S., & Hanchett, E. (2001). Human change and individuation in pivotal life situations: Development and testing the theory of enlightenments. *Visions, 9*(1), 6–19.	Enlightenment

Year	Full citation (APA)	Name of theory
2001	Engebretson, J., & Littleton, L. Y. (2001). Cultural negotiation: A constructivist-based model for nursing practice. *Nursing Outlook, 49*(5), 223–230.	Cultural negotiation
2001	Woods, S. J., & Isenberg, M. A. (2001). Adaptation as a mediator of intimate abuse and traumatic stress in battered women. *Nursing Science Quarterly, 14*(3), 215–221.	Adaptation as a mediator of intimate abuse and traumatic stress in battered women
2002	Barnes, S., & Adair, B. (2002). The cognition-sensitive approach to dementia: Parallels with the science of unitary human beings. *Journal of Psychosocial Nursing and Mental Health Services, 40*(11), 30–37.	The cognition-sensitive approach to dementia
2002	Smith, C. E., Pace, K., Kochinda, C., Kleinbeck, S. V. M., Koehler, J., & Popkess-Vawter, S. (2002). Care giving effectiveness model evolution to a midrange theory of home care: A process for critique and replication. *Advances in Nursing Science, 25*(1), 50–64.	Caregiving effectiveness
2002	Roux, G., Dingley, C. E., & Bush, H. A. (2002). Inner strength in women: Metasynthesis of qualitative findings in theory development. *Journal of Theory Construction and Testing, 6*(1), 86–93.	Inner strength in women
2002	Whittemore, R., & Roy, C. (2002). Adapting to diabetes mellitus: A theory synthesis. *Nursing Science Quarterly, 15*(4), 311–317.	Adapting to diabetes mellitus
2003	Lawson, L. (2003). Becoming a success story: How boys who have molested children talk about treatment. *Journal of Psychiatric and Mental Health Nursing, 10*, 259–268.	Becoming a success story
2003	Tsai, P. (2003). A middle-range theory of caregiver stress. *Nursing Science Quarterly, 16*(2), 137–145.	Caregiver stress
2003	Tsai, P., Tak, S., Moore, C., & Palencia, I. (2003). Testing a theory of chronic pain. *Journal of Advanced Nursing, 43*(2), 158–169.	Chronic pain
2003	Dorsey, C. J., & Murdaugh, C. L. (2003). The theory of self-care management for vulnerable populations. *The Journal of Theory Construction & Testing, 7*(2), 43–49.	Self-care management for vulnerable populations

(Continued)

TABLE A.1   (Continued)

Year	Full citation (APA)	Name of theory
2004	Walton, J., & Sullivan, N. (2004). Men of prayer: Spirituality of men with prostate cancer. *Journal of Holistic Nursing, 22*(2), 133–151.	Spirituality
2004	Dunn, K. S. (2004). Toward a middle-range theory of adaptation to chronic pain. *Nursing Science Quarterly, 17*(1), 78–84.	Adaptation to chronic pain
2005	Dunn, K. S. (2005). Testing a middle-range theoretical model of adaptation to chronic pain. *Nursing Science Quarterly, 18*(2), 146–156.	Adaptation to chronic pain
2004	Mefford, L. C. (2004). A theory of health promotion for preterm infants based on Levine's Conservation Model of Nursing. *Nursing Science Quarterly, 17*(3), 260–266.	Health promotion for preterm infants
2006	Register, M. E., & Herman, J. (2006). A middle range theory for generative quality of life for the elderly. *Advances in Nursing Science, 29*(4), 340–350.	Generative quality of life for the elderly
2006	Peters, R. M. (2006). The relationship to racism, chronic stress emotions, and blood pressure. *Journal of Nursing Scholarship, 38*(3), 234–240.	Chronic stress emotions
2006	Johnson, M. E., & Delaney, K. R. (2006). Keeping the unit safe: A grounded theory study. *Journal of the American Psychiatric Nurses Association, 12*(1), 13–21.	Violence prevention
2007	Bu, X., & Jezewski, M. A. (2007). Developing a mid-range theory of patient advocacy through concept analysis. *Journal of Advanced Nursing, 57*(1), 101–110.	Patient advocacy
2007	Penrod, J., Yu, F., Kolanowski, A., Fick, D. M., Loeb, S. J., & Hupcey, J. E. (2007). Reframing person-centered nursing care for persons with dementia. *Research and Theory for Nursing Practice: An International Journal, 21*(1), 57–72.	Need-driven dementia–compromised behavior
2007	Chen, H., & Boore, J. (2007). Establishing a super-link system: Spinal cord injury rehabilitation nursing. *Journal of Advanced Nursing, 57*(6), 639–648.	Super-link system for rehabilitation
2007	Shanley, E., & Jubb-Shanley, M. (2007). The recovery alliance theory of mental health nursing. *Journal of Psychiatric & Mental Health Nursing, 14*(8), 734–743.	Recovery alliance

Year	Full citation (APA)	Name of theory
2008	Christie, J., Poulton, B. C., & Bunting, B. P. (2008). An integrated mid-range theory of postpartum family development: A guide for research and practice. *Journal of Advanced Nursing, 61*(1), 38–50.	Postpartum parent development
2009	Hodges, H. F., Troyan, P. J., & Keeley, A. C. (2010). Career persistence in baccalaureate-prepared acute care nurses. *Journal of Nursing Scholarship, 42*(1), 83–91.	Career persistence
2009	Ryan, P., & Sawin, K. J. (2009). The individual and family self-management theory: Background and perspectives on context, process and outcomes. *Nursing Outlook, 57,* 217–225.	Individual and family self-management
2010	Davidson, J. E. (2010). Facilitated sensemaking: A strategy and new middle-range theory to support families of intensive care unit patients. *Critical Care Nurse, 30*(6), 28–39.	Facilitated sensemaking
2012	Dyess, S. M., & Chase, S. K. (2012). Sustaining health in faith community nursing practice: Emerging processes that support the development of a middle-range theory. *Holistic Nursing Practice, 26*(4), 221–227.	Sustaining health in faith communities
2012	Riegel, B., Jaarsma, T., & Strömberg, A. (2012). A middle-range theory of self-care of chronic illness. *Advances in Nursing Science, 35*(3), 194–204.	Self-care of chronic illness

Index